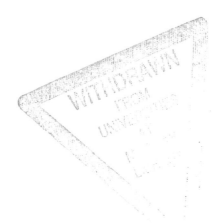

AGING PHENOMENA

**Relationships among Different
Levels of Organization**

ADVANCES IN EXPERIMENTAL MEDICINE AND BIOLOGY

Recent Volumes in this Series

Naito Symposium on Aging. 1978. Tokyo

AGING PHENOMENA
Relationships among Different
Levels of Organization

Edited by

Kunio Oota
Tokyo Metropolitan Institute of Gerontology
Tokyo, Japan

Takashi Makinodan
Veterans Administration
Wadsworth Medical Center
Los Angeles, California

Masami Iriki
Tokyo Metropolitan Institute of Gerontology
Tokyo, Japan

and

Lynn S. Baker
Veterans Administration
Wadsworth Medical Center
Los Angeles, California

PLENUM PRESS • NEW YORK AND LONDON

Library of Congress Cataloging in Publication Data

Naito Symposium on Aging, Tokyo, 1978.
    Aging phenomena.

    (Advances in experimental medicine and biology; v. 129)
    Includes index.
    1. Aging — Congresses. I. Oota, Kunio. II. Naitō Kinen Kagaku Shinkō Zaidan.
III. Title. IV. Series.
QP86.N34 1978   599.03'72   80-16223
ISBN 0-306-40460-5

Proceedings of the Naito Foundation Symposium
on Aging, held in Tokyo, Japan, August 27–29, 1978.

©1980 Plenum Press, New York
A Division of Plenum Publishing Corporation
227 West 17th Street, New York, N.Y. 10011

FOREWORD

The problem of senescence, as reflected in the history of reli-
gion and philosophy, has long been one of the greatest concerns of
humankind. In contrast, gerontology as a branch of science is still
comparatively young. During the past decade, concomitant with rapid
progress in our understanding of the basic life sciences, vast stores
of knowledge about biological aging have been accumulated. This
knowledge, however, arising from many scientific disciplines and
focused on varying levels of biologic organization, seems almost
random and covers everything from molecules to human societies.
Theories advanced to interpret the facts and to understand the mechanisms involved in senescence have remained in individual, rather
than general, territories.

It has long been felt by some gerontologists that it was time for
the various specialists to step back and take a generalist view of
gerontology, to reconsider and reevaluate the fruits of their analyt-
ical pursuits at different levels within a broader context. Some
others may think it still premature. It seemed, however, that the
majority of those who gathered in Tokyo on the occasion of the XIth
International Congress of Gerontology were of the opinion that there
was much to be gained in looking for interrelationships among the
facts and theories originated in the different levels of investigation in an attempt to observe and appreciate the biological drama of
senescence as an entity. In spite of the unusual late summer heat
and heavy schedules during the post-congress period, the Naito
Symposium was attended by no less than 170 people from a variety of
disciplines.

In the symposium, the organizer and participants tried to clarify
the status of our present knowledge in the individual areas, to determine exactly what the gaps are in our current understanding, and to
help point the way toward new paths for future research and, hope-
fully, our next breakthroughs. Thanks to the enthusiasm of colleagues
from all over the world, the Naito Symposium was felt to be a success:
a number of new facts were presented, some fresh strategic points
discussed, and certain new ways of reasoning proposed. Looking back,
however, the two full days were not enough time to arrive at a full
understanding of biological aging. They were sufficient, however,
for us to realize the importance of further attempts at unifying our
knowledge and to be optimistic that future efforts will, indeed, be
fruitful.

On behalf of the organizing committee, I would like to take this opportunity to express my deep-felt thanks to the Naito Foundation, both for sponsoring the project and for their warm hospitality, which was essential to the success of the meeting.

KUNIO OOTA, M.D.
August, 1979
Tokyo

INTRODUCTION: AN OVERVIEW

The theme of the Naito Symposium on Aging is "A Reevaluation of Interrelationships among Aging Phenomena in Different Levels of Organization." Inasmuch as aging is the most complex and multifaceted of all life processes, reevaluation must be performed recurrently and thoughtfully. The Naito Symposium contributes to this process by highlighting several new trends in biogerontological thinking and research.

Three speakers produce evidence against the somatic mutation hypothesis. Permanently tetraploid fibroblast clones produced by cell fusion had the same life span as diploid clones, tending to rule out any direct role of either recessive or dominant mutations in the aging processes of the diploid fibroblast cultures. The absence of any decrease with age of messenger RNA synthesis in most mouse brain regions, except for the specific decrease of mRNA/DNA ratios in the striatum, is consonant with other evidence about the distinctive aging pattern of the dopaminergic nigro-striatal system in mouse and man, and favors hypotheses of genetic program control of aging rather than hypotheses of mutational degradation. The discovery of methionine sulfoxide reductase in mammalian cells, and of its role in reversing peroxidative changes in proteins, tends to strengthen the role of postsynthetic changes in proteins as the basis for the loss of enzyme activity in old age, and to underline enzyme degradation as a major governing factor in the changes of enzyme levels with age. Consistent with these findings, evidence is given that the fidelity of RNA translation does not decrease with age. These lines of evidence imply, not that the somatic mutation hypothesis must be discarded, but rather that it is inadequate in its present form, and needs new kinds of data and a more refined theoretical formulation.

The relation of systemic aging processes to specific ultrastructural and molecular changes in the humoral and neural communication systems is documented in three papers. The almost linear decrease in number of steroid hormone receptors on cell surfaces with age, the decrement of immunological receptors, and the loss of dendritic processes and dendritic spines from cortical neurons suggest that the intercellular communication channels are particularly vulnerable to aging changes, but they also suggest the possibility of exciting new research efforts directed toward assessing the degree of reversibility of these changes.

The equivocal role of the immune system as both a life-sustaining and a senescence-engendering agent is examined from several viewpoints, but space allows me to note only one intriguing observation: the finding that some individuals with deficient immune competence are also deficient in the capacity for certain kinds of DNA repair.

The question of programmed versus random aging also arises in regard to animal cell populations in vivo. Certain body cells of developing animals have limited survival due to genetic programming, and genetically programmed cell death is also present in the adult stage. Continued work with exquisitely regulated systems may throw new light on the genetic control of cell proliferation and cell death.

The important problem of the impact of our industrial environment on the aging process is a recurrent theme. In addition to the studies on cellular systems mentioned above, the use of the medaka, or rice fish, Oryzias latipes, as a model system for investigating a variety of environmental problems is described, and the nature of the late injury produced in mammals by ionizing radiations is examined. The similarity of the cumulative radiation damage in cultured cells and whole animals is an especially valuable new insight.

This fragmentary account may dimly convey the exciting progress in biogerontological research today, but it cannot adequately convey the vigor and promise of the research being reported by the young Japanese investigators. The next such reevaluation will hear much more from them.

GEORGE A. SACHER
Division of Biological
and Medical Research
Argonne National
Laboratory
Argonne, IL 60439 USA

CONTENTS

IN VITRO CELL AGING

IN VIVO CELL AGING

CHANGES IN GENETIC INFORMATION AND AGING

AGING AND INTERCELLULAR COMMUNICATION

AGING IN THE HIGHER HIERARCHY

AGING: SOME PERSPECTIVES

PARTICIPANTS

Organizer:	K. Oota, Japan
Session Chairpersons:	L. Hayflick, United States
	M. Yamada, Japan
	H. Tauchi, Japan
	S. Fujita, Japan
	P. Ebbesen, Denmark
	D. Mizuno, Japan
	M.M.B. Kay, United States
	M. Iriki, Japan
	K. Oota, Japan
	S. Tsurufuji, Japan
	T. Makinodan, United States
	C. Finch, United States
	G. Sacher, United States
	N. Egami, Japan
Session Speakers:	A. Macieira-Coelho, France
	Y. Mitsui, Japan
	A. Shima, Japan
	K. Brizzee, United States
	Y. Hayashi (for M. Igarashi), Japan
	D. Gershon, Israel
	G. Martin, United States
	Y. Courtois, France
	G. Roth, United States
	T. Tada, Japan
	P. Ebbesen, Denmark
	W. Bondareff, United States
	M. Kay, United States
	Yu Nagai, Japan
	A. Ooshima, Japan
	C. Finch, United States
	A. Everitt, Australia
	T. Makinodan, United States
	T. Noumura, Japan
	R. Walford, United States
	N. Egami, Japan
	R. Cutler, United States

Discussants: E. Schneider, United States
                          T. Matsumura, Japan
                          M. Tomonaga, Japan
                          T. Yamaguchi, Japan
                          S. Goto, Japan
                          D. Mizuno, Japan
                          S. Aizawa, Japan
                          S. Kawashima, Japan
                          Yo Nagai, Japan
                          I. Yamashima, Japan
                          T. Ohno, Japan
                          S. Murota, Japan
                          T. Matsamura, Japan
                          K. Hirokawa, Japan
                          H. Imura, Japan
                          S. Kawashima, Japan
                          F. Bourliere, France
                          T. Sugahara, Japan
                          T. Yamakawa, Japan
                          T. Hidaka, Japan
                          T. Sado, Japan

Opening Remarks: H. Kumagai, Japan

Closing Remarks: G. Sacher, United States
                          K. Oota, Japan

KINETICS OF THE PROLIFERATION OF HUMAN FIBROBLASTS
DURING SERIAL SUBCULTIVATION IN VITRO

A. Macieira-Coelho

Department of Cell Pathology
Institut de Cancerologie et d'Immunogénétique
(INSERM U-50)
94800 Villejuif, France

INTRODUCTION

The studies of the kinetics of cell proliferation in vitro have
been plagued by the tendency to establish clear-cut limits to the
behavior of cells in regard to the division cycle. Investigators in
the field have predominantly thought in terms of compartments instead
of gradients, measured instants instead of variations during long
periods of time, and expressed the results in terms of means instead
of distributions.

Mean generation times aren't always valid because there can be
differences up to several days between the shortest and the longest
interdivision times; and cells considered arrested in certain periods
of the division cycle can actually be cells whose progress is merely
slowed down.

Inevitably, this led to overly simplified ideas, such as considering only cycling and non-cycling cells, or believing that the rates
of entrance into the cycle are constant. This type of thinking can
be particularly fallacious when analyzing the proliferation of human
fibroblasts during their life span in vitro.

We attempted to elucidate the kinetics of the proliferation of
human fibroblasts, taking into account the parameters mentioned above
(1-8). In 1966, when we first started to explore this virtually
unknown field, our aim was to find out which of the following three
hypotheses would fit the data (1): a) Only a small fraction of the
cell population in phase III cultures is dividing at unaltered rate,
but the majority of the cells are unable to divide. b) The entire

1

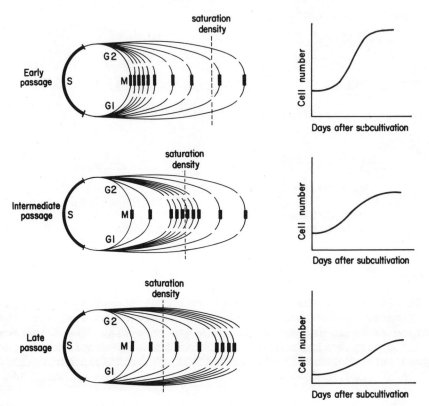

Fig. 1.   Illustration of a model of kinetics of the proliferation
           of human fibroblasts (see text below).

population is uniformly growing at a slow rate, possibly because of
selective interferences with one of the stages in the division
cycle. c) The cell population has become strongly heterogeneous, and
the cells show a spectrum between the two extremes, i.e., complete
inhibition and a normal division cycle.

RESULTS AND DISCUSSION

    The data collected favored the last hypothesis, and more recently
(8) we proposed a model that could explain our data and that of
others, while at the same time having the advantage of being free of
mathematical formulas. The model is illustrated in Figure 1, where
three different periods of the cell population life span are represented. On the left side of the figure, each circle and ellipse
represents the generation time of a cell. In early passages, most

cells in the population are postulated to have short division
cycles. Some cells already exist with long generation times (ellip-
ses) which are extended mainly at the expense of G1 and G2. There is
no gross prolongation of the S period and mitosis (4). Since the
saturation density is high (vertical dashed line), most cells are
able to complete their cycle before this density is reached. At this
stage, the growth curve of the population (right hand side of the
figure) has a short lag period, a phase of logarithmic growth with a
steep slope, and a high saturation density reached within 3-4 days.

Towards the middle of the life span (intermediate passage), there
are still cells with short generation times, but most cells have
division cycles between the two extremes. Since the saturation density is lower, an increased number of cells will not have time to
complete their cycle. Thus, during a prolonged labeling with tritiated thymidine (^{3}H-TdR), an increased number of cells will appear as
unlabeled. At this stage, the slope of the logarithmic portion of
the growth curve will be less steep and the cells will reach a lower
saturation density, although still within 3-4 days.

Towards the end of the life span (late passage), most cells have
very long generation times, and since the saturation density is very
low, a still greater number of cells do not have time to complete the
cycle between subcultivation and confluency. Thus, even more cells
will remain unlabeled after growing in the presence of ^{3}H-TdR. The
growth curve will be characterized by a long lag phase, a period of
short logarithmic growth with a shallow slope, and a low saturation
density reached only after 7-10 days.

In Figure 1, the prolongations of G1 and G2 are identical, but it
is possible that one is predominant. It should be emphasized that
when one speaks about the prolongation of G1 or G2, it applies only
to cells that are moving through the cycle. Since the cells that are
arrested due, for instance, to the effects of saturation density seem
to be all in G1, a distinction should and can be made when measuring
the prolongation of the G1 and G2 periods; otherwise, cells that are
arrested will be taken as prolonged in G1. This is particularly true
for the latter period, which is usually measured indirectly. Methods
that allow the analysis of cells in motion along the cycle should be
distinguished from those measuring only instants (5,6).

In addition, another important parameter becomes more pronounced
at higher population doubling levels: an increased heterogeneity in
the initiation of the cell cycle. The cells become more erratic with
aging in vitro (2). While in young cultures between subcultivation
and resting phase, the number of cells entering the S period
increases progressively to a maximum and then decreases to very low
levels, in old cultures there is a burst of cells entering S, then
the percentage of cells synthesizing DNA goes down and up again
before it decreases at confluency (2). This heterogeneity in the

initiation of division can lead an investigator to consider as non-dividers cells that still have the potential to enter the cell cycle in a more unpredictable way. This erratic behavior has been confirmed by direct examination of the cells with time lapse cinematography (9), and is suggested from measurements of the rate of entrance into the division cycle (10).

The model we described herein takes into consideration all the data previously published on the kinetics of the proliferation of human fibroblast populations, and may be helpful in understanding cell division during in vitro aging, as well as in other cell systems.

REFERENCES

1. A. Macieira-Coelho, J. Ponten, and L. Philipson, The division cycle and RNA synthesis in diploid human cells at different passage levels in vitro, Exp. Cell Res. 42:673 (1966).
2. A. Macieira-Coelho, J. Ponten, and L. Philipson, Inhibition of the division cycle in confluent cultures of human fibroblasts in vitro, Exp. Cell Res. 43:20 (1966).
3. A. Macieira-Coelho, Influence of cell density on growth inhibition of human fibroblasts in vitro, Proc. Soc. Exp. Biol. Med. 125:548 (1967).
4. A. Macieira-Coelho and J. Ponten, Analogy in growth between late passage human embryonic and early passage human adult fibroblasts, J. Cell Biol. 43:374 (1969).
5. A. Macieira-Coelho and L. Berumen, The cell cycle during growth inhibition of human embryonic fibroblasts in vitro, Proc. Soc. Exp. Biol. Med. 144:43 (1973).
6. A. Macieira-Coelho, Cell cycle analysis in mammalian cells, in: "Tissue Culture: Methods and Applications," P. F. Kruse, Jr. and M. K. Patterson, Jr., eds., Academic Press, New York (1973).
7. A. Macieira-Coelho, Are non-dividing cells present in ageing cell cultures? Nature 248:421 (1974).
8. A. Macieira-Coelho, Kinetics of the proliferation of human fibroblasts during their lifespan in vitro, Mech. Ageing Dev. 6:341 (1977).
9. P. M. Absher, R. G. Absher, and W. D. Barnes, Genealogies of clones of diploid fibroblasts. Cinematographic observations of cell division patterns in relation to population age, Exp. Cell Res. 88:95 (1974).
10. G. L. Grove and V. J. Cristofalo, The transition probability model and the regulation of proliferation of human diploid cell cultures during aging, Cell Tissue Kinet. 9:395 (1976).

NEW APPROACHES TO CHARACTERIZATION OF AGING HUMAN

FIBROBLASTS AT INDIVIDUAL CELL LEVEL

Youji Mitsui[1], Koji Matsuoka[1], Shinichi Aizawa[2], and Koichi Noda[3]

[1]Laboratory of Pharmacology, [2]Laboratory of Nutrition, and [3]Laboratory of Ultrastructure Research, Tokyo Metropolitan Institute of Gerontology 35-2 Sakaecho, Itabashiku, Tokyo-173, Japan

SUMMARY

Considering the heterogeneity of cell populations and other critcal problems in mass cultured senescent human fibroblasts, we proposed several new approaches for studying true cellular aging, as follows.

1)   To establish a correlation among aging indexes at the individual cell level, we demonstrated a relationship among ^{3}H-thymidine incorporation activity, nuclear size, cell volume, and DNA contents at individual cell level.

2)   To fractionate homogenous cell populations and examine the relationship between their life spans and aging indexes, we separated human cells into relatively homogenous populations by the sedimentation velocity method, and found that life span of fractionated cells was almost identical among various fractions, irrespective of their great differences in cell volume and ^{3}H-thymidine incorporation indexes. This suggests that some aging indexes, such as cell volumes and ^{3}H-thymidine incorporation activity, are reversible cell properties, and are not specific properties at the individual cell level.

3)   To find age-specific cell properties in fractionated senescent cell populations, we performed a quantitative analysis with an image analyzer on electromicroscopic pictures of fractionated small and large cell populations from young and senescent cultures. We discovered that the differences between young and senescent cultures in nuclear size, mitochonria size and number of lysosomes are due

solely to the presence of large cells in senescent cultures, and that
an increase in the constricted endoplasmic reticulum is a common
phenotype of fractionated senescent cell populations. This suggests
that there is some loss of function in endoplasmic reticulum or
changes in the membrane system.

4)   To examine age-specific changes in membrane system at the
individual cell level, we found that the amount of absorption of
concanavalin A-bound red blood cells to fibroblast surfaces increases
linearly with in vitro passage. Further examination of individual
cells indicated that this passage-related change in surface membrane
is not dependent on cell cycle phase, surface area, or metabolic age,
but certainly is dependent upon division age.

Finally, these findings should be confirmed by using cells from
human donors of different ages.

We conclude that our approaches are important for elucidating the
true mechanisms of cellular aging.

INTRODUCTION

The finite life span of cultured human diploid fibroblasts has
been suggested as a manifestation of aging at the cellular level
(1). The inverse relationship between human donor age and the in
vitro life span of skin fibroblasts has confirmed the validity of
using cultured diploid fibroblasts as a model system for human cellular aging (2,3). The precise characterization of senescent cells is
essential for the elucidation of the mechanisms of in vitro cellular
aging.

Phase III cells, a term originally used by Hayflick (1), usually
represent senescent cell populations, one of the characteristics of
which is a decrease in proliferation capacity. Phase III cells have
been called late passage cells, terminal phase cells, degenerative
phase cells, or senescent cells, depending on the research interest.
Although there have been extensive examinations of phase III cells, a
total integrated picture of the features of phase III cells remains
obscure. Phase III cells are not homogenous cell populations in
terms of proliferation capacity (4,5), cell volume (6), nuclear size
(7,8), or morphology (9). Therefore, some properties of phase III
cells are not necessarily characteristic of senescent cells, and rapidly dividing cell populations among phase III cells apparently look
like young cell populations (7,10). This finding calls for new
approaches to find more accurate indexes of cellular aging at the
level of the individual cells.

In this paper, we will first summarize the recent information on
the properties of phase III cells, and point out the crucial problems
involved in studying true senescent cells. Finally, we will propose

several approaches to these problems, capable of providing some
insights into the mechanisms of cellular aging.

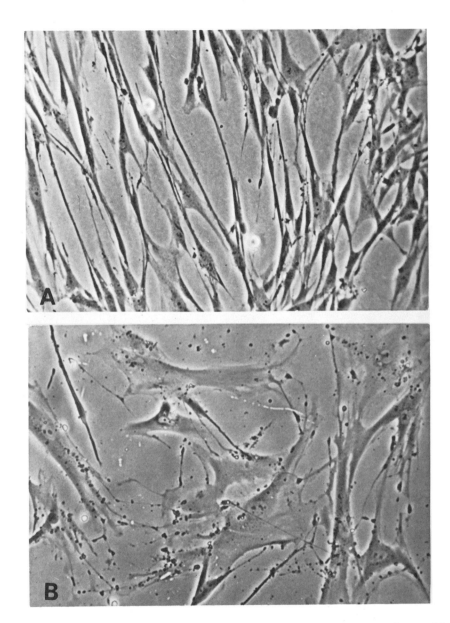

Fig. 1.   Morphological features of human fibroblasts under a light
           microscope.
                A: early passage cells (15 pdl)
                B: late passage cells (65 pdl)

SUMMARIZED FEATURES OF PHASE III CELLS

A typical example of the morphology of human diploid fibroblasts as revealed by an Olympus light microscope is seen in Figure 1. Most of the early passage cells (Fig. 1a) have a spindle shape and rapidly proliferate, resulting in a criss-cross cell layer. On the other hand, late passage cells (Fig. 1b) sometimes have an enlarged, flattened shape, and cease to proliferate at low cell density.

Although a considerable number of works comparing early passage cells and late passage cells have been published, efforts to integrate these observations with findings on cellular aging phenomena have been scarce. In Table 1, the biochemical and cytological changes in cell properties with passage are listed. In summary, the characteristics of phase III cells seem to be: 1) a decreased growth rate; 2) an increase in cell size; 3) a decreased cell function; and 4) an increase in abnormality. Since these studies have been performed on mass cultured cells, they reflect only average properties, which may vary widely in individual cells. Actually, as noted above (p. 6), an increase in heterogeneity is a fifth characteristic of phase III cells. Therefore, we lack knowledge about the correlation

Table 1. Changes in Cell Properties with in vitro Cell Aging

Colony formation	↓	Collagen: Synthesis, hydroxylation	
% labeled cell with ^{3}H-thymidine	↓	and degradation	↓
Duration of the G_1 phase	↑	Mucopolysaccharide synthesis	↓
Growth rate	↓	Glucose utilization	↑
DNA polymerase	↓	Lactate dehydrogenase	↓
Thymidine kinase	↓	Transaminases	↓
Cell volume	↑	Surface negative charge	↓
Surface area	↑	LETS protein content	↓
Nuclear size	↑	Cell movement	↓
Microfibril	↑	Neutral proteolytic enzyme	↓
Protein, glycogen, lipid contents	↑	Phagocytosis	↓
RNA synthesis	↓	Polyploidy	↑
Chromatin template activity	↓	Aneuploid cells	↑
Histone acetylation	↓	Abnormal G6PD cells	↑
RNA content	↑	Lysosomal enzyme	↑
		Chromatin associated degradation	
		enzymes	↑

correlation among these changes in cell properties at the individual cell level.

THE CORRELATION AMONG AGING INDEXES AT THE INDIVIDUAL CELL LEVEL

We have reported the close relationship between modal cell volume and population doubling time at various passage numbers (6). The fractionation by sedimentation velocity of small and large cells from the same culture has provided indirect evidence for the close correlation among cell volume, nuclear size, and proliferation capacity (7). As shown in Figure 2, cell nuclei are heterogenous in size, and a direct relationship between nuclear size and proliferation capacity can be examined in individual cells using autoradiography. Figure 3 shows the nuclear size distribution of labeled cells and unlabeled cells at middle and late passage cultures incubated with ^{3}H-thymidine for various time intervals, ranging from 17 hours to two weeks.

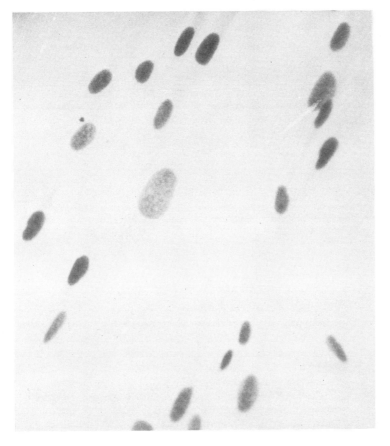

Fig. 2.   Nuclei of middle passage cells stained with giemsa. Note the heterogeneity in size.

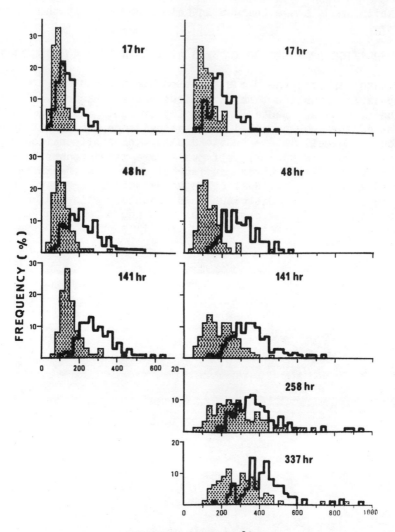

NUCLEAR SIZE (μ^2)

Fig. 3.   Nuclear size distribution of labeled cells and unlabeled
cells during continuous incubation with ^{3}H-thymidine.
Labeled nuclei: ▨ ; unlabeled nuclei: ▢ ; left column
of graphs: middle passage cells (35 pdl); right column of
graphs: late passage cells (53 pdl).
Cells were incubated with 0.01 µCi ^{3}H-thymidine for the
indicated periods. The percentage of labeled middle
passage cells was 84, 96, 99, and the percentage of
labeled late passage cells was 47, 70, and 91 at 17, 48,
and 141 hrs, respectively.

It is apparent that at any given incubation time, the unlabeled
cell nuclei are larger than labeled cell nuclei. Moreover, with
increasing incubation time, there is a definite shift in the nuclear
size distribution to larger sizes for both the labeled and unlabeled
cell populations. These findings, when one considers that unlabeled,
slowly dividing cells become labeled with increasing incubation time,
lead to the conclusion that the more slowly dividing cells have
larger nuclear sizes. Non-dividing cells were identified as the
cells with maximum nuclear size which remained unlabeled even after
the total number of unlabeled cells per dish ceased to decrease during incubation with ^{3}H-TdR. Non-dividing cells at terminal phase,
which remained unlabeled even after 10 days of incubation, had a mean
nuclear size of 430 μm^2, while the rapidly dividing cells at both
middle and terminal phase, which were labeled within 17 hours, had a
mean nuclear size of 100 μm^2.

Figure 4 shows the relationship between DNA content and the size
of individual, terminal phase cell nuclei. Since this terminal phase
culture was examined after it reached confluency at low cell density,
only a few S phase cells with an intermediate amount of DNA between
2C and 4C were observed. As can be seen in Figure 4, non-dividing
cells with nuclei of a maximum size of more than 400 μm^2 had 4C or 8C
DNA. On the other hand, small cells with a nuclear size smaller than
200 μm^2 had 2C DNA. We consider these small cells to be rapidly
cycling cells, as is indicated by their nuclear size distribution
when labeled within 17 hours.

Thus, we conclude that phase III cells can be divided into three
types of cell population in terms of proliferation capacity. These

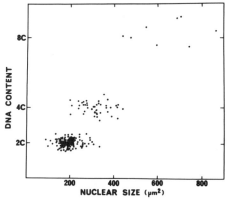

Fig. 4.   DNA content and nuclear size of individual cells at
terminal phase culture. The relative DNA content was
determined with a scanning microphotometer after Feulgen
staining.

types are terminal senescent cells (non-dividing), resting senescent cells (slowly dividing), and cycling senescent cells (rapidly dividing). However, cycling cells among phase III cells in our study were apparently identical to cycling cells in early passage cultures in terms of cell volume, nuclear size, and ^{3}H-TdR incorporating activity. Therefore, a question arises as to how cycling senescent cells are different from resting senescent cells, or from the cycling cells in early passage culture. Thus, our second approach was to examine aging indexes in relatively homogenous cell populations.

AGING INDEXES AND LIFE SPAN OF FRACTIONATED CELL POPULATIONS

We have previously reported that the cell separation method obtains relatively homogenous cell populations in terms of cell volume using sedimentation velocity (6,7,8). Figure 5 shows that the largest cell population (fraction 1) obtained using this technique had the highest percentage of unlabeled cells, while the smallest

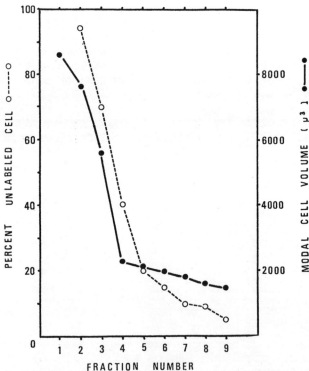

Fig. 5.   Cell volume and the percent of unlabeled cells in fractionated late passage cell populations. ^{3}H-thymidine was added to the culture for 24 hrs, and cells were fractionated by the sedimentation velocity method.

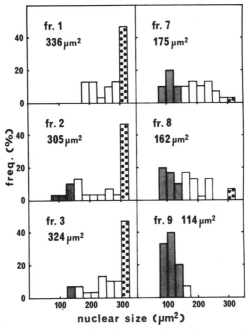

Fig. 6.   Nuclear size distribution of fractionated middle passage
          cell populations.
          Nuclear size was examined 24 hrs after the fractionated
          cell populations were reintroduced into cultures.
          Nuclei larger than 300 μm^2: ⊞ ; nuclei smaller than
          150 μm^2: ▨ . Note that there was no overlapping of
          nuclear size distribution between fractions 1 and 9.

cell populations (fraction 9) had the lowest percentage of unlabeled
cells.

     Due to the close correlation between cell volume and ^{3}H-thymi-
dine incorporation activity, we could obtain several cell populations
with various cell proliferation capacities. These fractionated cell
populations differing in size and proliferation capacity were
reintroduced into cultures, and their proliferation capacity and life
span thereafter were examined. Shortly after their reintroduction
into cultures, the nuclear size distribution of each fraction was
examined. As can be seen in Figure 6, fraction 1 had the largest
nuclear size distribution (mean: 336 μm^2), while fraction 9 had the
smallest nuclear size distribution (mean: 114 μm^2). It should be
noted that there was no overlapping in terms of nuclear size between
fractions 1 and 9. However, after 3 days in tissue culture, fractions that differed markedly at the time of fractionation returned to
a relatively uniform cell volume and proliferation capacity for both
early and late passage cultures (Fig. 7). Thus, the small rapidly

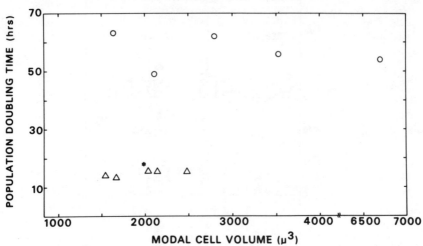

Fig. 7.   Growth rate of recultured cell populations as a function
          of cell volume at the time of fractionation. Fractionated
          cell populations from early (Δ) and late (O) passage
          cultures were reintroduced into cultures, and population
          doubling time was determined at the log phase of growth.
          Unseparated early passage control cells (*Δ) were also
          examined as above.

dividing cell population in the late passage culture was found not to
be identical with the small rapidly dividing cell population in the
early passage culture. Furthermore, in order to examine the life
span of fractionated cell populations, a middle passage cell culture
was fractionated first at the 29th population doubling level (pdl),
then both fraction 1 and 9 and the unseparated cells were recultured
for a further seven pdls. Fractions 1 and 9 were again fractionated
at the 36th pdl, yielding fractions 1, 2, and 3 from the recultured
fraction 1, and fractions 9 and 10 from the recultured fraction 9.
As can be seen in Figure 8, no significant difference between the in
vitro life span of each of the fractionated cell populations and the
parallel control culture was observed.

     These results indicate that: 1) rapidly dividing cell popula-
tions in late passage cultures have a much shorter life span than
rapidly dividing cells in early passage cultures, in spite of their
similarity on some aging indexes; and that 2) rapidly dividing cell
populations have almost the same life span as slowly dividing cell
populations in the same culture. These findings may suggest that the
proliferation capacity and the cell volume of individual cells in a
given culture are temporary properties. Thus, size and proliferative
capacity might be modifiable characteristics capable of changing with

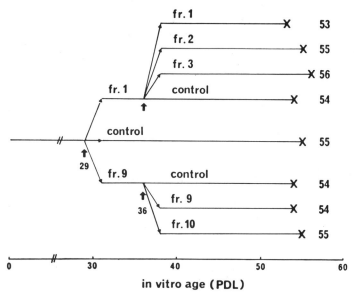

in vitro age (PDL)

Fig. 8.   Life span of fractionated cell populations.
After the separation of fractions 1 and 9 at the 29th pdl,
they were recultured for a further 7 pdls and fractionated
again at the 36th pdl.

cell division. These results support the program theory of aging
rather than the mutation or error theory.

We were next concerned to know how small and large cells in late
passage cultures are different from those in early passage cultures
in terms of cell properties other than ^{3}H-thymidine incorporation
capacity, cell volume and nuclear size. Therefore, our third
approach was to try to draw a common phenotype of aging from the
fractionated cell populations.

QUANTITATIVE ANALYSIS WITH AN IMAGE ANALYZER AND ELECTROMICROSCOPIC
PICTURES OF FRACTIONATED YOUNG AND OLD CELLS

Immediately after fractionating cells using the sedimentation
velocity method, small (fraction 8) and large (fraction 1) cell
populations from old cultures and a small cell population from young
cultures were fixed with osmic acid and processed for electromicroscopic observation.

The size of the nuclei of each fraction can be seen in Figure 9.
The largest cells had the largest nuclear size, and small cells from
old cultures had nuclei of the same size as those of small cells
from young cultures. Irregularity in nuclear size, which has been

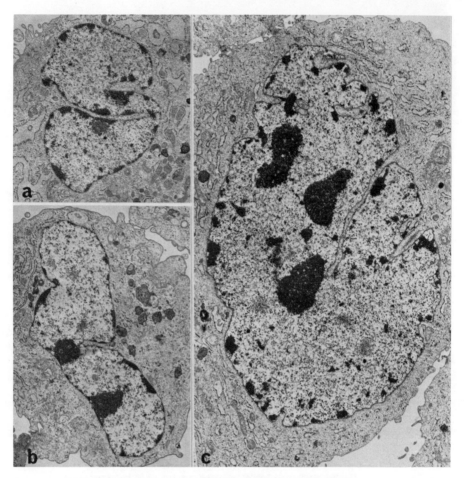

Fig. 9.   Electron microscopic pictures (x 6,000) of nuclei from
           fractionated cells.
             a. from fraction 8 of early passage cells;
             b. from fraction 8 of late passage cells;
             c. from fraction 2 of late passage cells.

suggested as a characteristic of old cultures, was determined by the
formula,

$$\frac{1}{2\sqrt{\pi}} \cdot \frac{L}{\sqrt{S}}$$

L, the length of the nuclear periphery, and S, the area of the
nucleus, were measured with an image analyzer and electron
microscopic pictures.

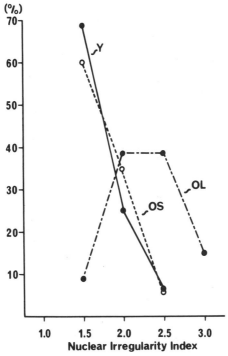

Fig. 10. Irregularity of nuclear shape.
Ordinate: percentage of cells with a given irregularity
index from the total number of cells examined (35 cells).
Abscissa: the nuclear irregularity index represented by
the formula

$$\frac{1}{2\sqrt{\pi}} \cdot \frac{L}{\sqrt{S}} \cdot$$

Y: fraction 8 of early passage cells; OS: fraction 8 of
late passage cells; OL: fraction 2 of late passage cells.

Figure 10 shows that passage-related differences in nuclear
irregularity are due solely to the presence of large nuclei with
increased irregularity. Thus, nuclear irregularity was found not to
be a common phenotype of senescent cells. Figure 11 gives the features of the mitochondria (M) and endoplasmic reticulum (ER) in young
small and old large cells. Swelling M were observed in 14% of each
group of small and large cells. The total area of M per cell was
much larger in old large cells than in young small cells. However,
the percentage of M area to area of cytoplasm showed no difference
among the different fractions (Fig. 12). A similar analysis was performed on the number and size of the fractions' lysosomes, which
indicated that the changes in M and lysosomes are a function of cytoplasm size and are not age-specific.

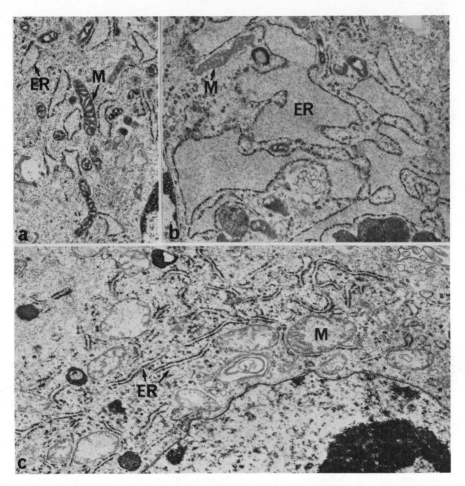

Fig. 11. Electron microscopic pictures (x 15,000) of cytoplasm from
          fractionated cells.
          M: mitochondria; ER: endoplasmic reticulum; a and b:
          fraction 8 of early passage cells; c: fraction 2 of late
          passage cells. Note the constricted ER and enlarged M in
          the late passage cells.

On the other hand, constricted ER were observed in both old small
and large cell fractions as compared with dilated ER in young small
cells (Fig. 11). In fact, an examination of the length of the short
axis of the largest ER in each cell (Fig. 13) suggested that ER
constriction in old cultures is an age-related change. This was
further confirmed by examining monolayer cultured young and old
cells. These facts suggest some loss of function on the part of ER
or changes in the membrane system. Therefore, our fourth approach
was to examine changes in the surface membrane of individual cells.

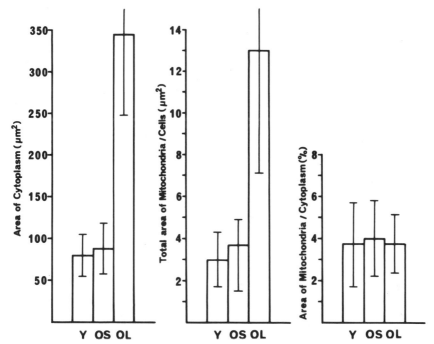

Fig. 12. The amount of area for cytoplasm and mitochondria in
          fractionated cells.
          The single line bar extending above each column represents
          standard deviation of the mean value of each index.
          Y, OS, and OL are as in Fig. 10.

AGE-RELATED CHANGES IN CELL SURFACE MEMBRANES

    The adsorption of Concanavalin A treated red blood cells to the
surface of fibroblasts can be examined at the individual cell level
(11). As can be seen in Figure 14, early passage cells adsorbed only
a few Concanavalin A-coated red blood cells, while, interestingly
enough, both small and large cells in senescent culture had a high
hemadsorption activity.

    Pulse labeled cells with ^{3}H-thymidine at the S phase had a hem-
adsorption almost identical to that of unlabeled cells at the G_1 or
G_2 cell cycle phase. Inhibitors of DNA and protein synthesis, as
well as a low serum concentration, had only slight effects on the
hemadsorption activity in contrast with their marked effects on
nuclear size.

    Three strains of human embryo lung fibroblasts (WI-38, IMR-90,
and TIG-1) showed a linear increase in hemadsorption per mg protein
of fibroblast as a function of population doubling level

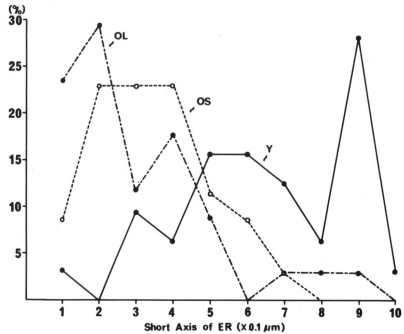

Fig. 13. Length of the short axis of ER of fractionated cells.
Ordinate: percentage of cells with a given ER short axis
from the total number of cells examined. Abscissa: the
length of the short axis of the largest ER in each cell.
There were few dilated ER per cell, if any, in some late
passage cells.

(see Fig. 15). Since the amount of ^{3}H-Concanavalin A binding to
fibroblast surfaces does not change throughout the life span of human
fibroblasts, the changes in the adsorption of Concanavalin A-coated
red blood cells to fibroblast surface was concluded to reflect a continuous change in the Concanavalin A receptor modulating system with
aging (12).

A linear progressive type of change, rather than a catastrophe
type of change, is very important for gaining insight into the cellular mechanisms of aging. In this sense, the clarification of the
molecular basis of surface changes is under extensive investigation
and is expected to reveal features important for our understanding of
cellular aging. However, we think that another examination we are
now carrying out, on the relation of the increased nuclear protein in
senescent cells to a decline in replication capacity (13,14), will
also provide an important key for disclosing the mechanisms of
cellular aging.

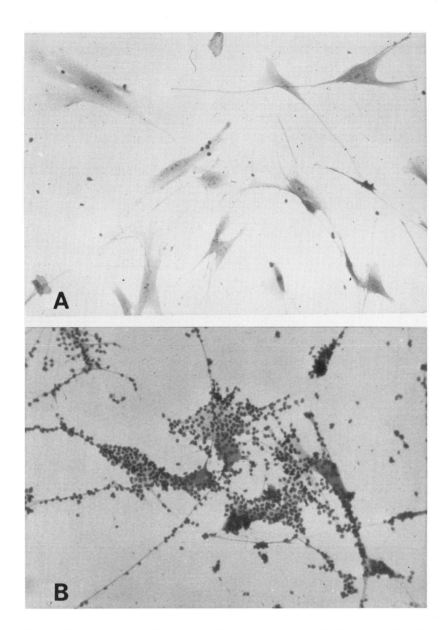

Fig. 14.   Adsorption of Concanavalin A-coated red blood cells to
           surfaces of human fibroblasts.

           A: early passage cells; B: late passage cells. Each round
           dot, or speck, on the cells shows a red blood cell.

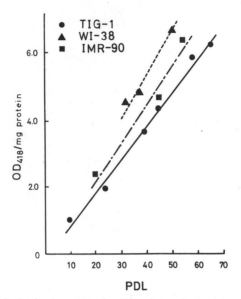

Fig. 15. Age-related changes in the hemadsorption activity of three
strains of human diploid fibroblasts.
The amount of adsorbed red blood cells was determined by
the absorbance of hemoglobin (O.D. 418) per mg of
fibroblast protein.

REFERENCES

1. L. Hayflick, The limited number of in vitro lifetime of human
    diploid cell strains, Exp. Cell Res. 37:614, 1965.
2. G. M. Martin, C. A. Sprague, and C. J. Epstein, Replicative
    lifespan of cultivated human cells: Effect of donor age,
    tissue, and genotype, Lab. Invest. 23:86, 1970.
3. E. L. Schneider and Y. Mitsui, The relationship between in vitro
    cellular aging and in vivo human age, Proc. Natl. Acad. Sci.
    USA 73:3584, 1976.
4. V. J. Cristofalo, Thymidine labelling index as a criterion of
    aging in vitro, Gerontology 22:9, 1976.
5. A. Macieira-Coelho, Kinetics of the proliferation of human
    fibroblasts during their lifespan in vitro, Mech. Ageing Dev.
    5:45, 1977.
6   Y. Mitsui and E. L. Schneider, Relationship between cell
    replication and volume in senescent human diploid
    fibroblasts, Mech. Ageing Dev. 5:45, 1976.
7. Y. Mitsui and E. L. Schneider, Increased nuclear sizes in
    senescent human diploid fibroblast cultures, Exp. Cell Res.
    100:147, 1976.

8. Y. Mitsui and E. L. Schneider, Characterization of fractionated
    human diploid fibroblast cell population, Exp. Cell Res.
    103:23, 1976.

9   J. J. Wolosewick and R. K. Porter, Observations on the
    morphological heterogeneity of WI-38, Am. J. Anat. 149:197,
    1977.

10. L. N. Kapp and R. R. Klevecz, The cell cycle of low passage and
    high passage human diploid fibroblasts, Exp. Cell Res.
    101:154, 1976.

11. Y. Mitsui, S. Aizawa, and K. Matsuoka, The relation of cell
    nuclei and surface membranes to the capacity of cell
    proliferation in human diploid fibroblasts, in:"Proceedings
    of XIth International Congress of Gerontology," Excepta
    Medica, The Netherlands, p. 149, 1979..

12. S. Aizawa, Y. Mitsui, and F. Kurimoto, Cell surface changes
    accompanying aging in human diploid fibroblasts. II. Two
    types of age-related changes revealed by Concanavalin
    A-mediated red blood cell adsorption, Exp. Cell Res., in
    press.

13. H. Sakagomi, Y. Mitsui, S. Murota, and Y. Yamada, Two
    dimensional electrophoretic analysis of nuclear acidic
    proteins in senescent human fibroblasts, Cell Struc. Funct.
    4:215, 1979.

14. Y. Mitsui, H. Sakagami, S. Murota, and Y. Yamada, Age-related
    decline in Hi histone fraction in human diploid fibroblast
    cultures, Exp. Cell Res., in press.

CHANGE OF RESPONSIVENESS TO GROWTH STIMULATION

OF NORMAL CELLS DURING AGING

Tadao Ohno

National Institute of Radiological Sciences
Anagawa, Chiba-shi
260 Japan

INTRODUCTION

The sole determinant of life span of normal diploid cells in vitro has been considered to be the intrinsic doubling number of the cells (1,2,3). Recent investigations, however, suggest that extra-cellular factors can affect the proliferative potential of the cells. For example, hydrocortisone (4) and epidermal growth factor (5) elongate the life span of fibroblasts and keratinocytes, respectively. In vivo experiments also suggest that the milieu in old animals reduces the growth potential of hematopoietic stem cells (6). However, quantitative relationships between cellular growth potential and factors which are supposed, or have been known, to influence cellular growth potential are obscure. This report describes the relationship between the amount of growth stimulating factors and cellular growth potential in the course of aging in vitro, and discusses a possible growth property of divergent cells in a cell population.

METHODS AND RESULTS

Response of Human Lung Fibroblasts to Dialyzed Serum

Figure 1 shows the growth rate of human lung fibroblasts (IMR-90) determined for various dialyzed serum concentrations at different population doubling levels (PDL) (7). By extrapolating the linear part to the level of 1 PDL-increase for 4 days and by plotting the extrapolated dialyzed serum concentrations versus the PDL, curve A in Figure 2 was obtained. The ordinate of Figure 2 is the log scale of the dialyzed serum concentration, and the curve slopes upward. Therefore, the cells require more and more dialyzed serum to maintain

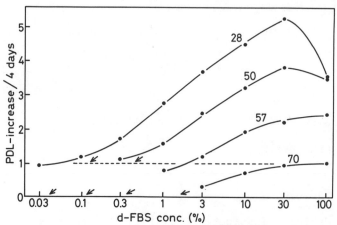

Fig. 1. Effect of dialyzed fetal bovine serum (d-FBS) concentration
on the growth rate of IMR-90 cells at different population
doubling levels (PDL).

Figures attached on each curve are PDLs of the cells
tested. Arrows indicate extrapolation of the linear part of
each curve to 1-PDL increase or no-PDL increase per 4 days
(Ohno, 1979).

a constant growth rate as the PDL increases. This means that the
cells must lose responsiveness to serum growth factors in an accelerated manner during aging in vitro.

    This property of the cells may provide a mechanism for the pre-
viously observed phenomenon that large-volume cells, which have been
supposed to be the non-dividing cells in the population, could divide
as well as the small-volume cells, which have been confirmed as act-
ively dividing cells (see Mitsui, this volume). If one part of a
population of cells divides more rapidly than others by consuming
serum growth factors, the former must lose their responsiveness to
serum growth factors before the latter does. The latter groups,
which have not divided, now get relatively more opportunities to respond to the serum growth factors. Since the large-volume cells are
considered to be the cells that remain in the intermitotic state for
a longer period and are, therefore, the cells that divide less
frequently than small-volume cells, the large-volume cells can divide
as well as, or rather better than, the small-volume cells when the
large-volume cells are separated and cultured in fresh medium
containing sufficient amounts of growth factors.

    By further extrapolating the linear part of the curves in Figure
1 to a no PDL-increase level, maximum dialyzed serum concentrations
incapable of promoting cell division were obtained (Fig. 2, Curve
B). Curve B has a slope similar to that of curve A, and suggests

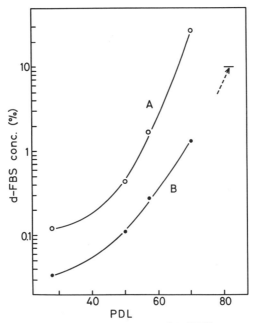

Fig. 2. Requirement of dialyzed serum (d-FBS) concentration for
maintenance of a constant growth rate of IMR-90 cells during
aging in vitro.

Curve A, 1 PDL-increase/4 days; Curve B, no PDL-increase/4
days. The arrow shows extrapolation to 10% d-FBS level
(Ohno, 1979).

that the cells will stop their growth at higher concentrations of
dialyzed serum as the cells age. Therefore, it is possible to predict the cellular life span in vitro when the cells are cultured at a
limited concentration of the dialyzed serum, e.g., addition of 0.3%
or 10% dialyzed serum will result in 58 or 80-85 PDL. The observed
life spans of the cells cultured at 0.3% and 10% dialyzed serum were
54 and 76 PDL, respectively, which corresponds well with the predicted life span. These facts suggest that the loss of cellular responsiveness to serum growth factors and the level of these growth factors in the milieu of the cells are the strict determinants of the
cellular life span in vitro.

Response of Normal Cells to Growth Factors

Cell populations in older animals must contain the cells with
more doubling experience than those in younger animals. If the
progressive cellular loss of responsiveness to growth promotors in
vivo takes place concomitantly with division of the cells, as in

vitro (Fig. 2), it offers a mechanism for aging, at least in proliferative cell populations. In support of this hypothesis, Swierenga
et al. (8) demonstrated that rat thigh muscle cells progressively
lost mitogenic responsiveness to rat plasma growth factors as the age
of the cell donor increased. Adult human fibroblasts showed lower
mitogenic responsivness to the platelet growth factor than fetal
fibroblasts (9). Binding of ^{125}I-labeled insulin and insulin-stimu-
lated glucose metabolism of primary cultured human skin fibroblasts
were reduced when the cells were taken from aged donors (10). Furthermore, Makinodan and Adler (11) reported that T cells showed
striking decline of mitogenic responsiveness to lectins in mice aged
from 3 months to 24 months.

CONCLUDING REMARKS

The relationship between the size of growth stimulation and cellular growth responsiveness in the course of aging in vitro has been
presented. Loss of responsiveness by normal cells concomitant with
an increase in doubling experiences provides an explanation for cellular aging in vitro and probably in vivo. Future studies should
focus on mechanisms for this decline in responsiveness by normal
cells to growth factors.

REFERENCES

1. L. Hayflick and P. S. Moorehead, The serial cultivation of
       human diploid cell strains, Exp. Cell Res. 25:585, 1961.
2. L. Hayflick, The limited in vitro lifetime of human diploid cell
       strains, Exp. Cell Res. 37:614, 1965.
3. R. T. Dell'Orco, J. G. Mertens, and P. F. Kruse, Jr., Doubling
       potential, calendar time, and senescence of human diploid
       cells in culture, Exp. Cell Res. 77:356, 1973.
4. V. J. Cristofalo, Metabolic aspects of aging in diploid human
       cells, in "Aging in Cell and Tissue Culture," E. Holeckova
       and V. J. Cristofalo, eds., Plenum Press, New York (1970).
5. J. G. Rheinwald and H. Green, Epidermal growth factor and the
       multiplication of cultured human epidermal keratinocytes,
       Nature 265:421, 1977.
6. J. W. Albright and T. Makinodan, Decline in the growth potential
       of spleen-colonizing bone marrow stem cells of long-lived
       aging mice, J. Exp. Med. 144:1204, 1976.
7. T. Ohno, Strict relationship between dialyzed serum concentra-
       tion and cellular life span in vitro, Mech. Ageing Dev.
       11:179, 1979.
8. S. H. H. Swierenga, J. F. Whitfield, and A. L. Boynton,
       Age-related and carcinogen-induced alterations of the
       extracellular growth factor requirements for cell
       proliferation in vitro, J. Cell Physiol. 94:171, 1978.

9. J. R. B. Slayback, L. W. Y. Cheung, and R. P. Geyer, Comparative
    effect of human platelet growth factor on the growth and
    morphology of human fetal and adult diploid fibroblasts, Exp.
    Cell Res. 110:462, 1977.
10. H. Orimo and H. Ito, Glucose intolerance in the aged, Jap. J.
    Geriat. 13:157, 1976.
11. T. Makinodan and W. Adler, The effects of aging on the
    differentiation and proliferation potentials of cells of the
    immune system, Fed. Proc. 34:153, 1975.

MULTINUCLEATION AND POLYPLOIDIZATION OF

AGING HUMAN CELLS IN CULTURE

Toshiharu Matsumura

Department of Cancer Cell Research
Institute of Medical Science
University of Tokyo
Shirokanedai, Minato-ku
Tokyo 108, Japan

INTRODUCTION

Multinucleated cells and polyploid cells appear widely in liver, salivary glands, and other mammalian organs. In liver, the multinucleation and polyploidization of hepatocytes are the functions of development, nutrition, regeneration and aging (1,2,3,4). A schematic genealogy of cells has been proposed for the development of multinucleation and polyploidization in rodent liver (2).

Multinucleation and polyploidization appear also in cultured cells. The subject of this paper will be limited to cultured cells from normal human donors that have limited life span (5), unless otherwise mentioned. This is because cells with infinite proliferation potential are different in many respects from cells with finite proliferation potential, and therefore cannot accurately reflect the process of cellular aging. Multinucleated cells have been observed in a human lung culture in its late passages (6). Polyploid cells were noticed both in early and late passages of human lung cell cultures (7,8,9) and in human kidney cell cultures (10).

In a previous study in which human lung cells were cultivated for weeks after the cessation of their rapid proliferation, multinucleated cells were observed to comprise around 50% of total cell population (11). In another study, in which epithelial-like cells from fetal human liver were proliferated in culture, multinucleated cells were noticed early in the primary and secondary cultures (12). The purpose of this short paper is to summarize the results obtained recently in the two systems of human lung cell culture and human

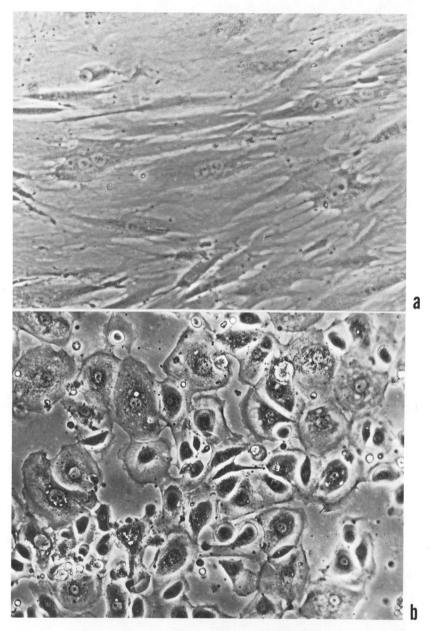

Fig. 1.   Phase-Contrast Micrographs of Cultured Human Lung WI-26
Cells (Fig. 1a, x280) and Cultured Human Liver Cells (Fig. 1b,
x480).   WI-26 cells were cultivated, after their rapid proliferation,
for 26 additional weeks without appreciable further proliferation.
The liver cells obtained from a human fetus were cultivated for 13
days in a primary culture. This population of the liver cells was
proliferating. Binucleated cells are noticeable in both Figures 1a
and 1b.

liver cell culture (details to be published elsewhere by Matsumura
and Nitta, and by Matsumura and Miyashita), to present a working
hypothesis by the author on the multinucleation and polyploidization
of cultured cells, and to try to make an assessment of the hypothesis
with special reference to cellular aging in culture.

MATERIALS AND METHODS

Lung Cell sytem and Liver Cell System

Human lung cells (WI-38 and WI-26) were cultivated for weeks
following the conclusion of their rapid proliferation phase, as described previously (11). These cells will subsequently be referred to
as senescent cells. Epithelial-like cells from fetal human liver
were cultivated in a chemically defined medium supplemented with 10%
fetal bovine serum, and in the presence of irradiated feeder cells
(12). Liver cells were passaged by trypsinization. These liver
cells produced colonies similar to those produced by keratinocytes
(13), and the proportion of clonogenic cells in a given cell population was small. Both the senescent human lung cells and the liver
cells in early passages were examined for the proportion of multinucleated cells, for their nuclear DNA content by Feulgen staining
and microspectrophotometry, and for their entrance into S phase by
continuous labelling with tritiated thymidine and autoradiography.
Detailed methods will be described elsewhere by Matsumura and Nitta,
and by Matsurmura and Miyashita.

MODE OF MULTINUCLEATION AND POLYPLOIDIZATION

Figure 1a shows the morphology of a typical senescent human lung
cell population. Multinucleated cells comprised around 30 to 50% of
the cell population. These were predominantly binucleated cells.
The nuclei in both mononucleated and binucleated cells contained DNA
levels of around one, two, or four times that of the usual amount.
The two nuclei in a single binucleated cell generally contained
equivalent amounts of DNA. With respect to the DNA content and the
number of nuclei, the senescent cells could be divided into six major
groups, as shown in Figure 2. Although detailed data are not
presented in this paper, the senescent cells showed the following
properties: the number of labelled mononucleated cells and labelled
binucleated cells increased during continuous exposure to tritiated
thymidine; the rate of entrance into S phase, however, was considerably slower than that of proliferating (phase II) cells; no clonogenic cells were found in the senescent population when the cells in
a given senescent population were kept for weeks or months and showed
a slight increase or decrease in cell number.

In a proliferating (phase III) cell population, a small proportion of multinucleated cells was detected. The proportion of these
cells increased with increasing population doubling levels. When

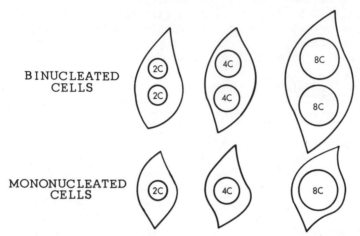

Fig. 2. Schematic presentation of major classes of senescent human
         lung cells. In a cell drawn in a spindle-like shape, there
         are one or two nuclei, drawn as circles. The number in a
         circle shows the amount of DNA in a nucleus. It should be
         noted that, in an actual cell population, a nucleus with a
         DNA content between, or more than, the amounts indicated in
         this figure can also be present. In addition, there are
         some cells with more than two nuclei, or with nuclei
         demonstrating irregular morphology, although they are in the
         minority.

proliferating (phase II) cells were grown in colonies for two weeks
in the presence of 10% serum, and then incubated in the presence of
0.5% serum, no appreciable cell proliferation occurred after the
first two weeks, but multinucleated cells comprising 10 to 20% of the
cell population appeared after 6 to 8 weeks. The proportion of multinucleated cells was higher in small colonies than in large colonies.

    Figure 1b shows the morphology of human liver cells in primary
culture. They are similar in morphology to those classified as
immature liver cells (14). Multinucleated cells comprised about 10%
of the total cell population. These were also predominantly binucleated cells. The two nuclei in a single binucleated cell contained
equivalent amounts of DNA. A nucleus in either a mononucleated or a
binucleated cell contained DNA levels that varied from the usual
quantity to twice the usual quantity. Labelled mononucleated cells
and binucleated cells accumulated during continuous exposure to tritiated thymidine. When liver cells were trypsinized and plated, a
small proportion of the cells formed colonies of varying sizes within
two weeks of incubation. The proportion of multinucleated cells was
higher in small colonies than it was in large colonies.

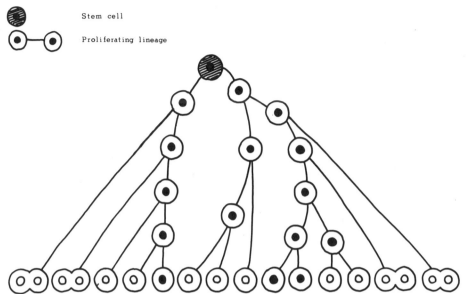

Fig. 3. A hypothetical scheme for the proliferation and multinucle-
         ation of cultured human liver cells. The cells at the
         bottom are the descendants of a single cell, shown at the
         top. Clonogenic cells are represented by cells with filled
         nuclei. Nonclonogenic cells are represented by cells with
         open nuclei.

DISCUSSION

Cell Cycle and "Cell Spiral" Model. Experimental studies using
pulse labelling and cinemicrography will tell much about the mode of
multinucleation and polyploidization in culture. While these studies
are in progress, this author would like to interpret the results summarized above by presenting a hypothetical model. In Figure 3, a
model of proliferation and multinucleation of human liver cells in
culture is described schematically. In this model, it is hypothesized that: a clonogenic cell is diploid; a nonclonogenic cell is a
descendent of a clonogenic cells; and that the latter cell contains
either a single nucleus or two nuclei. This model can qualitatively
explain all of the above results for both human liver and lung
cells. The quantitative terms in both systems, such as the proportion of clonogenic cells in a culture or the time required for a
direct descendant of a clonogenic cell in a cell population to become
a binucleated cell, may differ, however.

For senescent human lung cells, some of which are polyploid, a
further model of multinucleation and polyploidization is shown in

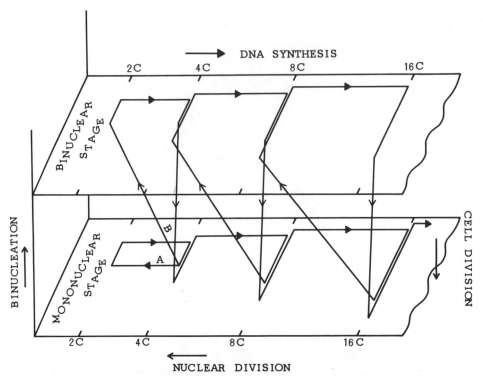

Fig. 4. Cell cycle and "cell spiral" model of in vitro cellular
        aging. A cell cycle in which a clonable cell remains is
        shown by "A" at the bottom left. When a cell leaves this
        cycle (by an unknown mechanism), it follows the path
        indicated by "B," referred to as "cell spiral" in the text.

Figure 4. In Figure 4, it is hypothesized that: a clonogenic cell
is diploid and proliferates by turning a cell cycle; that there is an
unknown mechanism by which a cell leaves the cycle, follows another
path, which is referred to as a "cell spiral," and never returns to
the cell cycle; and that the cell in the "spiral" shuttles back and
forth between a mononuclear and a binuclear stage, synthesizes DNA in
between, and moves up to a polyploid state. It should be noted that
there may be several ways other than that described in Figure 4 to
explain how a cell might shuttle between the mononuclear and the
binuclear stages, synthesizing DNA in between. Leaving the cell
cycle may not mean instant commitment, since commitment could possibly happen while a cell is still cycling. For senescent human lung
cells, spiralling cells may be destroyed or removed from a culture by
such outside influences as trypsinization. Removal of spiralling
cells from a senescent population may cause the loss of a culture.
No evidence was found that human liver cells undergo polyploidization

in culture. Possibilities were that the period of observation was
too short to detect polyploid cells, that polyploidizing cells were
removed from a culture by outside influences such as trypsinization,
or that there were mechanisms preventing a cell from spiralling further.

Previously reported observations of cultured rat liver cells support the present model. Richman et al. (15) found that a primary
culture of rat hepatocytes containing many binucleated cells did not
proliferate, but was able to synthesize DNA upon a hormonal stimulation. It is possible that those hepatocytes were not in cell cycle,
but in "cell spiral." Proliferating clones of liver epithelial-like
cells have been obtained in culture. They have some of the differentiated functions of hepatocytes (16). Careful studies permitted the
maintenance of diploid clones of mononuclear cells (17,18). Although
they should not directly be compared with human liver cells because
the former have infinite proliferation potential, one could speculate
that those diploid clones are transformed in such a way that they
remain in a permanently cycling state and never "spiral."

SUMMARY

In conclusion, evidence has been presented to show that multinucleation and polyploidization are common, if not ubiquitous,
phenomena observable both in proliferating human cell populations in
culture, and in cell populations which have already passed through
their proliferative phase in culture. A hypothetical model is presented, the essence of which postulates the existence of a regularly
controlled cell life, including DNA synthesis, out of cell cycle.

AKNOWLEDGEMENT

The author gratefully acknowledges Dr. L. Hayflick and Dr. H.
Katsuta for their kind introduction aging study in culture.

REFERENCES

1. H. Tauchi and T. Sato, Some micromeasuring studies of hepatic
    cells in senility, J. Gerontol. 17:254 (1962).
2. C. Nadal and F. Zajdela, Polyploidie somatique dans le foie de
    rat. I. Le role des cellules binucleees dans la genese des
    cellules polyploides, Exp. Cell Res. 42:99 (1966).
3. D. N. Wheatley, Binucleation in mammalian liver: Studies on the
    control of cytokinesis in vivo, Exp. Cell Res. 74:455 (1972).
4. W. Ya. Brodsky and I. V. Uryvaeva, Cell polyploidy: Its
    relation to tissue growth and function, Int. Rev. Cytol.
    50:275 (1977).
5. L. Hayflick and P. S. Moorhead, The serial cultivation of human
    diploid cell strains, Exp. Cell Res. 25:585 (1961).

6. A. Maciera-Coelho, J. Ponten, and L. Philipson, Inhibition of the division cycle in confluent cultures of human fibroblasts in vitro, Exp. Cell Res. 43:20 (1966).

7. E. Saksela and P. S. Moorhead, Aneuploidy in the degenerative phase of serial cultivation of human cell strains, Proc. Natl. Acad. Sci. 50:390 (1963).

8. M. C. Yoshida and S. Makino, A chromosome study of non-treated and an irradiated human in vitro cell line, Japan J. Human Gen. 5:39 (1963).

9. Z. K. Kadanka, J. D. Sparkes, and H. G. Macmorine, A study of the cytogenetics of the human cell strain WI-38, In Vitro 8:353 (1973).

10. R. C. Miller, W. W. Nichols, J. Pottash, and M. M. Aronson, In vitro aging: Cytogenetic comparison of diploid human fibroblasts and epitheliod cell lines, Exp. Cell Res. 110:63 (1977).

11. T. Matsumura, Z. Zerrudo, and L. Hayflick, Senescent human diploid cells in culture: Survival, DNA synthesis and morphology, J. Gerontol., (1977) (in press).

12. T. Matsumura and S. Miyashita, Characteristics of human liver epithelial-like cells proliferating in culture, Proc. Japan Cancer Assoc., 37th Annual Meeting 120 (1978).

13. J. G. Rheinwald and H. Green, Epidermal growth factor and the multiplication of cultured human epidermal keratinocytes, Nature 265:421 (1977).

14. H. Imai, Human embryonic liver cell in culture. A preliminary report, Okayama Igakkai Zasshi 89:237 (1977).

15. R. A. Richman, T. H. Claus, S. Pilkis, and D. L. Friedman, Hormonal stimulation of DNA synthesis in primary cultures of adult rat hepatocytes, Proc. Natl. Acad. Sci. USA 73:3579 (1976).

16. A. Ichihara, Relation of the characteristics of liver cells during culture, differentiation, and carcinogenesis, in: "Control Mechanisms in Cancer," W. E. Criss, T. Ono, and J. R. Sabine, eds., Raven Press, New York (1976).

17. J. Bausher and W. I. Schaeffer, A diploid rat liver cell culture. I. Characterization and sensitivity to alfatoxin B_1, In Vitro 9:286 (1974).

18. H. Masuji, H. Nakabayashi, and J. Sato, Long-term cultivation of two diploid epithelial cell lines derived from normal rat liver cells, Acta Med. Okayama 28:281 (1974).

MECHANISM OF AGE-DEPENDENT DECREASE IN SULFATION

OF CHONDROITIN SULFATE

Sei-itsu Murota[*], Atsushi Honda[*,**], Midori Abe[*],
and Yo Mori[**]

[*]Department of Pharmacology, Tokyo Metropolitan Institute
of Gerontology, Itabashi-ku, Tokyo 173 and
[**]Department of Biochemistry, Tokyo College of Pharmacy,
Hachioji-shi, Tokyo 192-03, Japan

INTRODUCTION

A number of investigators have been concerned with the relationship between extracellular substances and aging (1,2). It is generally recognized that the amount of hexosamine-containing substances
in tissue decreases with age, while the insoluble collagen content in
the tissue increases with age (3). Recently, it has been reported
that the decrease in elasticity of cartilage with age is related to
the content and structure of the proteoglycan in the matrix (4).

The main purpose of the present study was to determine what
causes these age-dependent alterations in both the amounts of hexosamine-containing substances in tissues and the changes in the
structure of chondroitin sulfate chains of proteoglycan macromolecules. This paper discusses the age-dependent decrease in sulfation
of chondroitin sulfate in rat costal cartilage. A part of this work
has been published elsewhere (5).

METHOD AND RESULTS

Changes in Glycosaminoglycan Content with Aging

The amount of glycosaminoglycan (GAG) in dry costal cartilage
tissue from Sprague-Dawley male rats of various ages (young, 3
months; middle, 12-18 months; and old, 23-24 months) decreased with
aging, while the GAG content in mg DNA (unit cartilage cell) remained
the same with aging. These results can be explained by the finding
that the total number of cartilage cells decreased with aging.

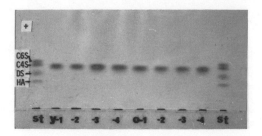

Fig. 1.   Electrophoresis of glycosaminoglycan from young (3 months;
           y-1 to y-4) and old (23 months; 0-1 to 0-4) rat costal
           cartilage.
           Electrophoresis was carried out in 0.3 M calcium acetate
           (pH 7.25) at a constant current of about 1 mA/cm for 3 hr
           (6). The strips were stained with 0.5% Alcian Blue in 3%
           acetic acid. Hyaluronic acid (HA), chondroitin 4-sulfate
           (C4S), chondroitin 6-sulfate (C6S), and dermatan sulfate
           (DS) were used as reference standards. Similar
           electrophoretic patterns were obtinted in the middle-aged
           (15 months) rat glycosaminoglycan samples.

Chondroitin Sulfate in Rat Costal Cartilage

Electrophoretic analysis demonstrated that chondroitin 4-sulfate
was the major glycosaminoglycan of rat costal cartilage irrespective
of age (3, 15, and 23 months), as shown in Figure 1. This result was
in agreement with that reported in the literature (7), but was quite
different from the results reported in the literature for human (8,9)
and rabbit (10) costal cartilage, i.e., there is an age-dependent
decrease in the ratio of chondroitin 4-sulfate to chondroitin 6-sul-
fate. This means that rat costal cartilage is suitable for examining
the influence of aging on the biosynthesis of chondroitin sulfate.

Age-Dependent Alteration in the Biosynthetic Activities of Cartilage

In an attempt to determine the cause of an age-dependent alteration in the tissue contents of GAG, we examined the influence of
aging on the biosynthetic activity of cartilage in the production of
hexosamine-containing substances. Rat costal cartilage of different
ages was incubated with radioactive precursors, ^{3}H-glucosamine or
^{35}S-sulfuric acid, and newly synthesized hexosamine-containing substances, i.e., glycosaminoglycan (GAG) and glycopeptide (GP), were
prepared and analyzed. The radioactivity uptake of GAG per mg dry
cartilage tissue indicated that there was an apparent decrease in the
incorporation of ^{35}S-sulfate into GAG with age (a statisticallv
significant difference existed between 100-day- and 350-day-old
rats: $p < 0.01$, but no significant difference existed between

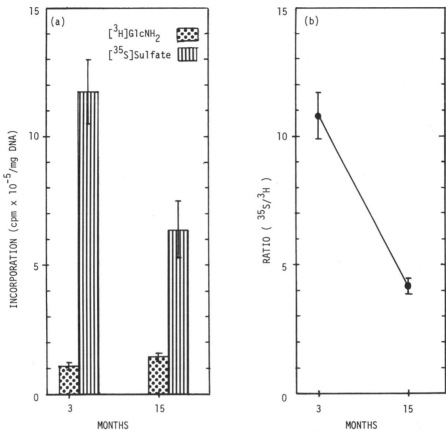

Fig. 2.   Effect of age on incorporation of ^{3}H-glucosamine and
           ^{35}S-sulfate into glycosaminoglycan. The cartilage
           slices were incubated in Ham's F-12 medium containing
           5 μCi of ^{3}H-glucosamine and 5 μCi of ^{35}S-sulfuric acid
           for 3 hr, and the doubly labeled glycosaminoglycan formed
           was used for subsequent analyses. Experimental details
           are described in reference (5). Results indicate mean
           $\pm$ S.E. (n = 3 or 4).

350-day- and 710-day-old rats), while the incorporation of
^{3}H-glucosamine into GAG did not show a change with age. On the
other hand, the incorporation of ^{3}H-glucosamine into GP occurred
only to a minor extent, and this level remained unchanged with age.
The incorporated ^{35}S-radioactivity level in GP was negligible.

To confirm the above mentioned findings, that the ^{35}S-sulfate
incorporation was much more affected by aging than the ^{3}H-glucos-
amine incorporation, a double isotope method was used. Rat costal

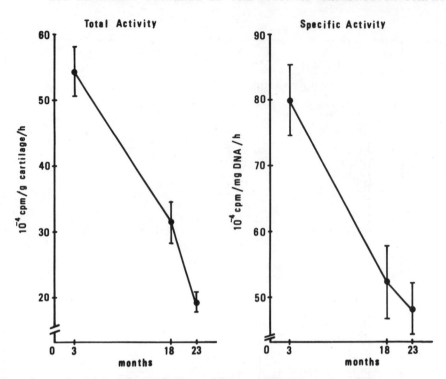

Fig. 3.   Changes of sulfotransferase activity with aging.
The enzyme activity using chondroitin as sulfate acceptor
was determined by the method of Habuchi et al. (11). For
further experimental details, see reference (5). Results
indicate mean ± S.E. (n = 3 or 4). The total activity
of sulfotransferase was defined as cpm/g cartilage/hr
incorporated into chondroitin. The specific activity of
sulfotransferase was defined as cpm/mg DNA/hr incorporated
into chondroitin.

cartilage was incubated in the presence of both ^{35}S–sulfuric acid
and ^{3}H–glucosamine at the same time, and the newly synthesized GAG
was prepared and analyzed. As shown in Figure 2a, there was a significant decrease in the specific radioactivity of ^{35}S–sulfate per
mg DNA (unit cartilage cell), whereas the specific radioactivity of
^{3}H–glucosamine per mg DNA (unit cartilage cell) did not change significantly in the young (3 months) and the middle-aged (15 months)
rats. The ratio of radioactivity of ^{35}S–sulfate to ^{3}H–glucosamine, then, decreased significantly between 3 months and 15 months of
age, as shown in Figure 2b.

The above result suggested that the biosynthesis of the repeating
disaccharide units in the chondroitin sulfate molecule was affected
little with aging, but the sulfation of the chondroitin sulfate chain

decreased with the process of aging.

Changes in Sulfotransferase Activity with Aging

Sulfation of chondroitin sulfate by 3'-phosphoadenosine 5'-phosphosulfate (PAPS) was first described by D'Abramo and Lipmann (12). Later, direct transfer of a sulfate group from ^{35}S-PAPS to both chondroitin sulfate and chondroitin by sulfotransferase was demonstrated _in vitro_ (13-16). DeLuca et al. (17) showed that sulfation occurred on the polysaccharide, along with, or immediately following, polymerization. In our laboratory, an attempt was made to examine the changes in sulfotransferase activity with aging. This enzyme is known to be responsible for the sulfation process in chondroitin sulfate biosynthesis. At present, however, the true sulfate acceptor of sulfotransferase in the biosynthesis of proteochondroitin sulfate has not been fully elucidated. Therefore, the enzyme activity was determined using chondroitin as sulfate acceptor (11). As was expected, both the total sulfotransferase activity and the specific activity per mg DNA (unit cartilage cell) decreased significantly with age, as shown in Figure 3. Similar results were also obtained when female rats were used. It is possible that this change can be attributed to a decrease in the enzyme activity of individual chondrocytes with aging. Furthermore, the decrease in sulfotransferase activity of cartilage cells with age was parallel to a reduction in the incorporation of ^{35}S-sulfate in chondrocytes with age. Recently, Hart (18) reported that the specific activity of glycosaminoglycan-sulfotransferase with each exogenous acceptor (e.g., keratan sulfate) changed only slightly during chick corneal development. It is interesting to note, however, that a difference exists in the activity of sulfotransferase between the processes of development and aging. Moreover, the analysis of disaccharide units formed after chondroitinase ABC digestion of ^{35}S-chondroitin or ^{35}S-endogenous acceptor, produced in the enzymic reaction mixtures (the enzyme source from 3-month-old rats), showed that the percentage of incorporation of ^{35}S sulfate into ΔDi-4S (ΔGlcUA-GalNAc-4S) was about 90% (Honda et al., unpublished data). Similar results were obtained when the enzyme source from old (23-month-old) rat costal cartilage was used. These results indicated that the sulfotransferase in rat costal cartilage specifically catalyzed the transfer of sulfate from ^{35}S-PAPS to position 4 of acetlygalactosamine residue of chodroitin or endogenous acceptor. It may then be said that chondroitin, used as a sulfate acceptor, behaved similarly to _in vivo_ rat costal cartilage, in that the sulfotransferase specified the position for introduction of a sulfate group.

Changes in Degree of Sulfation and Molecular Size of Chondroitin Sulfate with Aging

Analysis of disaccharide units, formed after chondroitinase ABC digestion (19) of ^{3}H-labeled GAG isolated from young (3 months) and

old (23 months) cartilage, showed that the percentages of incorporation of ^{3}H-glucosamine into ΔDi-0S (ΔGlcUA-GalNAc) increased
significantly (from 7.7% to 13.6%) with age. This result suggested
that the appearance of nonsulfated positions in the structure of the
chondroitin sulfate chain increased with age.

On the basis of gel chromatography on Bio-Gel A-1.5m, no significant difference in the approximate molecular size of chondroitin sulfate was observed between the young (3 months) and old (23 months)
samples. This finding suggested that aging did not affect the average chain length of chondroitin sulfate, and was consistent with the
findings of Inerot et al. (4) and S̄imůnek and Muir (20). It is,
therefore, not unreasonable to assume that the biosynthesis of the
repeating disaccharide units in the chondroitin sulfate chain is
affected little by the aging process.

DISCUSSION

Cartilage proteoglycan is composed of a protein core to which a
large number of highly negatively charged chondroitin sulfates and a
relatively small number of keratan sulfates are covalently attached,
in the model proposed by Heinegård and Hascall (21). Recently,
Inerot et al. (4) indicated that the structural change of proteoglycan macromolecules of articular cartilage with age was probably due
to a diminishing of the chondroitin sulfate-rich region, whereas the
hyaluronic acid-binding region and the keratan sulfate-rich region
remain comparatively constant. This change in the proteoglycan
macromolecular structure is believed to result in a decrease in the
elasticity of the older cartilage.

In our study, sulfation of the chondroitin sulfate chain was
found to decrease with age. Moreover, the number of non-sulfated
positions in the structure of the chondroitin sulfate chain of rat
costal cartilate proteoglycan increased with aging. The decrease in
sulfation may result from either defective sulfation enzymes or an
enhanced sulfatase activity, or a combination of both. At the
present time, however, there is little direct evidence for the
involvement of sulfatases in aging (22,23). The fact that the sulfotransferase activity decreased with aging, as shown in our study,
must be directly related to the decrease in the biosynthetic sulfation of chondroitin sulfate.

It is of biological significance to relate the decreased sulfation of chondroitin sulfate in aged rats to the change in the elastic
properties of cartilage with age, since negatively charged sulfate
groups of the chondroitin sulfate chains in the proteoglycan molecule
may play an important role for the interaction between proteoglycan
and collagen. It is also important to consider that the sulfate
group of proteochondroitin 4-sulfate binds with Ca^{2+} to function as
a store of Ca^{2+}, and prevents the cartilage from calcifying (24,25).

Further, the degree of sulfation of chondroitin sulfate chains in proteoglycan molecule must be one of the major factors in the organization of the multimolecular-structures in the cartilage matrix.

REFERENCES

1. H. G. Vogel, ed., "Connective Tissue and Ageing," Excerpta Medica, Amsterdam (1973).
2. D. A. Hall, ed., "The Aging of Connective Tissue," Academic Press, London (1976).
3. H. Boström, in: "Aging of Connective and Skeletal Tissue," A. Engel and T. Larson, eds., Nordiska Bokhandelsforlag, Stockholm (1969).
4. S. Inerot, D. Heinegård, L. Audell, and S.-E. Olsson, Articular-cartilage proteoglycans in aging and osteoarthritis, Biochem. J. 169:143 (1978).
5. A. Honda, M. Abe, S.-I. Murota, and Y. Mori, The effect of aging on the synthesis of hexomsamine-containing substances from rat costal cartilage: A decrease in sulfation of chondroitin sulfate with aging, J. Biochem. 85:519 (1979).
6. N. Seno, K. Anno, K. Kondo, S. Nagase, and S. Saito, Improved method for electrophoretic separation and rapid quantitation of isomeric chondroitin sulfates on cellulose acetate strips, Anal. Biochem. 37:197 (1970).
7. Y. H. Liau, N. I. Galicki, and M. I. Horowitz, Heterogeneity of rat rib chondroitin sulfate and susceptibility to rat gastric chondrosulfatase, Biochim. Biophys. Acta 539:315 (1978).
8. M. B. Mathews and S. Glagov, Acid mucopolysaccharide patterns in aging human cartilage, J. Clin. Invest. 45:1103 (1966).
9. H. Iwata, The determination and fine structures of chondroitin sulfate isomers of human cartilage and pathological tissues, J. Jap. Orthop. Assoc. 43:455 (1969).
10. H. J. Mankin and A. Z. Thrasher, The effect of age on glycosaminoglycan synthesis in rabbit articular and costal cartilages, J. Rheumatol. 4:343 (1977).
11. O. Habuchi, T. Yamagata, and S. Suzuki, Biosynthesis of the acetylgalactosamine 4,6-disulfate unit of squid chondroitin sulfate by transsulfation from 3'-phosphoadenosine 5'-phosphosulfate, J. Biol. Chem. 246:7357 (1971).
12. F. D'Ambramo and F. Lipmann, The formation of adenosine-3'-phosphate-5'-phosphosulfate in extracts of chick embryo cartilage and its conversion into chondroitin sulfate, Biochim. Biophys. Acta 25:211 (1957).
13. S. Suzuki and J. L. Strominger, Enzymatic sulfation of mucopolysaccharides in hen oviduct. I. Transfer of sulfate from 3'-phosphoadenosine 5'-phosphosulfate to mucopolysaccharides, J. Biol. Chem. 235:257 (1960).

14. S. Suzuki and J. L. Strominger, Enzymatic sulfation of mucopolysaccharides in hen oviduct. II. Mechanism of the reaction studied with oligosaccharides and monosaccharides as acceptors, J. Biol. Chem. 235:267 (1960).

15. S. Suzuki and J. L. Strominger, Enzymatic sulfation of mucopolysaccharides in hen oviduct. III. Mechanism of sulfation of chondroitin and chondroitin sulfate A, J. Biol. Chem. 235:274 (1960).

16. H. C. Robinson, The sulfation of chondroitin sulfate in embryonic chicken cartilage, Biochem. J. 113:543 (1969).

17. S. DeLuca, M. E. Richmond, and J. E Silbert, Biosynthesis of chondroitin sulfate: Sulfation of the polysaccharide chain, Biochemistry 12:3911 (1973).

18. G. W. Hart, Glycosaminoglycan sulfotransferases of the developing chick cornea, J. Biol Chem. 253:347 (1978).

19. H. Saito, T. Yamagata, and S. Suzuki, Enzymatic methods for the determination of small quantitites of isomeric chondroitin sulfates, J. Biol. Chem. 243:1536 (1968).

20. Z. Simůnek and H. Muir, Changes in the protein-polysaccharides of pig articular cartilage during prenatal life, development and old age, Biochem. J. 126:515 (1972).

21. D. Heinegård and V. C. Hascall, Aggregation of cartilage proteoglvcans. III. Characteristics of the proteins isolated from trypsin digests of aggregrates, J. Biol. Chem. 249:4250 (1974).

22. R. Silberberg and P. Lesker, Enzyme activity in aging articular cartilage, Experientia 27:133 (1971).

23. Å. Wasteson, U. Lindahl, and A. Hallén, Mode of degradation of the chondroitin sulfate proteoglycan in rat costal cartilage, Biochem. J. 130:729 (1972).

24. J. D. Salvo and M. Schubert, Specific interaction of some cartilage protein-polysaccharides with freshly precipitating calcium phosphate, J. Biol. Chem. 242:705 (1967).

25. R. D. Campo, C. D. Tourtellotte, and R. J. Bielen, The protein-polysaccharides of articular, epiphyseal plate and costal cartilages, Biochim. Biophys. Acta 177:501 (1969).

HYDRODYNAMIC PROPERTIES OF

COLLAGEN FIBRIL AND AGING

Toshiharu Matsumura

Department of Cancer Cell Research
Institute of Medical Science
University of Tokyo
Shirokanedai, Minato-ku, Tokyo 108
Japan

INTRODUCTION

One biochemical approach to aging research has been to isolate
bodily structural components, study their physiochemical properties,
and establish the molecular basis for bodily changes during the aging
process. This approach has been particularly fruitful in the field
of connective tissue research, ever since soluble collagen was first
isolated from tendon, and synthetic fibrils were reconstituted from
the soluble collagen in vitro (1). When, in addition to soluble collagens and soluble ground substances, connective tissue components
with high order structures, observable as collagen fibril, collagen
fiber, and collagen fiber bundle (2) are isolated and characterized,
such age-related changes as shrinkage temperature and tensile
strength of skin (3) may be able to be expressed in terms of the
physiochemical properties of their structural components.

Collagen fibril is one of those structural units in connective
tissue where collagen molecules assemble in a regular fashion. They
have an familar cross striation pattern when observed by an electronmicroscope. The fact that the average diameter, and the variability
of diameter, of collagen fibril increases during mammalian aging was
described by Banfield (4) and Schwarz (5). In the last ten years,
the presence of an intrafibrillar structural unit, tentatively called
either collagen filament or collagen microfibril, has been predicted
with evidence resulting from electronmicroscopy (6), sequence analyses (7), and X-ray diffraction (8). The structure of the predicted
microfibril consists of a five-fold helix of collagen molecules
related by a 1D (length of the unit striation pattern) stagger.

47

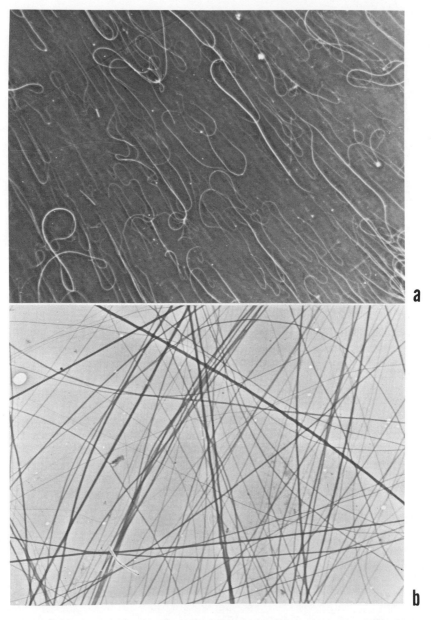

Fig. 1a. Phase contrast micrograph of sea cucumber (Stichopus
          japonicus) collagen fibrils. A drop of the fibril
          suspension was smeared and dried on a glass slide (x 310).

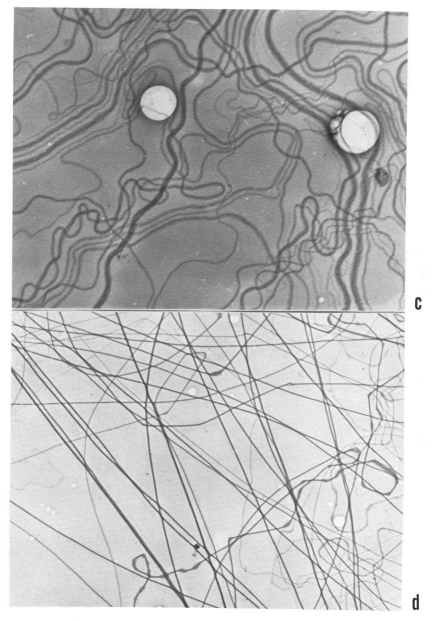

Fig. 1b-d.   Electron micrographs of native (b), denatured (c), and
             partially denatured (d) collagen fibrils. An aliquot
             of fibril suspension was kept in the cold without
             incubation (b), incubated at 55°C for 10 min (c), or
             at 47°C for 60 min (d), and processed for electron-
             microscopy following pseudo-replica technique and
             uranyl acetate staining (x 8000).

Since the difference between the denaturation temperature of collagen molecule (around body temperature for mammals) and the shrinkage temperature of skin (around 60°C for mammals, depending on age) predicts the presence of weak and cooperative interactions among collagen molecules, a hydrodynamic study of collagen fibril would provide information about its predicted structure and the thermodynamic properties of connective tissues.

Preparations of mammalian collagen fibril have been obtained by Banfield (9) and Steven (10). Those preparations, however, were not used for hydrodynamic studies, perhaps because the preparation process may have interrupted the intact structure. Preparations of collagen fibrils have also been obtained from various echinodermal animals (11,12,13). Figure 1a shows collagen fibrils with a spindle-like shape and heterogeneous sizes obtained from the sea cucumber, Stichopus japonicus (14). There are advantages in using the sea cucumber fibrils and other echinodermal fibrils for a hydrodynamic study: there is only a single collagen type, and no collagenase has so far been found in echinoderms; the fibrils are quite insoluble both in acid and neutral solutions; and the fibril can be kept in suspension for days without precipitation, which allows the investigators to handle a fibril suspension as though it were a solution of macromolecules. The disadvantages are that no laboratory-grown echinoderms are available, and that echinodermal collagens cannot directly be compared with mammalian collagens, even though they are very similar. However, the body size of Stichopus japonicus, which increases during development and aging, can be used as a parameter of aging (15).

In this short paper, some viscometric and electromicroscopic observations using prepartions of collagen fibril from Stichopus japonicus will be described. Although the results are preliminary, they are the first, to this investigator's knowledge, that show the hydrodynamic and thermal properties of isolated collagen fibril.

MATERIALS AND METHODS

Preparation of Collagen Fibril. Collagen fibril from the sea cucumber was prepared in a cold room by a method described previously (13). Briefly, tissue fragments were disaggregated in a neutral salt solution containing EDTA and β-mercaptoethanol, and then collagen fibril was isolated from soluble macromolecules and residual particles by centrifugation. The isolated fibril was resuspended in neutral salt solution, dialyzed against water with the pH adjusted to 8.0 with a trace amount of Tris-HCL buffer. For viscometry, the suspension of isolated fibrils was passed through a sintered-glass filter to remove remaining aggregates of fibrils.

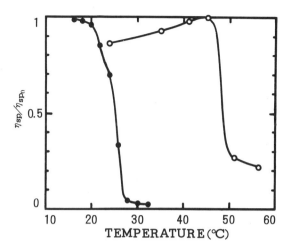

Fig. 2.   Viscosity changes of collagen fibril suspensions and of a
solution of solubilized collagen. The fraction of
specific viscosity at a temperature (η sp) to the maximal
value of the specific viscosity observed during the
experimental range of temperature (η sp_0) is shown as a
function of increasing temperature (ca. 0.12°C/min). A
fibril suspension was treated with Pronase (50 µg/ml) at
4°C overnight, and then the solubilized collagen was
isolated from Pronase solution by acid precipitation and
resolubilization (detailed methods to be described
elsewhere). Capillary viscometers with a flow of about
100^{-1} sec were used.

RESULTS

Thermal Denaturation of Collagen Fibril. Individual collagen
fibrils in the preparation obtained above show a striation pattern
under an electronmicroscope (Fig. 1b). After an incubation of the
fibril suspension at 55°C for 10 minutes the cross striation pattern
was completely lost and the fibrils were swollen (Fig. 1c). No
significant amount of collagen protein was lost from the denatured
fibril into the water following this short incubation. After a
60-minute incubation at 47°C, the collagen fibrils lost their cross
striation pattern in some areas, whereas it was retained in most
areas of the fibrils (Fig. 1d).

The viscosity of collagen fibril suspension decreased between
46°C and 50°C when the suspension was incubated with increasing temperature (Fig. 2). This temperature range is about 20°C higher than
that for the viscosity change of solubilized collagen (see legend for
Fig. 2). Profiles of the isothermal decline of viscosity varied to a
certain extent, depending on the preparations used. Some examples

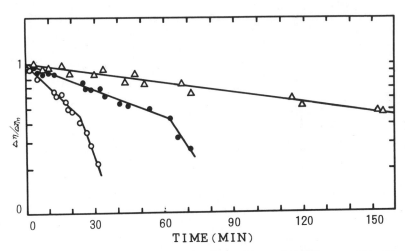

Fig. 3.   Isothermal decline of viscosity of collagen fibril
            suspensions. From the specific viscosities of the
            initiation of incubation (ηsp t = o), at an incubation
            time (η sp t), and after complete denaturation (ηsp d)
            which was attained by keeping the suspension at 50°C for
            10 min, the fraction of viscosity change to the total
            viscosity decrement ($\Delta\eta/\Delta\eta$o = $\dfrac{\eta\text{sp t} - \eta\text{sp d}}{\eta\text{sp t} = \text{o} - \eta\text{sp d}}$) is
            presented as a function of incubation time. The value
            ($\Delta\eta/\Delta\eta$o) was measured for a preparation of fibril
            suspension at 47°C (o———o) and at 46°C (●———●), and
            for another preparation at 48°C (△———△).

are shown in Figure 3. The profile consisted of one or two consecu-
tive phases, hereafter referred to as phase A and phase B. In both
phases, the difference between specific viscosity at time t and that
after full denaturation declined exponentially. The kinetic constant
for phase B was larger than that for phase A.

DISCUSSION

    The Structural Bases of Thermal Denaturation. The electron
microscopic and viscometric results as described above present
conclusive evidence that the thermal shrinkage of connective tissue
is an event happening within the collagen fibril, consisting of a
cooperative denaturation of the ordered structure within the fibril.
An isothermal profile of viscosity changes (Fig. 3) suggests that the
denaturation consists of one or two first-order reactions, depending
on the preparations used. Electronmicroscopic results show that, at
least for some preparations, the denaturation does not happen
throughout the entire fibril at once (Fig. 1c). A simple hypothesis
that can explain all of the above results is that there is a

subfibrillar structural unit which denatures in a first-order reaction with the kinetic constant of phase B, and that the accumulation in a fibril of a certain number of denatured subfibrillar units leads to the denaturation of the entire fibril. For other fibril preparations that showed only one phase of isothermal viscosity change, the subfibrillar units may be tightly packed by an interaction among the subfibrillar units within a fibril, so that the fibril denatures as a first-order reaction with the kinetic constant of phase A. If this is the case, then the size of a collagen fibril, which is known to be a function of age, will influence the kinetic constant and period of phase A, but not of phase B. The two-phase viscosity change for some preparations might also be indicative of a loss of structural intactness during fibril preparation. Substantiation of the above hypothesis awaits further experimental work, as does the determination of thermodynamic parameters of fibril denaturation.

ACKNOWLEDGEMENT

The assistance of Professor Haruhiko Noda is gratefully acknowledged.

REFERENCES

1. J. Nageotte, Coagulation fibrillaire in vitro du collagène dissous dans un acide dilué, Compt. Rend. Acad. Sci. 184:115 (1927).
2. A. J. Cruise, The structure and deformation of collagen fibers. II. The morphology of collagen fibers, J. Soc. Leather Chemists 40:321 (1965).
3. D. M. Rusmussen, K. G. Wakim, and R. K. Winkelmann, Effect of aging on human dermis: Studies of thermal shrinkage and tension, in: "Advances in Biology of Skin, Vol. VI, Aging," W. Montagna, ed., Pergamon Press, Oxford (1964).
4. W. G. Banfield, Width and length of collagen fibrils during the development of human skin, in granulation tissue and in the skin of adult animals, J. Gerontol. 10:13 (1955).
5. W. Schwarz, Morphology and differentiation of the connective tissue fibres, in: "Connective Tissue," R. E. Tunbridge, M. Keech, J. F. Delafresnaye, and G. C. Woods, eds., Blackwell Scientific Publications, Oxford (1957).
6. J. W. Smith, Molecular pattern in native collagen, Nature 219:157 (1968).
7. B. L. Trus and K. A. Piez, Molecular packing of collagen: Three-dimensional analysis of electrostatic interactions, J. Mol. Biol. 108:705 (1976).
8. A. Miller, Molecular packing in collagen fibrils, in: "Biochemistry of Collagen," G. N. Ramachandran and A. H. Reddi, eds., Plenum Press, New York (1976).

9. W. G. Banfield, Occurrence of tapered collagen fibrils from
    human sources with observations on mesenchymal neoplasms,
    Proc. Soc. Exp. Biol. Med. 81:658 (1952).

10. F. S. Stevens, he Nishihara technique for the solubilization of
    collagen: Application to the preparation of soluble
    collagens from normal and rheumatoid connective tissue, Ann.
    Rheum. Dis. 23:300 (1964).

11. T. Matsumura, M. Shinmei, and Y. Nagai, Disaggregation of
    connective tissue: Preparation of fibrous components from
    sea cucumber body wall and calf skin, J. Biochem. 73:155
    (1973).

12. T. Matsumura, M. Hasegawa, and M. Shigei, Collagen biochemistry
    and phylogeny of echinoderms, Comp. Biochem. Physiol. 62B:101
    (1978).

13. T. Matsumura, Shape, size and amino acid composition of collagen
    fibril of the starfish Asterias amurensis, Comp. Biochem.
    Physiol. 44B:1197 (1973).

14. T. Matsumura, Collagen fibrils of the sea cucumber, Stichopus
    japonicus: Purification and morophological study, Connective
    Tissue Res. 2:117 (1974).

15. K. Mitsukuri, "otes on the habits and life-history of Stichopus
    japonicus Selenka, Annot. Zool. Japan 5:1 (1903).

ALTERNATE CELLULAR MODELS

FOR AGING STUDIES

Edward L. Schneider[*]

Section on Cellular Aging and Genetics
Laboratory of Cellular and Molecular Biology
Gerontology Research Center
National Institute on Aging
National Institutes of Health
Baltimore, Maryland 21224, USA

Studies such as those described by Drs. Macieira-Coelho and
Mitsui lead to increased insight into the mechanisms of the limited
proliferative capacity of human diploid fibroblasts. While I suggest
that these elegant studies of the in vitro passage of human cells be
continued, I urge the development of alternate models for the study
of cellular aging. In our laboratory, we have examined human diploid
cells as a function of in vitro passage and the age of the donor of
these cells. The first studies in this latter area were conducted by
Drs. Hayflick, Goldstein, Martin, and their co-workers (1-3). These
investigators demonstrated the diminished proliferative potential of
cell cultures with the increasing age of the donor. At the Gerontology Research Center in Baltimore, we have been fortunate to be able
to conduct our studies on skin fibroblast cultures derived from young
and old volunteer members of the Baltimore Longitudinal Study. We
have examined the total replicative ability of these skin fibroblast
cultures, as well as many of the parameters analyzed by Drs. Mitsui
and Macieira-Coelho as a function of in vitro passage (4).

Our results confirm the findings of Dr. Martin that cell cultures
from young donors have greater numbers of total population replica-
tions and delayed onsets of senescence than parallel cultures
obtained from old donors (Table 1). The percent replicating cells
was determined by incubating cell cultures for 24 hours with

_____
[*]Dr. Schneider's current address: Davis Institute on Aging,
700 Delaware Street, Denver, Colorado 80204, USA.

55

Table 1.   Summary of Studies Conducted on Skin Fibroblast
           Cultures Derived from Young and Old Human Subjects[a]

Replication Parameter	Young Subjects (20-35 yrs)	Old Subjects (65 + yrs)
Onset of Senescent Phase (PD)[b]	35.2 ± 2.1 (23)[c]	22.5 ± 1.7 (21)
In Vitro lifespan (PD)	44.6 ± 2.5 (23)	33.6 ± 2.1 (21)
Cell population replication rate (hrs.)	20.8 ± 0.8 (18)	24.3 ± 0.9 (18)
Percent replicating cells[d]	87.7 ± 1.6 (7)	79.6 ± 2.5 (7)
Cell number at confluency (x 10^4 cells/cm^2)	7.31 ± 0.42 (18)	5.06 ± 0.52 (18)
Percent cells able to form colony > 16 cells[e]	69.0 ± 3.3 (9)	48.0 ± 4.4 (8)
Sister chromatid exchanges/cell[f]	67.9 ± 1.6 (7)	56.1 ± 1.4 (6)

[a]The results of these studies have been originally published in ref. 4, 5, and 7.

[b]PD = Population doublings

[c]Numbers within brackets indicate number of cell cultures examined, values are mean

± standard error of the mean.

[d]Determined by incubating cells for 24 hours with tritiated thymidine and then

measuring the frequency of labeled nuclei by autoradiography.

[e]Two weeks after plating at low cell densities

[f]Cell cultures were incubated for 48 hours with 7.5 ng/ml mitomycin C. Fifteen

cells from each culture were analyzed for SCE.

tritiated thymidine, and then determining the percent labeled nuclei
by autoradiography. Cell population doubling time and the cell
number at confluency were measured from cell culture growth curves.
For each measure of cell replication, cell cultures from old donors
had diminished capabilities when compared to parallel cultures from
young donors (Table 1).

Studies of individual cells have been conducted in collaboration
with Dr. James Smith and Olivia Pereira-Smith (5). Analysis of the
colony size distributions of young and old donor skin fibroblast cultures indicates that cells from young donors form larger colonies
more frequently than do cell cultures from old donors (Table 1).

We have recently completed studies of sister chromatid exchanges
(SCE). These studies indicate that mitomycin-C induced SCE are

diminished as a function of in vitro passage (6) and the age of the
cell culture donor (7) (Table 1). A number of other collaborative
studies have been completed on cell cultures from young and old donors, including studies of macromolecular synthesis using a viral
probe (8) and examination of insulin and EGF receptors (9).

In summary, a number of the alterations that are found as a function of in vitro passage can also be seen as a function of donor
age. At the Gerontology Research Center, we have 800 relatively
healthy volunteers who visit our Center every year and a half for a
comprehensive series of physiological and psychological testing.
Thus, we can examine the relationship between in vitro and in vivo
measurements.

Finally, I would like to urge the combination of in vitro and in
vivo studies. We have taken this approach in our studies of SCE
which have been conducted in vitro in human cells and well as in vivo
in rodent cell populations (10).

REFERENCES

1. L. Hayflick, The limited in vitro lifetime of human diploid cell
      strains, Exp. Cell Res. 37:614 (1965).
2. S. Goldstein, J. W. Littlefield, and J. S. Soeldner, Diabetes
      mellitus and aging: Diminished plating efficiency of
      cultured human fibroblasts, Proc. Nat. Acad. Sci. USA 64:155
      (1969).
3. G. M. Martin, C. A. Sprague, and C. J. Epstein, Replicative
      lifespan of cultivated human cells: Effect of donor age,
      tissue, and genotype, Lab. Invest. 23:86 (1970).
4. E. L. Schneider and Y. Mitsui, The relationship between in vitro
      cellular aging and in vivo human age, Proc. Nat. Acad. Sci.
      USA 73:3584 (1976).
5. J. R. Smith, O. M. Pereira-Smith, and E. L. Schneider, Colony
      size distributions as a measure of in vivo and in vitro
      aging, Proc. Nat. Acad. Sci. USA 75:1353 (1978).
6. E. L. Schneider and R. E. Monticone, Aging and sister chromatid
      exchange II. The effect of in vitro passage level of human
      fetal lung fibroblasts on baseline and mutagen-induced sister
      chromatid exchange frequencies, Exp. Cell Res. 115:269 (1978).
7. E. L. Schneider and B. Gilman, Sister chromatid exchanges and
      aging III. The effect of donor age on mutagen induced sister
      chromatid exchange, Hum. Genet., in press (1979).
8. D. B. Danner, E. L. Schneider, and J. Pitha, Macromolecular
      synthesis in human diploid fibroblasts: A viral probe
      examining the effect of in vivo aging, Exp. Cell Res. 114:63
      (1978).

9. M. D. Hollenberg and E. L. Schneider, Receptors for insulin and
    epidermal growth factor-urogastrone in adult human
    fibroblasts do not change with donor age, Mech. Ageing Dev.,
    in press (1979).

10. D. Kram, E. L. Schneider, R. R. Tice, and P. Gianas, Aging and
    sister chromatid exchange. I. The effect of aging on
    mitomycin-C induced sister chromatid exchange frequencies in
    mouse and rat bone marrow cells in vivo, Exp. Cell Res.
    114:471 (1978).

AGING OF HEPATOCYTES

Akihiro Shima

Department of Experimental Radiology
Shiga University of Medical Science
Ōtsu, Shiga 520-21
Japan

INTRODUCTION

The purpose of this paper is not to survey current knowledge on
aging of hepatic cells in general, but to summarize some of our own
results that are concerned with the age changes in DNA content-based
polyploidization of hepatocytes of three kinds of laboratory animals:
mouse (1), fish (2), and house shrew (3).

The major technique used throughout the experiment was a strictly
controlled Feulgen-DNA cytofluorometry combined simultaneously with
tritiated thymidine autoradiography (4,5,6). As a parameter of age
changes in hepatocytes, we measured the changes in DNA contents of
hepatocytes which had been suggested by the extensive micromorpho-
metric studies on human livers by Tauchi and Sato (7,8,9).

AGING OF MOUSE HEPATOCYTES

The C57BL/6 male mice used in our experiments had a mean life
span of 24 months and a maximum life span of 31 months under our laboratory conditions (1). Figure 1 summarizes the change in relative
frequency of each nuclear ploidy class as a function of animal age.
The nuclei in S phase are not included in this figure. All measurements were done without regard to binuclearity, which is well known
to occur in the liver of rodents and humans during aging. The
decrease in percentage of 2C (diploid) nuclei occurred as early as 1
month of age, and the reduction continued steadily up to 28 months.
This decrease in the percentage of 2C nuclei is accompanied by a
marked increase in the percentage of 4C nuclei after about 1 month of
age. However, the percentage of 4C nuclei stayed at almost the same

59

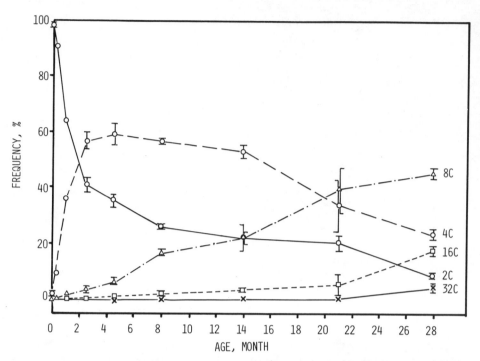

Fig. 1. Changes in relative frequency of mouse hepatocytes of
        various ploidy classes. Reproduced from Shima and Sugahara
        (1).

level from 2.5 months to 14 months of age, and thereafter it climbed
toward 24 percent at 28 months of age. The percentage increase in 8C
and 16C nuclei, and probably even in 32C nuclei, might be persistent
throughout the life of the mice.

The clear age dependency in hepatocyte polyploidization can be
shown in another, simpler, way by introducing the term, "Polyploidization Index," (P.I.), as shown in Figure 2. The Polyploidization
Index is defined by dividing the summation of percentage of polyploid
nuclei by percentage of diploid nuclei, because diploid (2C) nuclei
might be possibly regarded as the basic unit in somatic cells. A
straight line could be fitted between logarithms of age in months and
P.I., by least square method, with a correlation coefficient $r =
+0.892$. These results do not tell anything about the mechanism(s) of
the age-dependent polyploidization in mouse hepatocytes. However,
the present results could be of use as basic data for further
research into the mechanism(s).

As the next step following the phenomenalistic description of
age-dependent polyploidization of mouse hepatocytes, it would be

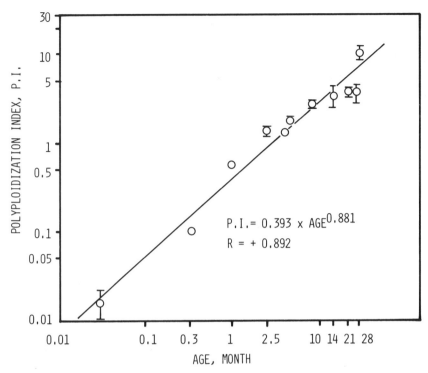

Fig. 2. Relationship between age in months and degree of
polyploidization of mouse hepatocytes. Polyploidization
Index (P.I.) = % polyploids/% diploids; r, correlation
coefficient. Reproduced from Shima and Sugahara (1).

quite natural for one to attempt to learn what the differences are
among hepatocytes of various ploidy classes. To begin with, we
compared the template-primer activities of DNA among hepatocytes of
various ploidy classes (10), by utilizing the enzymatic method
originally developed by Modak et al. (11-14). In the method they
originated, the paraffin sections of animal tissues were used to
react with exogenously added DNA polymerase. However, we used methanol-fixed smears of the liver in order to avoid possible artifacts
derived from routine histological procedures, and also to make it
possible to combine grain counting method with Feulgen-DNA cytofluorometry simultaneously. The details of the present procedures have
already been described (15). Briefly, methanol-fixed smears of the
liver were allowed to react with exogenously added DNA polymerase I
of E. coli in the presence of ^{3}H-TTP, three other dNTP's and other
co-factors. E. coli DNA polymerase can be utilized to nick DNA with
3'-OH end as well as the gapped DNA (16). The specimens were then
stained with Feulgen nuclear reaction and dipped into a nuclear emul-
sion to prepare autoradiographs. The DNA content measurement and

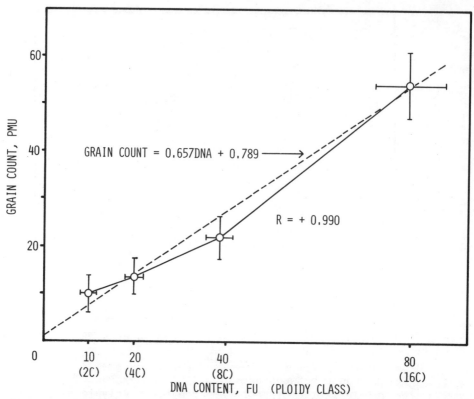

Fig. 3. Template-primer activity of 12-month-old mouse hepatocytes
of various ploidy classes detected by E. coli DNA polymerase
I. FU, fluorescence unit; PMU, photo-multiplier unit.
Reproduced from Shima, Egami and Sugahara (10).

grain counting were done simultaneously on each hepatocyte nucleus.
Since no grain could be found on nuclei wihout denaturing treatments
of the specimens, all preparations were treated with 0.01 N HCl at
25°C for 30 min prior to incubation with the reaction mixture.

The results shown in Figure 3 were obtained from livers of
12-month-old C57BL/6 male mice (10). The grain count was in an
almost linear relationship with the amount of DNA, i.e., nuclear
ploidy classes. However, if the grain count was divided by the DNA
content, something like "specific" template-primer activities could
be obtained, as shown in Figure 4 (10). It appears evident that no
principal difference in such "specific" activities could be found
among four ploidy classes of the hepatocytes. In summary, the number
of sites in the nucleus which were sensitive to 0.01 N HCl and which
could also react with exogenously added DNA polymerase I of E. coli
might be doubled when the ploidy class of hepatocyte ascends from one

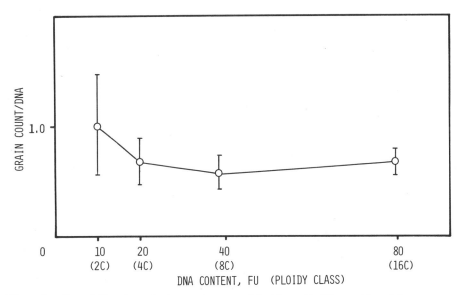

Fig. 4. Specific template-primer activity of 12-month-old mouse
hepatocytes of various ploidy classes detected by E. coli
DNA polymerase I. Reproduced from Shima, Egami and Sugahara
(10).

class to the next higher class, i.e., through polyploidization. In
addition, the type of DNA damage that can be detected by E. coli DNA
polymerase I might not be primarily responsible for age-dependent
polyploidization of mouse hepatocytes.

AGING OF FISH HEPATOCYTES

The age-related changes in the DNA contents of hepatocytes were
also examined using male Japanese killifish Medaka, Oryzias latipes,
which is one of the best known poikilothermal laboratory animals.
The life table of the fish has already been established with mean and
maximum life spans of 1000 days and 1838 days, respectively (17,18).
The results summarized in Figure 5 indicate that: (a) there is no
principal difference among the frequency distributions of nuclear DNA
contents of young (about 100-day-old), medium (about 450-day-old),
and old (about 1200-day-old) fish, and (b) the distributions of DNA
contents are continuous from 2C (= 10 FU) to 4C range, irrespective
of age (2). The first point indicates that no systematic polyploidization occurs in hepatocytes of the fish during aging, and the
second point suggests that almost the same fraction of hepatocytes
might be in S phase of 2C cell cycle in young, medium, and old fish,
at least judging from our previous data on mouse hepatocytes (1). In
order to examine the second point, the fish were injected with
tritiated thymidine and autoradiographs were prepared with the

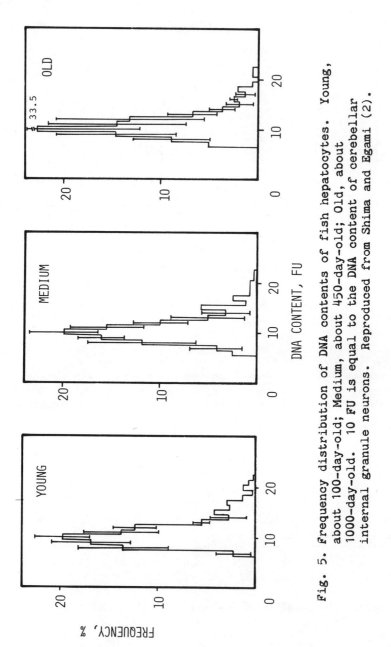

Fig. 5. Frequency distribution of DNA contents of fish hepatocytes. Young, about 100-day-old; Medium, about 450-day-old; Old, about 1000-day-old. 10 FU is equal to the DNA content of cerebellar internal granule neurons. Reproduced from Shima and Egami (2).

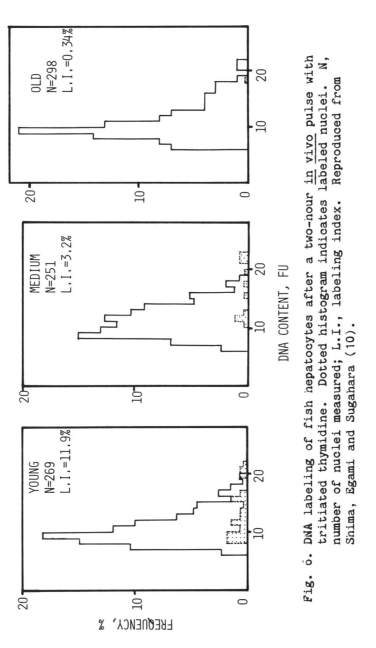

Fig. 6. DNA labeling of fish hepatocytes after a two-hour in vivo pulse with tritiated thymidine. Dotted histogram indicates labeled nuclei. N, number of nuclei measured; L.I., labeling index. Reproduced from Shima, Egami and Sugahara (10).

results shown in Figure 6 (10). The labeling index decreased, from
12 percent in young fish to 0.3 percent in old ones, with advancing
age of the fish. Another point which should be marked in Figure 6 is
that only the minor fraction of hepatocytes with intermediate DNA
contents between 2C and 4C could be labeled. This result is quite
different from that obtained from mouse hepatocytes (1). No answer
for this discrepancy is possible at the present time.

Another interesting property of fish hepatocytes is given in
Figure 7 (10). Since fish are poikilothermal vertebrates, the cell
cycle parameters can be easily changed by keeping fish at different
temperatures. Such alteration in cell cycle parameters has already
been reported for intestinal epithelium of the goldfish (19).
Therefore, we transferred old fish which were reared, during winter
days, under natural low temperature conditions to 25°C, and the fish
were warmed for 10 days. A remarkable increase in labeling index was
evident, and also many more fractions of hepatocytes with intermediate DNA contents between 2C and 4C were labeled, although considerable fractions still remained unlabeled. It has been well documented
that hepatocytes of rodents can undergo compensatory proliferation
after partial hepatectomy or CCl4 poisoning, particularly after
large-scale cell loss. As far as we observed, no detectable signs of
pycnosis could be found in livers of the warmed fish. These results
might indicate that hepatocytes in old fish still reserve high growth
potentials which could express themselves without cell death and
probably cell loss in the parenchyma. One could speculate that the
present findings could possibly be related to the initial response of
the warmed fish which are ready to grow, even though they are old.
Finally, it is interesting to this author that Comfort has concluded
that fish do age despite continued growth (20).

AGING OF SHREW HEPATOCYTES

As the third laboratory animal for experimental aging research,
we have just begun to use the house shrew, Suncus murinus. The
domestication of the house shrew is now in progress in the laboratory
of Professor Kondo of Nagoya University, the outline for which can be
found in reference 21. In brief, the house shrew, Suncus murinus,
belongs to the Family Soricidae of the insectivores; and insectivores
are generally accepted as the most primitive placental mammals. The
average life expectancy of Suncus murinus has been supposed to be 2
years or so with a maximum of 3 years (21).

Since the number of shrews which can be used for our experiment
is still small, only preliminary results on the DNA content distribution of hepatocytes and cerebellar internal granule neurons of 1- and
2-year-old males are now in our hands (3). In order to simplify the
comparison with mice, the liver and cerebellum of the house shrew
were stamped onto the same slide glass on which mouse cerebellum was

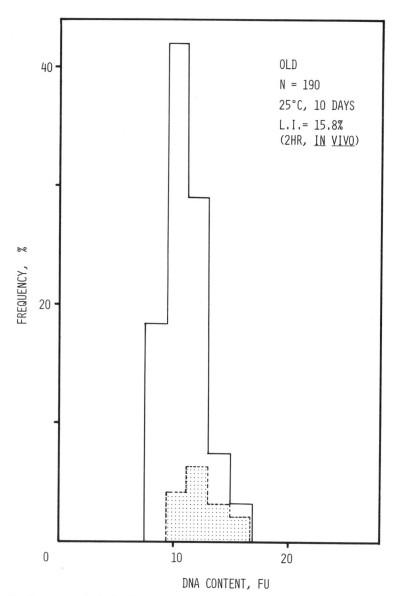

Fig. 7. Increased labeling of hepatocytes of old fish transferred
        from low temperature to 25°C. Dotted histogram, labeled
        nuclei. Reproduced from Shima, Egami and Sugahara (10).

stamped, which provided a standard. As shown in Figure 8, the mean
DNA content of cerebellar internal granule neurons of the house shrew
was 8.5 FU, while that of the mouse was 10.0 FU. This consistent

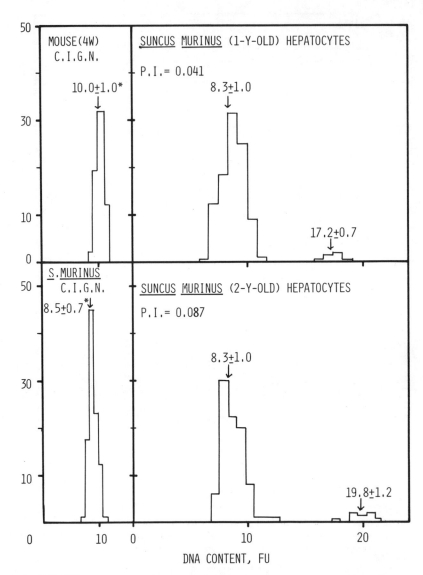

*: P<0.001

Fig. 8. Frequency distribution of DNA contents of neurons and
        hepatocytes of mouse and house shrew (Suncus murinus).
        C.I.G.N., cerebral internal granule neurons; FU,
        fluorescence unit. P.I., polyploidization index
        (= % polyploids/% diploids). Reproduced from Shima,
        Shinohara and Kondo (3).

difference (p < 0.001) indicates that the genome size of the house shrew is significantly smaller than that of the mouse.

Two other points should be made. The frequency distribution histograms of DNA contents of shrew hepatocytes, characterized by major 2C peak and minor 4C peak, are almost identical between two age groups; and the hepatocyte nuclei with intermediate DNA contents are equally almost absent. Whether the nuclei with DNA contents around 17 FU are G_2 nuclei of diploid cells or G_1 nuclei of tetraploids is not yet clear. Further studies utilizing larger numbers of the shrews of various ages and combining autoradiography are now in progress. There preliminary results indicate that, in the house shrew, almost all the hepatocytes seemed to be diploid, at least in 1- and 2-year-old animals; which is to say that few polyploids occur.

CONCLUSION

Judging from the DNA content measurements, mouse hepatocytes are most prone to undergo polyploidization with advancement of the animal age, while fish hepatocytes are the least likely to do so, and shrew hepatocytes are probably somewhere between the two. Our attempt to find uniformity in the aging of hepatic cell resulted in the finding of rather a marked diversity. However, further efforts to search for mechanism(s) responsible for the diversity might allow us to approach the uniformity.

REFERENCES

1. A. Shima and T. Sugahara, Age-dependent ploidy class changes in mouse hepatocyte nuclei as revealed by Feulgen-DNA cytofluorometry, Exp. Gerontol. 11:193 (1976).
2. A. Shima and N. Egami, Absence of systematic polyploidization of hepatocyte nuclei during the ageing process of the male Medaka, Oryzias latipes, Exp. Gerontol. 13:51 (1978).
3. A. Shima, S. Shinohara, and K. Kondo, Unpublished data.
4. S. Fujita, T. Ashihara, M. Fukuda, T. Hattori, and S. Yoshida, Combination of Feulgen cytofluorometry with 3H-thymidine autoradiography, Acta Histochem. Cytochem. 6:205 (1973).
5. S. Fujita and M. Fukuda, Irradiation of specimens by excitation light before and after staining with Pararosaniline Feulgen: A new method to reduce non-specific fluorescence in cytofluorometry, Histochemistry 40:59 (1974).
6. S. Fujita, T. Ashihara, and M. Fukuda, Simultaneous measurement of DNA content and grain count on an autoradiograph of Feulgen stained cells, Histochemistry 40:155 (1974).
7. H. Tauchi, On the fundamental morphology of the senile changes, Nagoya J. Med. Sci. 24:97 (1960).
8. T. Sato, T. Miwa, and H. Tauchi, Age changes in the human liver of the different races, Gerontolgia 16:368 (1970).

9. H. Tauchi and T. Sato, Effect of environmental conditions upon age changes in human liver, Mech. Ageing Dev. 4:71 (1975).

10. A. Shima, N. Egami, and T. Sugahara, Comparative study on the polyploidization of hepatocytes of mouse and fish during ageing, in:"Liver and Aging-1978," K. Kitani, ed., Elsevier/North-Holland Biomedical Press, Amsterdam (1978).

11. S. P. Modak, R. C. von Borstel, and F. J. Bollum, Terminal lens cell differentiation II. Template activity of DNA during nuclear degeneration, Exp. Cell Res. 56:105 (1969).

12. S. P. Modak and F. J. Bollum, Terminal lens cell differentiation III. Initiator activity of DNA during nuclear degeneration, Exp. Cell Res. 62:421 (1970).

13. S. P. Modak and F. J. Bollum, Detection and measurement of single-strand breaks in nuclear DNA in fixed lens sections, Exp. Cell Res. 75:307 (1972).

14. G. B. Price, S. P. Modak, and T. Makinodan, Age-associated changes in the DNA of mouse tissue, Science 171:917 (1971).

15. M. Matsui, A. Shima, and N. Egami, Autoradiographic detection of the template-primer activities of DNA by exogenous DNA polymerases in fixed mouse tissues, J. Fac. Sci., Univ. Tokyo, Sec. IV, 13:399 (1976).

16. R. B. Kelly, N. R. Cozzarelli, M. P. Deutscher, I. R. Lehman, and A. Kornberg, Enzymatic synthesis of deoxyribonucleic acid XXXII. Replication of duplex deoxyribonucleic acid by polymerase at a single strand break, J. Biol. Chem. 245:39 (1970).

17. N. Egami and H. Etoh, Life span data for the small fish, Oryzias latipes, Exp. Geront. 4:127 (1969).

18. N. Egami, Further notes on the life span of the teleost, Oryzias latipes, Exp. Geront. 6:379 (1971).

19. Y. Hyodo-Taguchi and N. Egami, Development of gastrointestinal radiation injury and recovery at different temperatures in fish, in:"Comparative Cellular and Species Radiosensitivity," V. P. Bond and T. Sugahara, eds., Igaku-Shoin, Tokyo (1969).

20. A. Comfort, The effect of age on growth-resumption in fish (Lebiste) checked by food restriction, Gerontologia 4:177 (1960).

21. K. Kondo, S. Oda, H. Takahashi, and R. Izeki, The house shrew: A new laboratory animal for comparative study of aging, in:"Abstracts for Plenary Sessions and Symposia of the XIth International Congress of Gerontology," Tokyo (1978).

THE AGING PROCESS IN THE NEURON*

Kenneth R. Brizzee[1] and Craig Knox[2]

[1]Department of Neurobiology
Delta Regional Primate Research Center
Tulane University Medical Center
Covington, Louisiana 70433

[2]Department of Anatomy
Tulane University Medical Center
New Orleans, Louisiana 70122

INTRODUCTION

The neuron as the ultimate anatomical and physiological unit of the nervous system, and the archetype of postreplicative cells of the body, has perhaps received a greater amount of attention as a model for the study of aging processes than any other cell type. Additional interest in the neuron as a subject for aging studies stems from the view that that these elements, in strategic locations in the nervous system, may function as pacemakers, or the central control elements, of the "time clocks" of aging which may determine the onset and rate of senescence (1).

Several topics pertaining to aging in the neuron, including neurotransmitters, hormonal receptors, age changes in dendritic organization, and neuroendocrine factors, will be covered by other authors in this volume. The present chapter therefore will be confined to a consideration of age changes in neuron cell populations, synapses and synaptic end bulbs, and structural and cytologic changes in these postreplicative cells with age.

CHANGES IN NEURONAL POPULATIONS AND THE NEURON-TO-GLIA RATIO WITH AGE

General Considerations

Of the many age-related structural changes in the brain which

*Supported by NIH RROO164

have attracted the attention of experimental gerontologists, probably
none has excited greater interest than the possibility of neuronal
"fall-out" (2) with age. Although opinions still differ with regard
to the magnitude, rate, and even the occurrence of neuronal loss,
there appears to be a consensus among most experimental gerontologists that neuron loss with age does indeed occur in certain regions
of the mammalian central nervous system.

Changes in Total Cell Populations in Whole Brain

One investigation of neuron populations in the whole brain of the
mouse using the "sonification" technique revealed no significant
decline in the numbers of neurons from young adulthood to 24 months
of age. However, by 29 months the neuron population decreased
significantly to approximately one-third of the original number,
while the glial population appeared to increase (3). It was
concluded that the shape of the neuron survival curve resembled the
shape of the mouse survival curve, and both tended to correspond to
the exponential Gompertz plot.

In another recent investigation of possible changes in neuronal
number in the whole body employing the "DNA method" in mice, no
change in total number of neurons with age was observed (4).

Cerebral Cortex

In a series of human brains, without demonstrable pathology,
ranging in age from newborn to 95 years of age, Brody (5) reported a
decrease in neurons with age in several regions of the cerebral
cortex.

In another study involving an analysis of neuron populations in
the brains of two "elderly" men, without any major disease known to
be associated with cell loss, a decrease of 44% in neuron number was
reported (6). In yet another investigation comparing neuron
populations in cerebral cortex in young and old human subjects, a
decrease of 22% in the number of neurons in Brodman's area 6, 28% in
area 10, 23% in area 21, and 29% in the subiculum was observed (7).

Quantitative histological studies in the cerebral cortex of young
adult and aged rhesus monkeys have also revealed a similar but less
severe decrease in the packing density in cerebral cortex, especially
in area 3 (8). The greatest loss was observed in the granule cell
population in lamina IV. Wisniewski et al. (9) also described a loss
of neurons in the cerebral cortex in aged rhesus monkeys. In our
study (8), it was also shown that the number of glial cells per mm^3
of tissue and the glia/neuron ratio increased significantly with age.

In the cerebral cortex of the albino rat, a quantitative histological study using an automated technique (Leitz Texture Analyzing

These symposium proceedings attempt to identify and fill in gaps in the current understanding of ~~the~~ ageing and particularly to integrate knowledge from ~~different~~ different fields of study. The first sections deal with cell aging _in vitro and in vivo_, and succeeding ones with the effects of aging on genetic information and intercellular communication. The final sections look at ~~the~~ role of the immune and neuroendocrine systems, and ~~some~~ some broader perspectives on aging such as environmental factors and longevity potentials.

Category C

The proceedings of a symposium held in 1978 consisting of some twenty five papers. The main two sections are concerned with cell aging in vitro and cell aging in vivo. It is possible that this thriving area of research has progressed well beyond these papers and that they are background reading. The remaining sections are concerned with aging in terms of changes in genetic information, inter cellular communication, the higher hierarchy. The last section has some intriguing data on maximum life potentials — some perspectives.

System) revealed a significant decrease in neurons in the visual cortex (area 17) (10). It was not possible in that investigation, with the automated equipment, to differentiate vascular cell nuclei from glial nuclei. Hence the "small cell" population included both glial and vascular cell counts. These did not appear to change with age. Earlier studies carried out by manual methods of cell enumeration in our laboratory showed that no neuron loss occurred in the somatosensory area of cerebral cortex of aged as compared with young adult Long-Evans rats (11). In that investigation, a significant increase in the glial population with a concomitant reduction in the neuron-to-glia ratio with age was observed. Such glial increases with age have been observed in cerebral cortex of various species by several workers, including Wahal and Riggs (12), Timiras and Vernadakis (13), Vaughan and Peters (14), Uemura and Hartmen (15,16), and Sturrock (17). It is noteworthy that Sturrock, in an earlier study (18), found a decrease in total numbers of glia in the anterior commissure with age. He tentatively suggested that part of the reason for the differences in glial counts in different structures might be gradual migration of neuroglia from white to gray matter with increasing age (17). We concur with this postulate.

The possibility of subspecies differences in the rate and intensity of the aging process, as evidenced by the difference in neuron loss between Long-Evans (11) and albino (10) rats, clearly indicates a need for additional aging studies giving special attention to subspecies comparisions in relation to the median and maximum life span of each, as well as to environmental conditions during the rearing of the animals.

Cerebellum

In the cerebellum of man, apes, dogs and cats, a decrease in the number of Purkinje neurons per unit volume of tissue has recently been observed in aged as compared to young adult animals (19,20). More recently, Tarnowska-Dziduszko (21) reported atrophy of all 3 layers of the cerebellar cortex, patchy cell losses in the granular layer, and marked loss of Purkinje neurons in aged human tissues. The most recent investigations by Hall et al. (22), which employed automated techniques, also reported a loss of Purkinje neurons in the cerebellum with age.

Basal Ganglia and Thalamus

An 18% decrease in number of neurons in the human anterior thalamic nucleus with age was reported (23). Neuroglial cell populations, reported as mean number of cells per field of view, did not appear to change significantly from age 24 to 64 years in man in various thalamic nuclei (23). Quantitative data on age differences in glial populations in the thalamus at older age levels have not yet been reported.

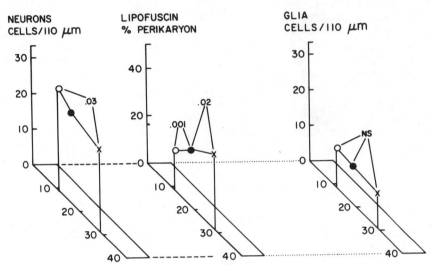

Fig. 1.   Age differences in neurons, lipofuscin and glia in
          hippocampus CA-1 zone. (Brizzee and Ordy, Mech. Ageing
          Dev., in press, 1978). Reprinted with the permission of
          the publisher.

In the striatum, Gellerstedt (24) described a loss of small
neurons. A recent report (25) supports this finding and, in
addition, describes a loss of large neurons in the 65-year-old human
putamen with concurrent loss of putamen volume.

Hippocampus

Quantitative histological studies on the CA-1 zone of the hippocampus of Fisher 344 rats of 11, 17, and 29 months of age revealed a
significant decrease in number of neurons per unit area of the pyramidal layer between the 11th and 29th months (26) (Fig. 1). Quantitative estimates of the lipofuscin in the neurons increased significantly in the same tissues. Although there is no apparent increase
in the glial packing density in the aged rat (26) or human (27), hippocampus, astroglial hypertrophy and increased oligodendroglial
satellitosis are prominent features of the hippocampus of the aged
rat (28,29).

Brain Stem

No loss in total number of neurons was observed in the ventral
cochlear nucleus in man, but the total volume decreased significantly
in old age (30). The human abducens nucleus was also observed to
exhibit no neuron loss in advanced age (31). A significant decrease

in neuronal populations of the substantia nigra (32) and locus
coeruleus (33), however, may indicate dysfunction of central
monoaminergic systems in aged persons.

Conflicting results on changes in total numbers of neurons in the
main nucleus of the human inferior olive have been reported in recent
years. Monagle and Brody (34) observed no decrease in number of
neurons, while Sandoz (35) reported a significant loss of neurons in
this nucleus with age.

Spinal Cord

An investigation of the changes in the total number of large
cells in the spinal cord of mice revealed no significant differences
at 6, 25, and 50 weeks (37). However, at 110 weeks the number of
cells was decreased by 15 to 20%. A loss of up to 38% of ventral
horn neurons was described in the aged rat (38).

Nucleus

A decrease in the size of nuclei of cerebellar granule cells in
aged chinchillas was reported by Cammermeyer (39), and a similar
observation was made with respect to mean nuclear volume in the

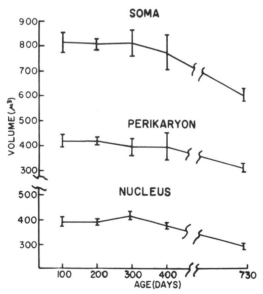

Fig. 2.   Decrease in mean soma, perikaryal and nuclear volume in
          neurons of somatosensory cerebral cortex with age in
          albino rats. (Brizzee et al., 1962, Pergamon Press).
          Reprinted with permission of the publisher.

somatosensory area of the rat cerebral cortex by Brizzee et al. (40)
(Fig. 2). Lin et al. (41) reported that nuclear volume in female
rats decreased with age in several hypothalamic nuclei or areas.

It has been reported by some authors that the neuron nucleus in
aged mammals is characterized by a darkening of the culeoplasm,
increased basophilia and accumulation of Feulgen-stainable chromatin
(42,43). Other authors (23) have described increased pallor of
neuron nuclei and a diminution in the amount of Feulgen-stained
chromatin in cerebellar granule cell neurons of aged, as compared
with young, rabbits and chinchillas (39).

The differentiation between the nucleus and cytoplasm was sharp
in neurons of young animals but much less so in some neurons in aged
subjects (Fig. 3). The same tendency was noted in human tissues, but
the variation was greater than in animals. A loss of regularity of
cell outline and absence of a sharp demarcation between nucleus and
cytoplasm was observed in senile rhesus monkeys (44) and humans (45).

Fine structural studies have also revealed nuclear inclusions
(Fig. 4) which appear to increase in number with age in lateral
vestibular nucleus neurons of rats (46). Other studies have
indicated that increased numbers of nuclear invaginations (28,46)
and decreased numbers of perichromatin granules in pyramidal neurons
of the central cortex and in cerebellar granule cells (47) may also
be age-related changes in neuronal nuclei.

Perikaryon

Chromidial (Nissl) substance, rough surface endoplasmic reticulum
(RER) and free ribosomes. The Nissl material observed at light
microscope levels, and the RER as observed in electron micrographs,
have long been implicated in protein synthesis in neurons. It
appears reasonable to assume that a decrease in this material must
result in a decreased ability on the part of a neuron to carry out
the vital function of protein synthesis. Such a decrease has been
observed in neurons of "old" mammalian brains by many investigators
(39,48,49,50).

In our own studies, we have observed reduced basophilia in
pyramidal neurons of the motor cortex and neurons of spinal ganglia
(44) in aged as compared with young adult rhesus monkeys (Fig. 3A,B;
Fig. 5A,B). Our studies, as well as those of Mann and Yates (48),
showed that neuronal chromidial substance apparently decreased with
age, as the amount of lipofuscin increased. It was also observed, in
another study, that the neuronal cytoplasm of neurons of the lateral
vestibular nucleus in aged (18 months) rats contained fewer patches
of granular endoplasmic reticulum than in young adults (Figs. 6,7)
and that the small patches do not consist of parallel cisternase in
the older rats (46).

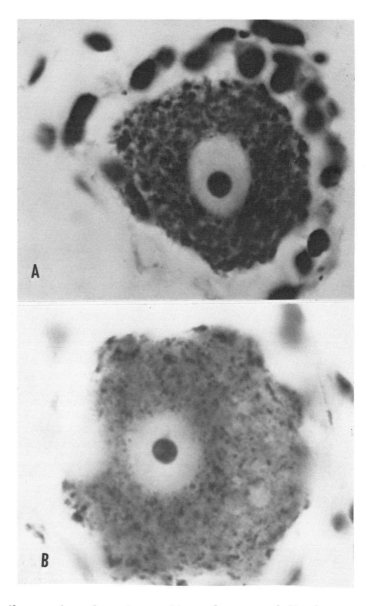

Fig. 3A. Neuron dorsal root ganglion of young adult rhesus monkey
showing relatively large densely packed Nissl bodies and marked
basophilia. Toluidine blue.
Fig. 3B. Neuron of dorsal root ganglion of aged rhesus monkey showing
sparse, relatively fine Nissl bodies and apparent early stage in the
formation of vacuoles (arrow). The relatively sharp distinction
between the nucleus and cytoplasm observed in the young adult is not
seen in the aged animal. Toluidine blue. (Brizzee et al., 1975,
Plenum Press). Reproduced with the permission of the publisher.

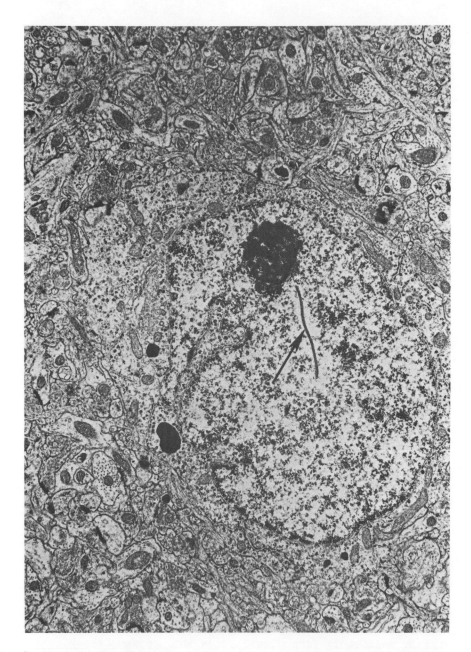

Fig. 4. Nuclei of cerebral cortical neurons in 7-year-old squirrel
       monkey showing nuclear rodlet inclusion (arrow). X 13,650.
       Reproduced with the permission of Dr. J. E. Johnson, Jr.,
       National Institute on Aging.

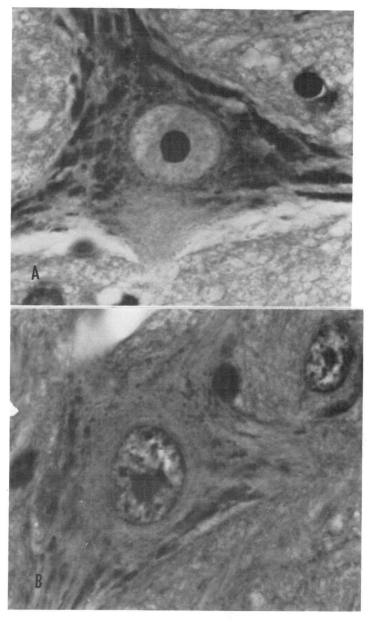

Fig. 5A. Neuron in lamina V of motor cortex of young adult rhesus monkey, showing marked basophilia of Nissl bodies. Toluidine blue.

5B. Neuron of lamina V of motor cortex of aged rhesus monkey showing reduced basophilia and sparcity of the Nissl bodies. Toluidine blue. (Brizzee et al., 1975, Plenum Press.) Reprinted with the permission of the publisher.

Golgi complex and smooth surface endoplasmic retiuclum (SER).
The neuronal Golgi apparatus in adult mice, as observed at light
microscope magnifications, appears as a discrete, reticulated
structure composed of coarse threads. In old mice, it has been
described as a mass of argentophilic granules of varying shapes and
sizes distributed irregularly in the cell (51).

Ultrastructural studies in cerebral cortex have shown that Golgi
vesicles as well as those of the SER and RER become dilated with age,
as do the cisterns of the RER (50).

Mitochondria. The mitochondria of the nucleus gracilis in aged
mice were observed to exhibit a loss of the outer unit membrane,
accompanied by vesiculation of cristae and the formation of
multivesicular bodies (52). The single unit membrane of the
multivesicular body apparently disintegrated, leaving a mass of
vesicular material. The author was of the opinion that the latter,
through a process of aggregation and joining, gave rise to large
reticular masses which were commonly observed in the nucleus gracilis.

Metals and calcifications. Copper content has been observed to
increase with age in the mammalian brain (53). Copper granules were
most consistently associated with glia which did not manifest TPPase
activity in the brain of the aged dog and rhesus monkey (54). Copper
has also been localized in the hippocampal fimbria, habenular nucleus
and periventricular regions of the hypothalamus in mature and
senescent rats (53).

Iron content also increases with age in the human brain (55).
Some of the brain cells which contain iron have been identified as
oligodendroglia (24). According to Barden (54), there appears to be
no correlation between the presence of copper, iron and neuromelanin
in any given region of the brain in rats. He concluded that the
accumulation of each substance is independent of either of the other
two.

Calcium, together with iron, has been identified in the brains of
aged horses and cattle, as well as in the human brain (56,57).
Bilateral symmetrical calcified deposits have also been observed in
the thalamus of old mice. These deposits did not contain iron and
were believed to arise in relation to blood vessels (58).

Eosinophilic bodies. The presence of protein-containing
eosinophilic bodies in perikarya of thalamic neurons of old mice has
been reported by Fraser et al. (59). These elements were characterized by sharply defined contours and were most frequently spherical,
though some appeared ovoid, rod- , saucer- , or disc-shaped.

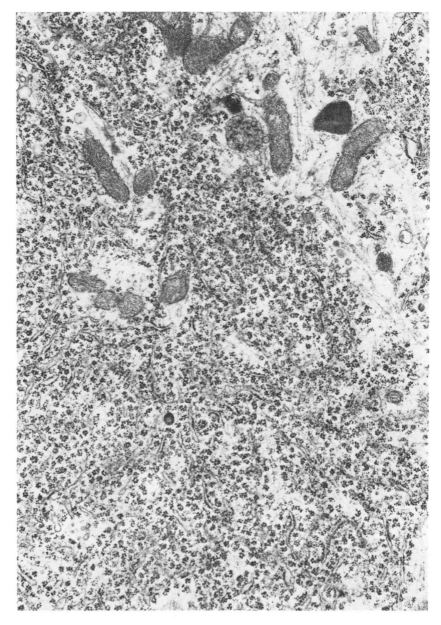

Fig. 6. The rough surface of endoplasmic reticulum (RER) in a neuron
of the lateral vestibular nucleus of a 1-month-old albino
rat consists of heavy patches of granular cisternae.
X 20,500 (Johnson and Miquel, Mech. Ageing Dev. 3:203,
1974). Reprinted with the permission of the publisher and
author.

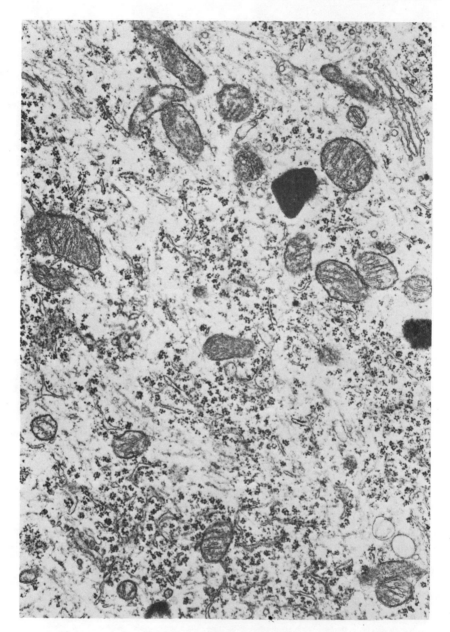

Fig. 7. The rough surface endoplasmic reticulum (RER) in this neuron
of the lateral vestibular nucleus in an aged rat exhibits
small patches of granular cisternae. X 20,500. (Johnson
and Miquel, Mech. Ageing Dev. 3:203, 1974). Reprinted with
the permission of the publisher and authors.

Electron micrographs of the eosinophilic bodies revealed arrays of parallel fibrillar crystalline material with a substructure consisting of longitudinal and transverse striations (Fig. 8).

These authors have suggested that the eosinophilic bodies originate from the union of identical macromolecules, and represent an expression of some normal cell activity, accumulating during aging as a normal metabolite or as a result of a reduction in metabolic mechanisms which catalyze their removal. They also suggested that such bodies might arise as a result of reduced cell function with age, unaccompanied by a commensurate reduction in synthesis of the particular macromolecule (59).

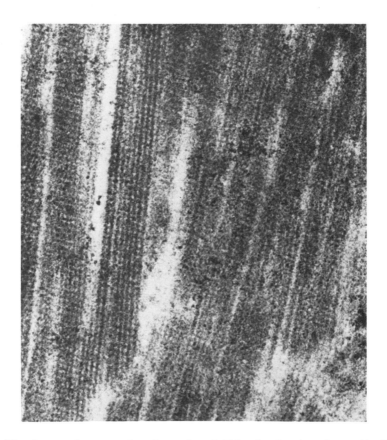

Fig. 8. Electron micrograph of eosinophilic inclusion in a thalamic neuron in an aged mouse, showing transverse and longitudinal striations. (Fraser et al., J. Neurol. Sci. 11:127, 1979). Reproduced with the permission of the publisher and the authors.

Lipofuscin pigment. Hueck (60) was the first to apply the term "lipsofuscin" to the yellow pigment which numerous authors had observed to increase in amount in neurons with age. At light microscope magnifications, this pigment appears to be composed of fine granules (1 to 3 μm in diameter) or clumped masses of variable size. it is easily visualized in PAS, Sudan black, Zielh-Nielson and Nile blue A or B-stained sections. The pigment appears a bright yellow-orange color in adult and aged neurons in blue light fluorescence at an approximate wave-length of 420 μμm, with appropriate filters. In neurons of younger subjects, however, the pigment is a lighter yellow or green color (61,62). The appearance of lipofuscin, as visualized in blue light fluorescence, is shown in neurons of the oculomotor nucleus in young adult, middle-aged, and aged rhesus monkeys in Figure 9A,B,C.

It has been demonstrated in histochemical studies that acid phosphatase, cathepsin type-C esterase, and acid deoxyribonuclease II activity occur at the same sites at which lipofuscin is identified by fluorescence (63).

Ultrastructural studies of liposfuscin pigment have generally shown it to be present in much larger amounts in aged mammalian neurons than in young neurons. The lipofuscin bodies, as seen in electron micrographs, are generally composed of a granular electron dense component and a vacuolar or vesicular electron lucent component (Fig. 10). The entire granule, consisting of a variable number of such components, is ensheathed in a single limiting membrane (64). The vacuolar component has been observed to increase in size with age, with some of the vacuoles attaining a diameter of 1 μm or more (63).

A number of investigators have classified lipofuscin according to morphological types, patterns of distribution or types of components. The classification proposed by Glees and Hasen (65) appears to coincide very closely to the patterns we have observed in our own investigations. These authors divided the lipofuscin patterns into six types, including homogeneous, finely granular, vacuolated, lamellated or banded, coarsely granular, and compound or heterogeneous. From our investigations in rats and rhesus monkeys, it appears that the first three types predominate in young neurons while the last two are commonly observed in aged neurons. The lamellated type was only rarely observed in our preparations, in agreement with the observations of Glees and Hasen (65).

In quantitative studies on regional differences in the accumulation of lipofuscin pigment in rhesus monkeys, it was noted that the nucleus with the highest neuronal pigment content was the inferior olive (61). In marked constrast to that nucleus, the neurons of the medial nucleus of the superior olive exhibited only very fine, widely scattered pigment even in the oldest animals. The

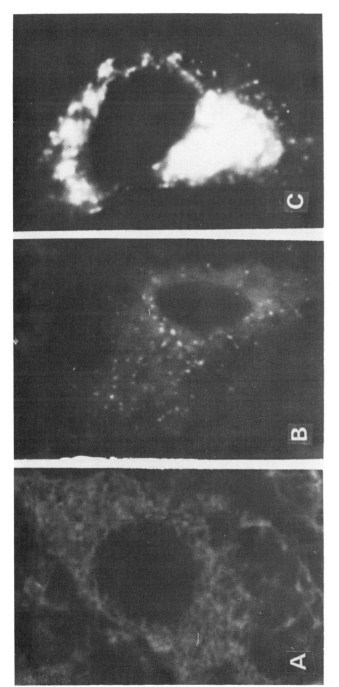

Fig. 9A. Photomicrograph of formalin-fixed unstained section of oculomotor
          nucleus in newborn rhesus monkey (age 5 days), showing absence of
          autofluorescent pigment.
       B. Photomicrograph of oculomotor neuron of middle-aged rhesus monkey
          (age about 10 years), showing scattered autofluorescent pigment
          granules in perikaryon.
       C. Photomicrograph of oculomotor neuron in aged rhesus monkey (age
          estimated to be greater than 22 years), showing heavy accumulation
          of autofluorescent lipofuscin material in perikaryon.

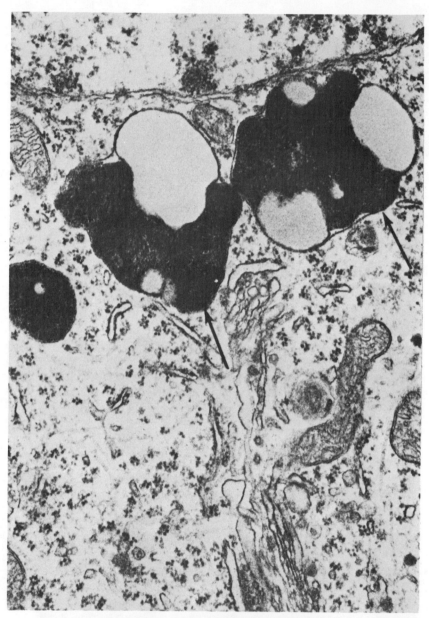

Fig. 10. Electron micrograph of typical lipofuscin body (arrow) in
          cytoplasm of pyramidal neuron of somatosensory cerebral
          cortex of aged albino rat, showing granular and vesicular
          components and limiting membrane. (Brizzee and Cancilla,
          Gerontologia 18:1, 1972). Reprinted with the permission
          of the publisher.

relative amounts of lipofuscin pigment in the above nuclei and 15
other CNS structures are shown in a rank order diagram in Figure 11.

Distinct regional differences in the accumulation of lipofuscins
have also been observed in glia cells. The glia surrounding the
Purkinje neurons of the cerebellum (61,66) and those of the medial
nucleus of the superior olive (61) have been shown to exhibit high

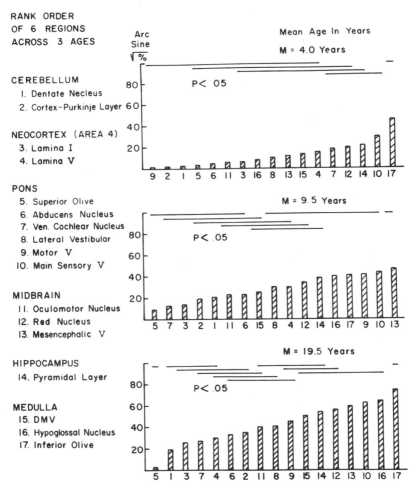

Fig. 11. Differential pattern of accumulation of lipofuscin in 17
          areas of the brain, shown at 3 age levels. The horizontal
          bars at the top of each of the 3 graphs indicate the
          number of subsets of related data at each age level
          (Brizzee et al., J. Gerontol. 29:366, 1974).

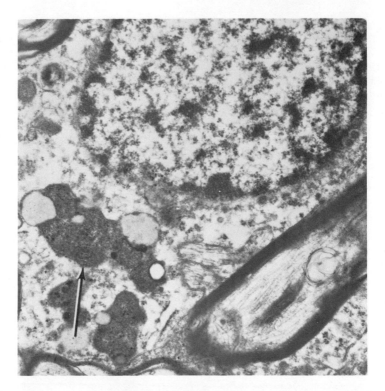

Fig. 12. Electron micrograph showing typical lipofuscin body
          (arrow) in astrocyte of the medial nucleus of the superior
          olive in aged rhesus monkey. X 9,200.

concentrations of lipofuscin in aged humans and rhesus monkey brains
(Fig. 12). The neurons of these structures are the most lipophobic
of all CNS neurons. This suggests the possibility that the glia
cells in those nuclei and other structures composed of lipophobic
neurons, may be particularly active in removing the lipofuscin from
the neurons. It seems equally plausible, however, in agreement with
the suggestion of Friede (66), that the oxidative activity in
lipophobic neurons may be lower than that of lipophilic neurons
(e.g., those of the inferior olive), and that the high oxidative rate
in the latter promotes relatively greater formation of lipofuscin
throughout the life span, regardless of its mode of removal from
neurons.

While the accumulation of lipofuscin throughout the life span
obviously occurs at different rates in different regions of the
brain, within a given region and type of neuron it appears to
increase normally as a linear function (64). It has been shown,
however, that under laboratory conditions, the rate of pigment
accumulation may be inhibited, and the amount of pigment may be

decreased. Injection of centrophenoxine (meclophenoxate, Lucidril), i.p. or i.m. into guinea pigs (80 mg/kg/day) for 4 to 12 weeks resulted in a marked decrease in the amount of lipofuscin in many areas of the CNS (67). In the same studies it was observed that the drug also reduced the activity of succinic dehydrogenase, lactic dehydrogenase, cytochrome oxidase and monoamine oxidase enzymes in the same tissues, and it was concluded that the pigments were eliminated by a possible shunting of glucose metabolism into the pentose cycle. More recently, studies utilizing morphometric techniques have shown that centrophenoxine is effective in reducing the amount of lipofuscin in aged neurons in the rat brain (68).

In view of its widespread phylogenetic ocurrence (69) and its progressive accumulation in organs composed mainly of postmitotic cells, such as the heart (70) and brain (64), lipofuscin deposition with age has been proposed as a basic "law of cellular aging" (71).

Melanin pigment. Cytophotometric studies in the locus coeruleus and substantia nigra in the human brain revealed that melanin granules first appeared in the constituent neurons at birth (49). This pigment then continued to increase in a linear manner until middle age, after which the levels decreased. This decrease in melanin content was thought to be caused by the selective atrophy of the most highly pigmented neurons rather than as a result of a general pigment loss from all such cells.

Neuropil

Axonal and synaptic changes. Alterations in axons characterized by focal swelling and thickening of pericellular baskets of Purkinje neurons have been described in the cerebellum of old human brains (24). Oval or round enlargements (spheroids) of axons in tissues from aging individuals have also been reported (72). Marked variations in size, shape and granularity were observed, and these were especially prevalent in the nucleus gracilis. They have also been observed, though to a lesser degree, in other brain stem structures and basal ganglia.

In aged mice (C57BL/10 up to 32 months of age), myelin sheaths in the pyramidal tracts were reported to be thicker than in young animals (73). Plots of regression curves of ratios between axon circumference and number of myelin lamellae in the sheath revealed a decreasing slope with increasing age, the ratios being linear for all sizes of unmyelinated fibers at each age level. In the same study it was shown that there was a significant decrease in the number of neurofilaments and an increase in the number of microtubules per fiber from 8 to 26 months of age. A statistically significant decrease in mitochondria in axons was observed in the same animals.

Ultrastructural studies in mice revealed neuroaxonal dystrophy (NAD) in the nucleus gracilis in some eight-month animals, and the condition was reported to increase with age. The NAD was characterized by enlarged profiles containing patches of smooth reticular networks and groups of vesicles (52). Degenerative changes in mitochondria were observed, apparently resulting in the formation of multivesicular bodies as intermediate stages, and numerous dense bodies of variable size and configuration were also seen. It was also noted that degenerative changes occurred in axons and synaptic terminals, and by 23 months of age a large number of nerve fibers in the nucleus gracilis had degenerated. The nucleus cuneatus exhibited similar changes, but to.a lesser extent.

A decrease in the number of vesicles in boutons of axon terminals in aged rhesus monkeys was reported, although the synaptic clefts were well preserved (83). In the rat hippocampus, axosomatic synapses were observed less frequently in old than young rats (28). Quantitative studies have revealed a decrease in the number of synapses in the molecular layer of the rat dentate gyrus (74,75) and in the human cerebral cortex (76) in the aging brain.

Dendrite changes. In the hippocampus of aged rats, there appeared to be an increase in the incidence of dendritic profiles and dendro-dendritic contacts without intervening glial fibers as compared with those of young adult rats (28). These authors emphasized the possible importance of such data in explaining decremental changes in integration of complex motor skills and decreased responsiveness of motor pathways which occur during old age. They also observed increased numbers of dendritic neurotubules and neurofilaments in aged animals.

Recent morphometric studies in cerebral cortical dendrites in old rats revealed a 35% decrease in the number of dendritic spines, and some of the dendrites appeared aspinous (77). Dendritic diameters also decreased by 12%. In auditory cortex of aged rats, the density of the dendritic arborization was noticeably decreased, but the extent of the arborization did not change (78). Morphological aging changes in dendritic processes, characterized by a loss or distortion of such processes in neurons of human cerebral cortex, have been described by Mann and Yates (48) and Scheibel and Scheibel (43).

In the mouse spinal cord and lower brain stem, Machado-Salas et al. (79) noted that early changes with age included irregular swelling and "lumpiness" of cell bodies and initial portions of dendrites, followed by increasing nodularization of the dendrite tree, and loss of whatever kinds of postsynaptic specializations may have been present in the young adult.

Similar studies of the hypothalamus in aging mice by these workers (80) showed progressive disruption of hypothalamic architecture paralleled by deterioration and loss of dendritic surface. They postulate that the observed dendritic changes in the hypothalamus contribute to the physiological phenomena associated with aging in the decline in the brain-gonadal functions in old individuals.

NEUROFIBRILLARY CHANGES IN AGING

Neurofibrillary tangles constitute a characteristic feature of the cytological changes in the brain in Alzheimer's disease, but are also found, though in lesser numbers, in the human brain in the course of "normal" aging (81). Neurofibrillary tangles are observed predominantly in the frontal and temporal cerebral cortex and hippocampus, but occasionally may be seen in the mesencephalon and rostral rhombencephalon. These elements are observed mainly in the perikaryon, but they may also occur in dendrite and synaptic terminals (81).

At light microscope magnifications, neurofibrillary tangles are characterized by neurofibrils in compact clusters producing abnormal intraneuronal configurations. They are argyrophilic and exhibit birefringence in polarized light. Ultrastructural studies have revealed that the neurofibrillary material consists of masses of modified microtubules. The microtubules measure 200 to 220 $\overset{\circ}{A}$ in width (as compared with normal microtubules of about 240 $\overset{\circ}{A}$ in diameter), and display periodic constrictions every 800 $\overset{\circ}{A}$. The tubules are actually in the form of paired helical filaments (PHF).

The abnormal tubules seen in the PHF are argentophilic, and are well preserved after direct osmic fixation. Normal neurotubules generally are not observed after osmication, and are not argentophilic (81). PHF have also been observed in neurons of aged rhesus monkeys, but periodicity is somewhat different from that in the human brain (9).

Amyloid and senile plaques

Amyloid is generally described in relation to disease conditions, but it also occurs in "normal" aging. While individual variation in amyloid content in the brain is very great, the amount of this substance in the brain of a given individual tends to increase progressively with age.

In the central nervous system, amyloid in "normal" aging commonly occurs in relation to senile plaques, although this is not the only pattern of distribution. Recent ultrastructural studies have shown that "classical" plaques, as illustated in Figure 13, consist of degenerative neuronal processes, an amyloid core and reactive cells (82). These authors concluded that degenerating neuronal processes constitute the primary source of the plaques. In 50% of "normal"

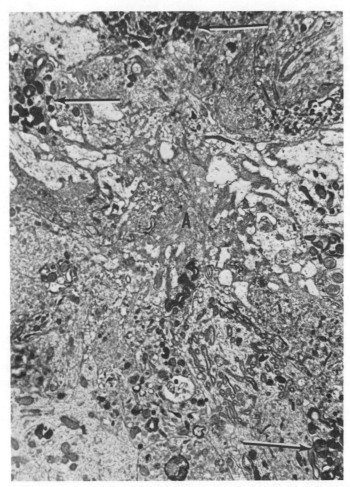

Fig. 13. Senile plague of the "classical" type with central core
          and amyloid (A) surrounded by clusters of dystrophic
          neurites (arrows). (Wisniewski et al., J. Neuropath. Exp.
          Neurol. 32:570, 1973). Reprinted with the permission of
          the authors and publishers.

aged brains, senile plaques are observed and are reported to increase
in numbers with age (72). In studies of large numbers of hospital
patients without evidence of dementia, the incidence of plaques was
small in middle-aged patients, but increased markedly in older
subjects (24,83). Senile plaques are also seen in the CNS of aged
mice (38), dogs (84), and monkeys (9).

Neurosecretory neurons

A study of the neurosecretory neurons of the human hypothalamus reported that a marked argentophilia occurred, with an increased density of the neurofibrillary apparatus with age (85,86). Vacuolization of such cells, as well as "retraction" of the cytoplasm, was also described, but there was no evidence of nuclear pyknosis, calcification, pigment accumulation or a decrease in volume of these neurons.

Age changes in glia cells. Aging changes in glia in the brain are reported to be greatest in the ependymal and submeningeal regions, fornix, optic chiasma, mammillary nuclei, and reticular formation, in that order (83).

Ultrastructural studies of age changes in glia in the rat hippocampus have revealed increased oligodendroglial satellitosis, binucleated cells or fusion of oligodendroglia, and invagination of oligodendroglial nuclear membranes with marked marginal condensation of nuclear chromatin (28). Obvious changes in astrocytes were not observed in this study, but numerous lipid vacuoles were seen in microglia.

In the nuclei of Bergmann astrocytes in the cerebellum of chinchillas, it has been shown that nuclear membranes were commonly indented and invaginated, with the tip of each invagination ending near a nucleolus (39). Deep pink PAS-stained bodies of varying shape (irregular rods, bars, spheres, or faceted bodies) were seen within astrocyte nuclei, in $145\frac{1}{2}$-month-old animals.

Degenerative changes have been observed in astrocytes in olfactory bulb tissue of aged human subjects (87). These alterations are characterized by a homogenization of the soma and gradual loss of processes, resulting in a round, homogeneous, dark-staining body with no resemblance to a cell.

REFERENCES

1. A. V. Everitt, and J. A. Burgess, eds., "Hypothalamus, Pituitary and Aging," Charles C. Thomas, New York (1976).
2. T. Hanley, Neuronal "fall-out: in the aging brain: A critical review of the quantitative data, Age and Ageing 3:133 (1974).
3. H. A. Johnson and S. Erner, Neuron survival in the aging mouse, Exp. Gerontol. 7:111 (1972).
4. L. M. Franks, P. D. Wilson, and R. D. Whelan, The effects of age on total DNA and cell number in the mouse brain, Gerontologist 20:21 (1974).
5. H. Brody, Organization of the cerebral cortex. III. A study of aging in the human cerebral cortex, J. Comp. Neurol. 102:511 (1955).

6. E. J. Colon, The elderly brain: A quantitative analysis in the
    cerebral cortex of two cases, Psychiatria, Neurologia,
    Neurochirurgia (Amst.) 75:261 (1972).
7. B. G. Shefer, The absolute number of nerve cells in cortical
    depth in normals and in patients with dementia, Pick's and
    Alzheimer's disease, Z. Nevropathol. i Psikhiatrii Imen S.S.
    Korsakova (Moskva) 72:1024 (1972).
8. K. R. Brizzee, J. M. Ordy, J. Hansche, and B. Kaack,
    Quantitative assessment of changes in neuron and glia cell
    packing density and lipofuscin accumulation with age in the
    cerebral cortex of a nonhuman primate (Macaca mulatta),
    in:"Neurobiology of Aging," R. D. Terry and S. Gershon, eds.,
    Raven Press, New York (1976).
9. H. M. Wisniewski, B. Ghetti, and R. D. Terry, Neuritic (senile)
    plaques and filamentous changes in aged rhesus monkeys, J.
    Neuropath. Exp. Neurol. 32:566 (1973).
10. J. M. Ordy, K. R. Brizzee, B. Kaack, and J. Hansche, Age
    differences in short-term memory and cell loss in the cortex
    of the rat, Gerontology 24:267 (1978).
11. K. R. Brizzee, N. Sherwood, and P. S. Timiras, A comparison of
    cell populations at various depth levels in cerebral cortex
    of young adult and aged Long-Evans rats, J. Gerontol. 23:289
    (1968).
12. K. M. Wahal and H. E. Riggs, Changes in the brain associated
    with senility, AMA Arch. of Neurol. Psychiat. 2:151 (1960).
13. P. S. Timiras and A. Vernadakis, Structural, biochemical and
    functional aging of the nervous system, in: "Develomental
    Physiology and Aging," P. S. Timiras, ed., Macmillan
    Publishing Co., New York (1972).
14. D. W. Vaughan and A. Peters, Neuroglial cells inthe cerebral
    cortex of rats from young adulthood to old age: An electron
    microscope study, J. Neurocytol. 3:405 (1974).
15. E. Uemura and H. A. Hartman, Age-related changes in RNA content
    and volume of the human hypoglossal neuron, Brain Res. Bull.
    3:207 (1978).
16. E. Uemura and H. A. Hartman, RNA content and volume of nerve
    cell bodies in human brain: I. Prefrontal cortex in aging
    normal and demented patients, J. Neuropath. Exp. Neurol.
    37:487 (1978).
17. R. R. Sturrock, Quantitative and morphological changes in
    neurons and neuroglia in the indusium griseum of aging mice,
    J. Gerontol. 32:642 (1977).
18. R. R. Sturrock, Changes in neuroglia and myelination in the
    white matter of aging mice, J. Gerontol. 31:513 (1976).
19. R. S. Ellis, Norms for some structural changes in the human
    cerebellum from birth to old age, J. Comp. Neurol. 32:1
    (1920).
20. T. Inukai, On the loss of Purkinje cells with advancing age,
    from the cerebellar cortex of the albino rat, J. Comp.
    Neurol. 45:1 (1928).

21. E. Tarnowska-Dziduszko, Morphological picture of the cerebellum in the course of the aging process, Neuropathol. Pol. 11:199 (1973).

22. T. C. Hall, A. K. H. Miller, and J. A. N. Corsellis, Variations in the human Purkinje cell population according to age and sex, Neuropath. Appl. Neurobiol., 1:267 (1975).

23. K. J. Hempel and M. Namba. Die involution des Supranucleus medialisdorsalis, soie der Lamella medialis und der Lamells interna thalami, J. Hirnforsch. 4:43 (1958).

24. N. Gellerstedt, "Zue kenntuis der Hirveranderungen bei der Normalen Altersunvolution," Almquist and Wiksells Boktryckeri - A -B, Uppsala (1933).

25. O. Bugiani, S. Salvarani, F. Perdelli, G. I. Mancardi, and A. Leonardi, Nerve cell loss with aging in the putamen, Europ. Neurol. 17:286 (1978).

26. K. R. Brizzee and J. M. Ordy, Age pigments, cell loss and hippocampal function, Mech. Ageing Dev., in press (1978).

27. V. F. Shefer, Hippocampal pathology as a possible factor in the pathogenesis of senile dementias, Neuropath. Exp. Neurol. 8:236 (1977).

28. M. Hansan and P. Glees, Ultrastructural age changes in hippocampal neurons, synapses and neuroglia, Exp. Gerontol. 8:75 (1973).

29. P. W. Landfield, G. Rose, L. Sandles, T. C. Wohlstadter, and G. Lynch, Patterns of astroglial hypertrophy and neuronnal degeneration in the hippocampus of aged, memory-deficient rats, J. Gerontol. 228:1335 (1970).

30. B. W. Konigsmark and E. A. Murphy, Neuronal populations in the human brain, Nature 228:1335 (1970).

31. N. Vijayashankar and H. Brody, A Study of aging in the human abducens nucleus, J. Comp. Neurol. 173:433 (1977).

32. P. L. McGeer, E. G. McGeer, and J. S. Suzuki, Aging and extrapyramidal function, Arch. Neurol. 34:33 (1977).

33. H. Brody, An examination of cerebral cortex and brain stem aging, in:"Neurobiology of Aging," R. D. Terry and S. Gershon, eds., Raven Press, New York (1976).

34. R. D. Monagle and H. Brody, The effects of age upon the main nucleus of the inferior olive in the human, J. Comp. Neurol. 155:61 (1974).

35. P. Sandoz, Age-related loss of nerve cells from the human inferior olive and unchanged volume of its grey matter, IRCS J. Med. Sci. 5:376 (1977).

36. E. A. Wright and J. M. Spink, A study of the loss of nerve cells in the central nervous system in relation to age, Gerontolgia (Basel) 3:277 (1959).

37. W. Andrew, and M. A. Bari, Some aspects of age changes in the spinal cord compared with those in other parts of the nervous system, in:"Proceedings of the Fifth International Congress of Neuropathology," Excerpta Medica Fdn., New York, Internat. Cong. Ser. No. 100 (1965).

38. J. Cammermeyer, Cytological manifestations of aging in rabbit and chinchilla brains, J. Geront. 18:41 (1963).

39. K. R. Brizzee, X. Kharetchko, and L. A. Jacobs, Effects of fetal X-irradiation on aging changes in cerebral cortex, in:"Some Aspects of Internal Irradiation," Pergamon Press, New York (1962).

40. K. H. Lin, Y. M. Peng, and M. T. Peng, Changes in the nuclear volume of rat hypothalamic neurons in old age, Neuroendrocrinology 21:247 (1976).

41. I. Klatzo, Uber das verhaltern des nukleolarapparates in den menschlichen pallidumzellen, J. Hirsforsch. 1:47 (1954).

42. F. Sanides, Untersuchumgen uber die histologische struktur des mandelkerngebietes, J. Hirnforsh. 3:56 (1957).

43. K. R. Brizzee, P. Klara, and J. E. Johnson, Changes in microanatomy, neurocytology and fine structure with aging, in:"Neurobiology of Aging: An Interdisciplinary Life Span Approach," J. M. Ordy and K. R. Brizzee, eds., Plenum Press, New York (1975).

44. P. Timiras, Degenerative changes in cells and cell death, in: "Developmental Physiology and Aging," P. S. Timiras, ed., Macmillan Publishing Co., New York (1972).

45. J. E. Johnson and J. Miquel, Fine structural changes in the lateral vestibular nucleus of aging rats, Mech. Ageing Dev. 3:203 (1974).

46. V. Zs-Nagy, C. Bertoni-Freddari, I. Zs-Nagy, C. Pieri, and G. Guili, Alterations in the numerical density of perichronatin granules in different tissues during ageing and cell differentiation, Gerontology 23:267 (1977).

47. D. M. A. Mann and P. O. Yates, Lipofuscin pigments--their relationship to ageing in the human nervous system. I. The lipofuscin content of nerve cells, Brain 97:481 (1974).

48. D. M. A. Mann and P. O. Yates, Lipofuscin pigments--their relationship to ageing in the human nervous system. II. The melanin content of pigmented nerve cells, Brain 97:489 (1974).

49. S. S. Sekhon and D. S. Maxwell, Ultrastructural changes in neurons of the spinal anterior horn of ageing mice with particular reference to the accumulation of lipofuscin pigment, J. Neurocytol. 3:59 (1974).

50. W. Andrew, The Golgi apparatus in the nerve cells of the mouse from youth to senility, Am. J. Anat. 64:351 (1937).

51. J. E. Johnson, W. R. Mehler, and J. Miquel, A fine structural study of degenerative changes in the dorsal column nuclei of aging mice. Lack of protection by vitamine E, J. Gerontol. 30:395 (1975).

52. N. Kaneta, Histochemical studies on the diencephalon of senescent rats, Tohoku J. Exp. Med. 90:249 (1966).

53. H. Barden, The histochemical distribution and localization of copper, iron, neuromelanin and lysosomal enzyme activity in the brain of aging rhesus monkey and the dog, J. Neuropath. Exp. Neurol. 30:650 (1971).

54. B. Hallgren and P. Sourander, The effect of age on the nonhaemin iron in the human brain, J. Neurochem. 3:41 (1958).

55. E. W. Hurst, Calcification of the brains of Equidae and bovidae, Am J. Path. 10:795 (1934).

56. G. Strassman, Iron and calcium deposits in the brain: Their pathologic significance, J. Neuropath. Exp. Neurol. 8:428 (1977).

57. H. Fraser, Bilateral thalamic calcification in aging mice, J. Path. Bact. 96:220 (1968).

58. H. Fraser, W. Smith, and E. W. Gray, Ultrastructural morphology of cytoplasmic inclusions within neurons of ageing mice, J. Neurol Sci. 11:123 (1970).

59. W. Hueck, Pigmenstudien, Beitrag. Path. Anat. 54:68 (1912).

60. K. R. Brizzee, J. M. Ordy, and B. Kaack, Early appearance and regional differences in intraneuronal and extraneuronal lipofuscin accumulation with age in the brain of a nonhuman primate, J. Gerontol. 29:366 (1974).

61. K. Nandy, Properties of neuronal lipofuscin pigment in mice, Acta Neuropath. (Berl.) 19:25 (1971).

62. T. Samorajski, J. R. Keefe, and J. M. Ordy, Intracellular localization of lipofuscin age pigments in the nervous system, J. Gerontol. 19:262 (1964).

63. K. R. Brizzee, and F. A. Johnson, Depth distribution of lipofuscin pigment in cerebral cortex of rat, Acta Neuropathol. 16:205 (1970).

64. P. Glees and M. Hasan, Lipofuscin in neuronal aging and diseases, Norm. Pathol. Anat. (Stuttg.) 32:1 (1933).

65. R. L. Friede, The relation of formation of lipofuscin to the distribution of oxidative enzymes in the human brain, Acta Neuropath. (Berl) 2:113 (1962).

66. K. Nandy, Further studies on the effects of centrophenoxine on the lipofuscin pigment in the neurons of senile guinea pigs, J. Gerontol. 23:83 (1968).

67. S. Riga and D. Riga, Effects of centrophenoxine on lipofuscin pigments on the nervous system of old rats, Brain Res. 72:265 (1974).

68. A. D. Dayan, Comparative neuropathology of ageing--studies on the brains of 47 species of vertebrates, Brain 94:31 (1971).

69. B. L. Strehler, D. D. Mark, A. S. Mildvan, and M. V. Gee, Rate and magnitude of age pigment accumulation in the human myocardium, J. Gerontol. 14:430 (1959).

70. B. L. Strehler and C. H. Barrows, Senescence: Cell biological aspects of aging, in: "Cell Differentiation," O. A. Schjeide and J. DeVellis, eds., Van Nostrand, New York (1970).

71. J. H. Sung, Neuroaxonal dystrophy in aging, in:"Proc. 5th Int. Congr. Neuropathol., Zurich," Excerpta Medica Fdn, New York, Interat. Contr. Ser. No. 100 (1966).

72. J. Samorajski, R. L. Friede, and J. M. Ordy, Age differences in the ultrastructure of axons in the pyramidal tract of the mouse, J. Gerontol. 26:542 (1971).

73. W. Bondareff, and Y. Geinisman, Loss of synapses in the dentate gyrus of the senescent rat, Am. J. Anat. 145:129 (1976).

74. Y. Geinisman and W. Bondareff, Decrease in the number of synapses in the senescent brain: A quantitative EM analysis of the dentate gyrus molecular layer in the rat, Meh. Ageing Dev. 5:11 (1976).

75. B. G. Cragg, The density of synapses and neurons in normal, mentally defective and ageing human brains, Brain 98:81 (1975).

76. M. L. Feldman, Degenerative changes in aging dendrites, Gerontolgist 14:34 (1974).

77. D. W. Vaughan, Age-related deterioration of pyramidal cell basal dendrites in rat auditory cortex, J. Comp. Neurol. 171:601 (1977).

78. M. E. Scheibel and A. B. Scheibel, Structural changes in the aging brain, in: "Aging," vol. 1, H. Brody, D. Harman, and J. M. Ordy, eds., Raven Press, New York (1975).

79. J. Machado-Salas, M. E. Scheibel, and A. B. Scheibel, Neuronal changes in the aging mouse. Spinal cord and lower brain stem, Exp. Neurol. 54:504 (1977a).

80. J. Machado-Salas, M. E. Scheibel, and A. B. Scheibel, Morphologic changes in the hypothalamus of the old mouse, Exp. Neurol. 57:102 (1977b).

81. H. M. Wisniewski and R. D. Terry, Morphology of the aging brain, human and animal, Progr. Brain Res. 40:167 (1973).

82. R. D. Terry and M. Wisniewski, Some structural and chemical aspects of the aging nervous system. Proc. IVth European Symposium on Basic Research in Gerontology, Scand. J. Clin. Lab. Invest. 34:(Suppl. 141)13 (1974).

83. B. E. Tomlinson, Morphological brain changes in non-demented old people, in:"Aging of the Central Nervous System. Biological and Psychological Aspects, H. H. van Praeg and A. F. Kalverboer, eds., DeErven F. Bohm, N.V. Hoarlem (1972).

84. A. Wisniewski, A. B. Johnson, C. S. Raine, W. J. Kay, and R. D. Terry, Senile plaques and cerebral amyloidosis in aged dogs. A histochemical and ultrastructural study, Lab. Invest. 23:287 (1970).

85. J. E. Azcoaga, Modificaciones gliales del hipotalamo senil, Archivos de Histologia Normal y Pathologica 8:278 (1963).

86. J. E. Azcoaga, Senilidad de las neuronas de los nucleos magnocellulares del hipotalamo, Archivo de Histologia Normal y Pathologica (Buenos Aires) 9:40 (1965).

87. L. Liss and F. Gomez, The nature of senile changes of the human olfactory bulb and tract, AMA Aidi 67:167 (1958).

HYPERTENSION, VASCULATURE AND AGING

Akira Ooshima and Yukio Yamori

Department of Pathology
Shimane Medical University
Izumo 693, Japan

INTRODUCTION

Essential hypertension develops with age, and its complication, arteriosclerosis, seems to be an accelerated form of aging process in blood vessels. With advancing age, the blood vessels lose elasticity and become stiff. This may be due in part to an increase in vascular connective tissue components. Special attention will be given in this report to the cardiovascular connective tissue and especially to the fibrils of collagen, which is known to be the major protein of connective tissue. The experiments were undertaken to elucidate an interrelationship between hypertension and vascular collagen metabolism. This report is a summary of experiments conducted during the past several years.

METHODS

Two different types of hypertensive animals were used as experimental animals. Hypertension was induced in a group of uninephrectomized, 8-week-old, male Wistar rats by twice-weekly subcutaneous injections of deoxycorticosterone acetate (DOCA) (5 mg/rat) and maintenance on 1% NaCl. The other hypertensive model was spontaneously hypertensive male rat (SHR) developed by Okamota and Aoki (1). As a control for SHR, genetically related male Wistar-Kyoto rats were used. All the animals were fed on regular stock chow diet and given either tap water or 1% NaCl throughout experiments.

The availability of methods in our laboratory for measuring a number of biochemical markers of collagen metabolism made it possible to determine the effects of hypertension on vascular collagen synthesis. Activities of prolyl hydroxylase and lysyl oxidase were

99

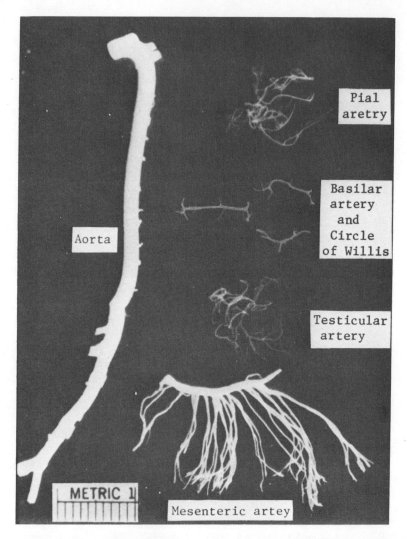

Fig. 1   The preparation of blood vessels used for assay. Samples
          are taken from a 4-month-old, male rat.

measured by the tritium release assays of Hutton et al. (2) and
Seigel et al. (3), respectively. Incorporation of labeled proline
into collagen was measured as described elsewhere (4). The amount of
net collagen deposition was determined by hydroxyproline assay (5).
Protein concentration was determined by the method of Lowry et al.
(6), with bovine serum albumin as the standard. DNA was determined
by the method of Burton (7). Blood vessels were isolated and prepared for assay as previously reported (4) (Fig. 1). Brain microvessels were neatly isolated without loss of metabolic activity

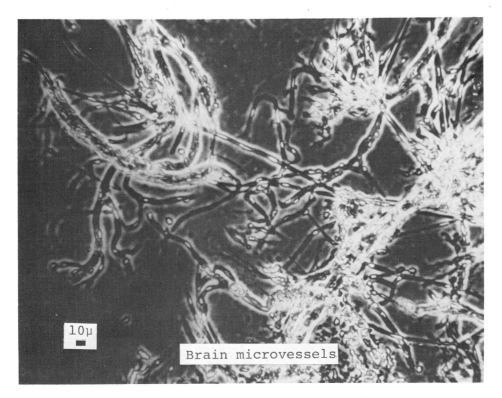

Fig. 2.   A portion of brain microvessels from a 4-month-old, male
          rat is shown in phase contrast microphotograph.

by a modification (8) of the method of Brendel et al. (9) (Fig. 2).
For the immunohistochemical demonstration of prolyl hydroxylase, the
immunoperoxidase method, using monospecific antibody against this
enzyme prepared from newborn rat skins, was utilized (10,11).

RESULTS

     Initial experiments were conducted with deoxycorticosterone ace-
tate (DOCA)-salt hypertensive rats, which developed severe hypertension within 4 to 6 weeks. As shown in Figure 3, prolyl hydroxylase
activities in DOCA-salt hypertensive rats was increased as compared
to normotensive controls in blood vessels of different diameters.
The other two indicators of collagen biosynthesis, ^{14}C-proline
incorporation into collagen and net deposition of collagen in the
tissues, were also shown to be elevated in DOCA-salt hypertensive
rats (not shown). To determine whether the increase in collagen
biosynthetic activity was related to the hypertension or to the DOCA-
salt treatment itself, the antihypertensive agent, reserpine (0.75
mg/kg, i.p.), was administered to a subgroup of the experimental

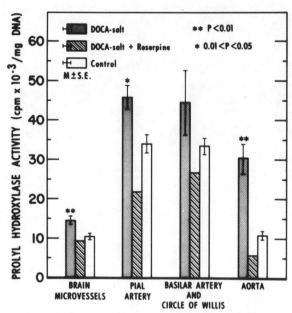

Fig. 3.   Prolyl hydroxylase activities of blood vessels in
           DOCA-salt treated rats with and without reserpine, and
           normotensive controls.
           Uninephrectomized, 8-week-old male rats were given
           deoxycorticosterone acetate (DOCA) (5 mg/rat) twice-weekly
           and maintained on 1% NaCl. Concomitant with DOCA-salt
           treatment, reserpine (0.75 mg/kg, i.p.) was administered
           daily by intraperitoneal injection for 4 to 6 weeks.
           Final blood pressures were DOCA-salt treated hypertensive
           rats, 210 ± 2 mmHg. From Ooshima et al. (8).

animals at the time of initiation of DOCA-salt treatment. Administration of reserpine prevented or reversed the increase in vascular
collagen biosynthesis comcomitant with the reduction of blood
pressure (Fig. 3).

     The effects of hypertension on vascular collagen biosynthesis
were also investigated in spontaneously hypertensive rats (SHR)
(Fig. 4). The blood pressure of SHR was greatly elevated over that
of controls. Two results were obtained by the prolyl hydroxylase
levels. First, the level of prolyl hydroxylase fell with age. The
second, and more important, was that the SHR consistently showed
higher enzyme activity when compared with normotensive controls. In
addition to these results, it was observed that when SHR yielded
severe arterial damage (such as periarteritis nodosa of mesenteric
artery, which is often observed in severe and prolonged hypertension)
the level of prolyl hyroxylase activity rose markedly. Since there

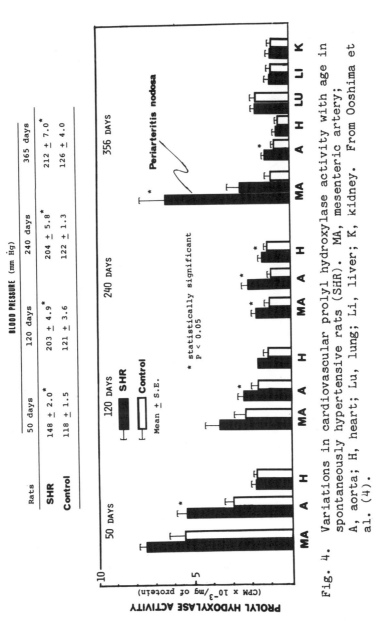

Fig. 4. Variations in cardiovascular prolyl hydroxylase activity with age in spontaneously hypertensive rats (SHR). MA, mesenteric artery; A, aorta; H, heart; Lu, lung; Li, liver; K, kidney. From Ooshima et al. (4).

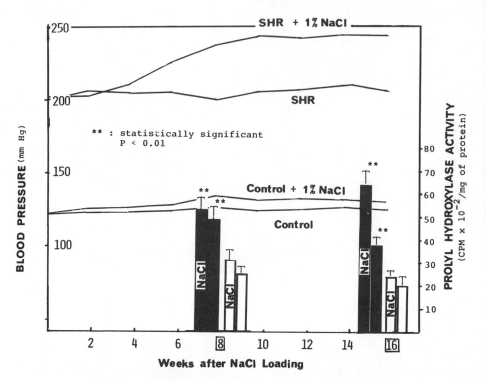

Fig. 5.   Effects of NaCl loading on blood pressure and vascular
               prolyl hydroxylase activity in spontaneously hyperten-
               sive rats (SHR). Some of the animals were given 1%
               NaCl as a source of drinking water in place of tap
               water at the age of 8 weeks.

is no difference in prolyl hydroxylase activity of the lung, liver
and kidney between SHR and controls, the increase observed here is
very specific for the cardiovascular system.

    When the SHR were given 1% NaCl in place of tap water at the age
of 8 weeks, their blood pressure became even more elevated. The
level of vascular prolyl hydroxylase activity increased concomitant
with the elevation of blood pressure after NaCl loading, suggesting a
close relationship between the level of blood pressure and the synthesis of vascular collagen (Fig. 5). The same close relationship
was observed when various antihypertensive agents were injected into
DOCA-salt hypertensive rats. Along with DOCA-salt treatment, antihypertensive agents with different pharmacologic effects (reserpine
0.75 mg/kg, chlorothiazide 10 mg/kg, hydralazine 5 mg/kg, α-methyl
DOPA 40 mg/kg, phentolamine 5 mg/kg, propranolol 5 mg/kg) were administered intraperitoneally on a daily basis. Figure 6 shows that the
development of hypertension in these animals was suppressed by the

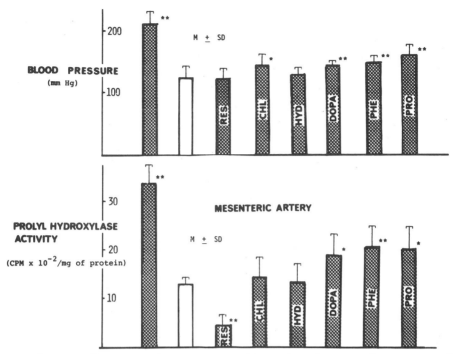

Fig. 6.   Effects of various antihypertensive agents on vascular
           prolyl hydroxylase activity and blood pressure in
           DOCA-salt treated rats. Hypertension was induced by
           DOCA·salt treatment for 4 weeks. Refer to Fig. 3.
           Concomitant with the DOCA-salt treatment, various
           antihypertensive agents (RES, reserpine 0.75 mg/kg;
           CHL, chlorothiazide 10 mg/kg; HYD, hydralazine 5 mg/kg;
           DOPA, α-methyl DOPA 40 mg/kg; PHE, phentolamine 5
           mg/kg; PRO, propranolol 5 mg/kg) were injected daily
           for 4 weeks intraperitoneally.
           *,**, Statistically significant compared to control:
           *, 0.01 < P < 0.05; **, P < 0.01.

administration of antihypertensive agents, and that the level of
prolyl hydroxylase activity was decreased as compared to those of
non-treated DOCA-salt hypertensive rats.

    In Figure 7, vascular lysyl oxidase activity and the effects of
lathyrogens, β-aminopropionitrile and D-penicillamine on blood pressure and vascular collagen deposition are presented. Lysyl oxidase
activity of blood vessels in DOCA-salt hypertensive rats was
increased as compared to that of controls. The daily injection of
reserpine 0.75 mg/kg, β-aminopropionitrile 150 mg/kg or D-penicil
lamine 150 mg/kg, i.p, decreased lysyl oxidase activity. Concomitant

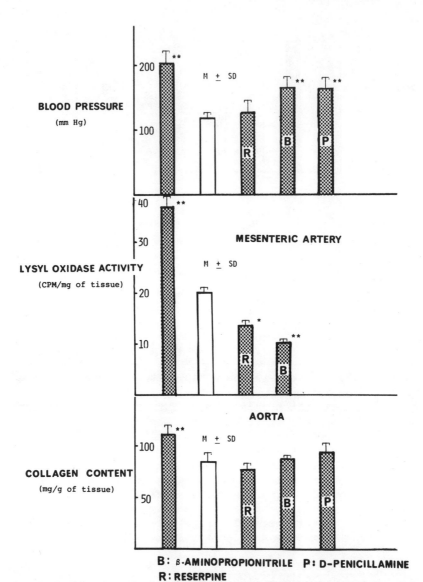

B: β-AMINOPROPIONITRILE   P: D-PENICILLAMINE
R: RESERPINE

Fig. 7. Effects of lathyrogen on blood pressure, vascular lysyl
oxidase activity and collagen content in DOCA-salt treated
rats. Hypertension was induced by DOCA-salt treatment for 4
weeks. Refer to Fig. 3. Concomitant with the DOCA-salt
treatment, reserpine (R) 0.75 mg/kg, β-aminopropionitrile
(B) 150 mg/kg or D-penicillamine (P) 150 mg/kg was administered daily for 4 weeks by intraperitoneal injection. From
Ooshima and Midorikawa (16).
*,**, statistically significant compared to control.
*, 0.01 < P < 0.05, **, P < 0.01.

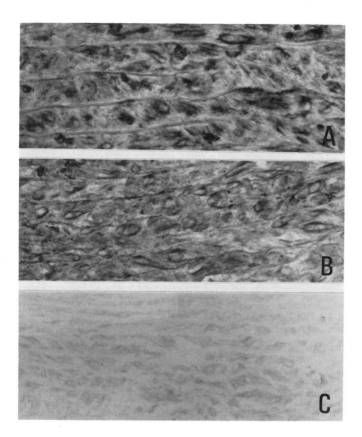

Fig. 8.   Immunohistochemical localization of prolyl hydroxylase
                 in aortas of 4-month-old spontaneously hypertensive
                 rats (SHR) (A) and age-matched normotensive rats (B).
                 Note more intense immunostaining in SHR (A) as compared
                 to normotensive rats (B). No specific staining is seen
                 in control section reacted with preimmune serum (C).
                 x 200. See reference (11) in detail.

with the reduction of the enzyme activity, the increase in vascular
collagen deposition was prevented. Histopathologically, DOCA-salt
animals treated with lathyrogens showed a lower incidence of vascular
damage and arteriosclerosis as compared to non-treated DOCA-salt
DOCA-salt hypertensive rats. It is of interest that along with the
reduction of these parameters, the development of high blood pressure
was partially prevented.

    The last part of the experiments focused on identifying the col-
lagen-producing cells in the cardiovascular tissues by an immunohistochemical localization of prolyl hydroxylase using monospecific

antibody against this enzyme (10,11). As shown in Figure 8, aortic medial smooth muscle cells in 4-month-old SHR (A) showed more intense immunoreaction as compared to age-matched normotensive controls (B). Control sections treated with preimmune serum did not show a non-specific reaction (C). The same was true in mesenteric artery and other blood vessels (not shown). It was of interest that brain microvessels from SHR yielded more intense immunostaining when compared to those from normotensive controls (11).

DISCUSSION

It has been demonstrated, by using various biochemical markers, that hypertension does induce an increased biosynthesis of collagen in blood vessels. When hypertensive rats were treated with anti-hypertensive agents, the increase in vascular collagen synthesis reverted to normal values, indicating that the vascular collagen synthetic activity is closely related to the level of blood pressure. It is likely that blood vessels produce collagen in response to hypertension, which acts as a physical insult or injury to the vessel walls. However, when deposition of collagen fibers in blood vessels was prevented by the administration of lathyrogens, β-amino-propionitrile and D-penicillamine in deoxycorticosterone acetate (DOCA)-salt treated rats, the development of hypertension and arter-iosclerotic changes was partially prevented. This may suggest that the increased accumulation of collagen also has an effect of initi-ation and progression of hypertension and arteriosclerosis.

Since prolyl hydroxylase is an important enzyme involved in an initial step of collagen biosynthesis (12), the immunohistochemical demonstration of this enzyme is assumed to be a sensitive indicator for cellular fibrogenetic activity in cardiovascular tissues. Using the immunoperoxidase method, it was demonstrated that medial smooth muscle cells yielded the most prominent immunostaining in the vascu-lar wall. The immunoreaction for prolyl hydroxylase was more intense in SHR as compared to normotensive controls. This result supports previous findings by other workers, who showed that medial smooth muscle cells in culture actually produce connective tissue compon-ents, including collagen (13,14,15), and may play a principal role in the pathogenesis of vascular diseases, particularly atherosclerosis.

SUMMARY

Essential hypertension is the most common disease which develops with advancing age, and its complication, arteriosclerosis, seems to be an exaggerated form of aging process in the mesenchymal tissues. Our present investigation demonstrated that deposition of collagen fibers in vessel wall may represent one aspect of the aging phenome-non occurring in normal vasculature.

ACKNOWLEDGEMENT

The authors wish to express their gratitude to Miss M. Kameda for her excellent assistance with this manuscript.

REFERENCES

1. K. Okamoto and K. Aoki, Development of a strain of spontaneously hypertensive rats, Jap. Circ. J. 27:282 (1963).

2. J. J. Hutton Jr., A. L. Tappel, and S. Udenfriend, A rapid assay for collagen proline hydroxylase, Anal. Biochem. 16:384 (1966).

3. R. C. Giegel and G. R. Martin, Collagen cross-linking. Enzymatic synthesis of lysine-derived aldehydes and the production of cross-linked components, J. Biol. Chem. 245:1653 (1970).

4. A. Ooshima, G. C. Fuller, G. J. Cardinale, S. Spector, and S. Udenfriend, Increased collagen synthesis in blood vessels of hypertensive rats and its reversal by antihypertensive agents, Proc. Natl. Acad. Sci. USA 71:3019 (1974).

5. K. I. Kivirriko, O. Laitinen, and D. J. Prockop, Modification of a specific assay for hydroxyproline in urine, Anal. Biochem. 19:249 (1967).

6. O. H. Lowry, N. J. Rosebrough, A. L. Farr, and R. J. Randall, Protein measurement with the Folin phenol reagent, J. Biol. Chem. 193, 265 (1951).

7 K. Burton, A study of the conditions and mechanism of the diphenylamine reaction for the colorimetric estimation of deoxyribonucleic acid, Biochem. J. 62:315 (1956).

8. A. Ooshima, G. C. Fuller, G. J. Cardinale, S. Spector, and S. Udenfriend, Collagen biosynthesis in blood vessels of brain and other tissues of the hypertensive rat, Science 190:898 (1975).

9. K. Brendel, E. Meezan, and E. C. Carlson, Isolated brain microvessels: A purified, metabolically active preparation from bovine cerebral cortex, Science 185:953 (1974).

10. A. Ooshima, Immunohistochemical localization of prolyl hydroxylase in rat tissues, J. Histochem. Cytochem. 25:1297 (1977).

11. A. Ooshima, Localization of prolyl hydroxylase by the immunoperoxidase method in cardiovascular tissues of hypertensive rats, Jap. Circ. J. 42:971 (1978).

12. G. J. Cardinale and S. Udenfriend, Prolyl hydroxylase, Adv. Enzymol. 41:245 (1974).

13. R. Ross and S. J. Klebanoff, The smooth muscle cell. I. In vitro synthesis of connective tissue proteins, J. Cell Biol. 50:159 (1971).

14. R. Ross, The smooth muscle cell. II. Growth of smooth muscle in culture and formation of elastic fibers, J. Cell Biol. 50:172 (1971).

15. R. Ross and J. A. Glomset, The pathogenesis of arteriosclerosis,
     New Engl. J. Med. 295:369 (1976).
16. A. Ooshima, and O. Midorikawa, Increased lysyl oxidase activity
     in blood vessels of hypertensive rats and effect of
     β-aminopropionitrile on arteriosclerosis, Jap. Circ. J.
     41:1337 (1977).

AGING OF IN VIVO CARTILAGE CELL

Mitsuo Igarashi and Yasufumi Hayashi

Department of Orthopedic Surgery
Tokyo Metropolitan Geriatric Hospital
Sakae-cho 35-2, Itabashi-ku, Tokyo
Japan

INTRODUCTION

A characteristic of cartilage cells is that, in vivo, small numbers of cartilage cells are present in a large volume of matrix composed of such substances as collagen, glycosaminoglycan, and glycoprotein. So, the metabolic behavior of in vivo cartilage cells, especially of in vivo aged cartilage cells, can be investigated by studying the nature of the products of cartilage cells, such as the biochemical and morphological natures of the matrix Only molecular studies on cartilage collagen that accounts for 60 to 70% of the organic matrix of cartilage can show the change of metabolic behavior of cartilage cells associated with aging.

Therefore, the changes in cartilage collagen of aged, fibrillated, and osteoarthritic cartilage were investigated in order to distinguish the effect of physiological versus pathological aging on the behavior or metabolism of in vivo cartilage cells.

MATERIALS AND METHODS

Samples of cartilage were obtained from 7 normal adults, 6 aged individuals, 7 patients with osteoarthritis, and 6 with rheumatoid arthritis. The samples were obtained at autopsy or on surgical treatment for total joint replacement. Age of donor and site from which sample materials were taken are summarized in Table 1. Samples of cartilage were carefully cut away to avoid contamination with subchondral bone, perichondrium or fibrous tissue. They were examined histologically to classify the pathological findings of hyaline cartilage and also to eliminate any possible contamination

111

Table 1. Materials of Articular Cartilage

	Number	Age (Mean)	Location
Young and adult	7	13 - 33 (23.9)	Shoulder j., 2 Knee j., 1 Ankle j., 4
Aged	6	72 - 82 (79.2)	Hip j., 6
Osteoarthritic	7	52 - 80 (73.3)	Hip j., 7
Rheum. Arthritic	6	51 - 84 (66.3)	Knee j., 6

with subchondral bone and fibrous tissue. Pieces of the hyaline cartilage embedded in paraffin were stained with hematoxyline and eosine, and toluidine blue.

Pepsin-soluble collagen and pepsin-insoluble collagen were obtained from different parts of normal and pathological cartilage by the method of Miller (1). A portion of the pepsin-insoluble collagen was reduced in vitro with sodium borohydride as described by Tanzer (2). Insoluble collagen, both reduced and untreated (not reduced) in vitro, was hydrolyzed. Quantitative analysis of aldimine cross-links were performed by the method of Masuda (3). A portion of the soluble collagen was cleaved with cyanogen bromide, and the collagen types were analyzed by calculation from the disc electrophoretic pattern of CNBr peptides (4).

Pepsin-insoluble collagen was extracted with 50% phenol to check the strength of hydrophobic bonds between collagen molecules. The procedure is summarized in Figure 1. This technique was originally devised for the separation of connectin, elastic protein in muscle fiber (5).

RESULTS

Solubilities of collagens from articular cartilage and fibrocartilage of the meniscus of the knee joint with pepsin at 40°C for 48 hours are shown in Figure 2. The solubility of collagen is calculated from the ratio of dry weight of solubilized collagen to original collagen before pepsin digestion. Although 7 to 70% of the collagen

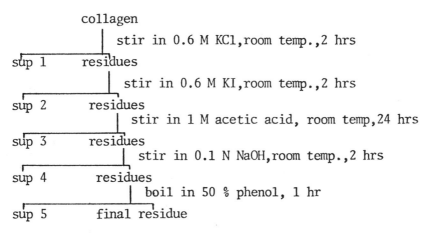

Fig. 1. Procedure of phenol extraction to check the strength of the
        hydrophobic bond between collagen molecules.

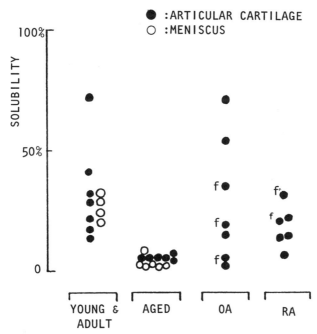

Fig. 2.   Solubility of collagens from articular cartilages and
          menisci following pepsin digestion (calculated from the
          ratio of dry weight of solubilized collagen to original
          collagen before digestion). OA, osteoarthritis; RA,
          rheumatoid arthritis; F, fibrillated cartilage.

Table 2. The Amount of Aldimine Cross-Links in Insoluble Collagen
          from Human Articular Cartilage

		Young and adult	aged
Number of sample		7	6
aldimine cross-links			
DHLNL	reduced	0.1810 + 0.0832	0.2321 + 0.1071
	non-reduced	0.1121 ∓ 0.0708	0.1716 ∓ 0.0603
HLNL	reduced	0.2554 + 0.1769	0.5035 + 0.2322
	non-reduced	0.2256 ∓ 0.0560	0.3343 ∓ 0.1078
LNL	reduced	0.0095 + 0.0054	0.0030 + 0.0008
	non-reduced	0.0000 ∓ 0.0000	0.0030 ∓ 0.0021
sum of cross-links			
	reduced	0.4459 + 0.2323	0.7386 + 0.4555
	non-reduced	0.3377 ∓ 0.2034	0.5089 ∓ 0.2876

Each cross-links is calculated from the color yield of
lysine and expressed as mean of residues ± standard
error per 1,000 amino acid residues.
DHLNL ; dihydroxylysinonorleucine, HLNL ; hydroxylysinonorleucine, LNL ; lysinonorleucine.

was solubilized in the adult group, only 4% was solubilized in the
aged group. Open circles indicate the solubility of fibrocartilage
of the meniscus of the knee joint. Similar solubilities can be seen
for both fibrocartilage and hyaline cartilage. On the other hand,
solubilities of osteoarthritic and rheumatoid arthritic cartilage
were higher than those of aged cartilage, although the mean ages of
the three donor groups were not significantly different. There was
no difference in solubility between fibrillated cartilage and the
other cartilages.

The analysis of cross-links indicated that at least three different kinds of aldimine cross-links, dihydroxylysinonorleucine,
hydroxylysinonorleucine, and lysinonorleucine, were present in the
insoluble collagen of aged cartilage. Some aldimine cross-links are
present even in adult cartilage collagen not reduced in vitro. The
total number of aldimine cross-links increased in both reduced and
untreated collagens from aged cartilage, in comparison with those
from normal adult cartilage, as shown in Table 2.

Figure 3 shows the extractibility of insoluble collagen of various tissues from aged donors using neutral salt, weak acid, weak
alkaline solution, and 50% phenol to study the strength of hydrophobic bonds. Extractability is calculated from the dry weight of each
extract per that of the original collagen. In comparison with skin

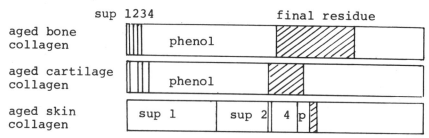

Fig. 3.   Extractability of pepsin insoluble collagens (dry weight
          of each extract per original collagen). Sup 1, extract of
          0.6 M KCl; sup 2, extract of 0.6 M KI; sup 3, extract of 1
          M acetic acid; sup 4, extract of 0.1 N NaOH solution,
          phenol or p, extract of 50% phenol.

collagen, a large portion of cartilage collagen was found in the
phenol extract, and a final residue remained which was not extracted
by any of the procedures. These results suggested that aged cartilage collagen contained a large number of hydrophobic bonds soluble
only in phenol. As shown in Table 3, the amino acid composition of
both extracts and final residues were unchanged from those of the
original collagen before the extraction.

A large number of aldimine cross-links were lost in each step of
the extraction procedure, and only a small number of aldimine cross-
links were present in the final residue (Table 4). This shows that
hydrophobic bonds are as important as aldimine cross-links for the
stability of aged cartilage collagen.

The disc electrophoretic patterns and their densitograms of CNBr
(cyanogen bromide) peptides of authentic type I collagen, normal aged
cartilage collagen, rheumatoid arthritic cartilage collagen, and
authentic type II collagen are shown in Figures 4 and 5, respectively. The characteristic α2CB3,5 peak of type I collagen is present and is shown as a black peak in Figure 5 A. The characteristic
α1(II)CB10 peak of type II collagen is present, and is shown as a
shaded peak in Figure 5, D. The characteristic peak of type I collagen, α2CB3,5, can be seen in the middle two densitograms of Figure 5,
which show the cyanogen bromide peptides of normal aged and rheumatoid arthritic cartilage collagens. The ratio of type I collagen to
type I plus type II collagens can be calculated from the ratio of the
density of the α2CB3,5 peak to that of the α1(II)CB10 peak.

On microscopic examination, all the cartilage studied was found
to be composed of hyaline cartilage uncontaminated with fibrocartilage, fibrous tissue, and bone. With toluidine blue staining, a
change of metachromasia was seen in the osteoarthritic cartilage,
especially in the fibrillated and osteophytic cartilage (Fig. 6).

Table 3.   AMINO ACID COMPOSITION
            Procedure 1--pepsin insoluble collagen from aged human
            cartilage (residues/1,000 total residues)

	pepsin insol. collagen before phe. ext.	50% phenol extract	final residue
Hydroxyproline	76.27	76.98	96.75
Aspartic acid	50.45	48.10	45.10
Threonine	24.15	23.89	18.68
Serine	30.98	23.50	22.75
Glutamic acid	94.14	94.56	84.23
Proline	105.08	98.27	112.01
Glycine	327.35	356.40	364.89
Alanine	93.93	93.92	90.16
Valine	25.04	23.60	19.81
Methionine	9.21	8.70	8.29
Isoleucine	11.99	14.12	11.43
Leucine	33.39	30.77	28.32
Tyrosine	7.81	6.17	3.70
Phenylalanine	19.19	21.22	17.42
Histidine	5.03	4.60	2.89
Hydroxylysine	12.47	12.73	13.18
Lysine	21.06	19.11	16.41
Arginine	52.45	46.60	43.91

To observe the relation between the type of collagen and the
classified lesions of pathological cartilage, the type of collagen in
the remaining hyaline areas was compared with those in fibrillated
and osteophytic areas (Fig. 7). Although cartilage from the remaining hyaline areas contained only type II collagen, hyaline cartilages
from fibrillated and osteophytic areas contained two types of collagen giving various ratios. The ratio of type I collagen to type I
plus type II collagens in fibrillated cartilage was not lower than
that found in the other pathological cartilage. The ratio of type I
collagen to type I plus type II collagens is correlated with the severity of degenerative changes in pathological cartilage, and is not
correlated with aging.

DISCUSSION

It was concluded from these results that the pepsin solubility
decreased and the number of aldimine cross-links increased in the
cartilage from aged donors; and the types of collagen present also
changed in aged cartilage.

Table 4.

The Amount of Aldimine Cross-links
Aged human cartilage collagen (pepsin insol.)

aldimine cross-links	pep.insol. coll.before phe. ext.	usp 1 (KCl)	sup 2-4	sup 5 (phenol)	final residue
DHLNL	0.000	0.000	-------	0.359	0.000
HLNL	0.470	1.650	-------	0.762	0.084
LNL	0.000	0.000	-------	0.000	0.000
total (res./1,000 amino acid residues)	0.470	1.650		1.121	0.084
percentage to original collagen (A)	100 %	3 %	3 %	41 %	15 %
total aldimine cross-links X $\frac{A}{100}$	0.470	0.050	-------	0.460	0.013

With respect to glycosaminoglycan, the amount of chondroitin sulfate present does not change significantly following maturation, but
the amount does decrease during the developmental period (6).

Using the fixed charge density method to estimate the total glycosaminoglycan content in tissue, the amount of glycosaminoglycan in
normal cartilage does not change with age, but the amount decreases
in fibrillated cartilage in a process unrelated to that of aging
(7). In the cartilage of pig knee joint, the percentage or uronic
acid and the ratio of molar galactosamine to glucosamine does not
change between 3 and 5 years of age, although the percentage and
ratio are very different prior to maturity, in the developmental
period up to 25 weeks of age. Age has not been found to influence
the concentration, nor the chain length, of chronodroitin sulfate (8).

Cellularity of human articular cartilage in the femoral condyle
does not change after 20 years of age, although many differences can
be seen between newborn and adult cartilages (9). Cartilage cells of
normal appearance do not change their number of nuclei during aging,
but the number decreases in cells of the superficial layer of fibrillated cartilage (10). The cell size of cartilage, rate of cell
division, oxygen utilization, total amount of expressible fluid content, and extractable lipid are unaffected by aging.

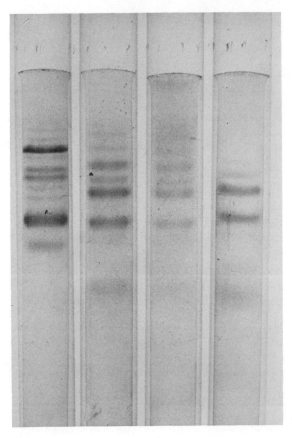

Fig. 4.   Disc electrophoretic pattern of cyanogen bromide peptides
           of authentic type 1 collagen in the left gel, normal aged
           cartilage in the second gel, rheumatoid arthritic carti-
           lage collagen in the third gel, and authentic type 2
           collagen in the right-most gel.

It is very interesting to find out whether these various changes
of the matrix of articular cartilage result from the change of the
matrix of cartilage cells in vivo associated with aging. Figure 8
summarized our hypothesis.

First, the decrease of solubility is not influenced directly by
in vivo cartilage cells, but is influenced by the amounts of glycosaminoglycan surrounding the cartilage collagen, the numbers of aldimine cross-links and of hydrophobic bonds. The strength and the
amount of hydrophobic bonds depend on the alignment and tertiary
structure of collagen molecules in the extracellular environment.
The quantitative and qualitative changes of glycosaminoglycan cannot
be seen in aged cartilage of normal appearance.

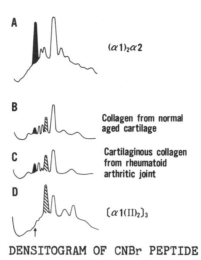

A $(\alpha 1)_2 \alpha 2$

B   Collagen from normal
                               aged cartilage

C   Cartilaginous collagen
                               from rheumatoid
                               arthritic joint

D $[\alpha 1(II)_2]_3$

DENSITOGRAM OF CNBr PEPTIDE

Fig. 5.   Densitogram of disc electrophoretic bands shown in
           Figure 7. Characteristis of type 1 collagen are the
           presence of α2CB3,5 peak, as shown as black peak in A.
           Characteristic peak of type 2 collagen is α1(II)CB10, as
           shown as shadow peak in D. Characteristic peak of type 1
           collagen, namely α2CB3,5, can be detected in the middle
           two figures of normal aged and rheumatoid arthritic
           cartilage collagens.

     Second, the number of aldimine cross-links is influenced by the
activity of lysyl oxidase and extracellular formation of Schiff's
base to derive ε-amino groups and aldehyde groups, derivatives of
lysine and hydroxylysine in collagen molecular sequences.

     Third, the type of collagen is influenced by the gene expression
of cartilage cells. Type I collagen which is not included in normal
cartilage is synthesized in aged cartilage and pathological cartilage
from disease processes associated with aging. In these last two
types of cartilage, chondrocytes change their gene expression. This
change is not irreversible, however, because in cartilage cells of a
pathological area, syntheses of both type I and type II collagens
were observed at the same time by immunofluorescent study. It is
also recognized that the change of collagen type is reversible and is
influenced by the amount of environmental calcium ions in an in vitro
study of a cell culture. Therefore, the change of collagen type is
due to changes in the environment surrounding cartilage cells rather
than to the aging phenomena intrinsic to the cells (11,12).

     Although we cannot recognize the irreversible changes in articu-
lar cartilage cells, various biochemical changes of collagen occur in

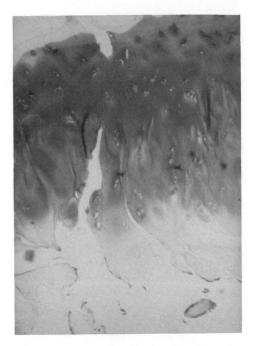

Fig. 6.   Histological finding of fibrillated cartilage with
          toluidine blue staining. Change of metachromasia is
          recognizable. (x 100).

the cartilage matrix associated with aging once maturation has occurred. The role of a cartilage cell in the joint is to maintain the
constancy of the cartilage acquired during the maturation period
thoughout the whole life. Our investigation of collagen indicated,
however, a disturbance of constancy in articular cartilage following
maturation. Also, in advanced stages of aging, normal articular
cartilage becomes osteoarthritic. From this, we question the occurrence of physiological aging in articular cartilage.

SUMMARY

    It can be seen from our results that, in aged cartilage: (1)
pepsin solubility of collagen increases; (2) the number of aldimine
cross-links of insoluble collagen increases; and (3) the type of collagen changes.

    Quantitative and qualitative changes of glycosaminoglycan cannot
be recognized, and cellularity does not change after 20 years of age,
or maturation. Only molecular research on cartilage collagen, which
accounts for 60 to 70% of the organic matrix in cartilage, can show
the changes in metabolic behavior of cartilage cells that are associated with aging.

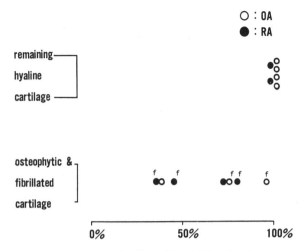

type 2 collagen/type 1 + type 2 collagen

PERCENTAGE OF TYPE 2 COLLAGEN IN SOLUBLE COLLAGENS
FROM VARIOUS ARTICULAR CARTILAGES

Fig. 7.   Relation between the type of collagen and the classified
           lesions of pathological cartilages. "f" indicates
           fibrillated cartilage. Cartilage of remaining area
           contains only type 2 collagen, but hyaline cartilages of
           fibrillated and osteophytic areas contain two types of
           collagens in various ratios.

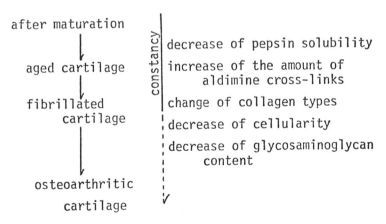

Fig. 8.   Changes of cartilage associated with aging.

REFERENCES

1. E. J. Miller, Isolation and characterization of a collagen from chick cartilage containing three identical α-chain, Biochem. 10:1652 (1971).
2. M. L. Tanzer and G. Meckanic, Collagen reduction in sodium borohydride: Effects of reconstruction, maturation and lathyrism, Biochem. Biophys. Res. Comm. 32:885 (1968).
3. M. Masuda, S. Karube, Y. Hayashi, H. Shindo, and M. Igarashi, Direct measurement of collagen cross-links with automatic amino acid analyzer - Identification of peaks due to cross-links, FEBS Letters 63:245 (1976).
4. H. Furthmayer and R. Timpl, Characterization of collagen peptides by sodium dodecylsulfate-polyacrylamide electrophoresis, Anal. Biochem. 41:510 (1971).
5. K. Maruyama, S. Matsubara, R. Natori, Y. Nonomura, S. Kimura, K. Ohashi, F. Murakami, S. Handa, and G. Eguchi, Connectin, an elastic protein of muscle - Characterization and function, J. Biochem. 82:317 (1977).
6. R. Kyselka, Biochemical alteration of hip joint cartilage in aged subject, Z. Alternsforsch. 20:279 (1967).
7. C. Ficat and A. Maroudas, Cartilage of the patella. Topographical variation of glycosaminoglycan content in normal and fibrillated tissue, Ann. Rheum. Dis. 34:515 (1975).
8. C. A. McDevitt, Biochemistry of articular cartilage. Nature of proteoglycans and collagen of articular cartilage and their role in aging and in osteoarthrosis, Ann. Rheum. Dis. 32:364 (1973).
9. R. A. Stockwell, The cell density of human articular and costal cartilage, J. Anat. 101:753 (1967).
10. G. Meachims and D. H. Collins, Cell count of normal and osteo-arthritic articular cartilages in relation to the uptake of sulphate ($^{35}SO_4$) in vitro, Ann. Rheum. Dis. 21:45 (1962).
11. S. Gay, P. K. Muller, C. Lemmen, K. Remberger, K. Matzen, and K. Kuhn, Immunohistological study on collagen in cartilage-bone metamorphosis and degenerative osteoarthrosis, Klin. Wschr. 54:969 (1976).
12. K. Deshmukh and B. D. Sawyer, Synthesis of collagen by chondrocytes in suspension culture: Modulation by calcium, 3':5'-cyclic AMP, and prostaglandins, Proc. Natl. Acad. Sci. USA 74:3864 (1977).

AGING AND CHANGES IN GENETIC INFORMATION[*]

R. W. Hart[+] and S. P. Modak[‡]

[+]Professor of Radiology, Pharmacology and Preventive
Medicine, The Ohio State University College of Medicine
410 W. 10th Ave., Columbus, Ohio 43210, USA

[‡]Visiting Professor in Radiology

INTRODUCTION

Although all placental mammals are characterized by similar
morphological, physiological, and biochemical parameters, they differ
from one another in maximum achievable life span by approximately
fifty-fold (1,2). Even within closely associated families of recent
evolutionary occurrence, such as the primates and Myomorph rodents,
e.g., Mus musculus and Peromyscus leucopus, life spans vary by more
than twenty fold (3) and three fold (4), respectively. Thus, it
appears that whatever governs the life span of a species must be able
to be modified rapidly. This imposes strong constraints on the
possible genetic mechanisms for the evolution of longevity-assurance
systems (4). Two ways by which rapid evolution of longevity could
occur, and yet be consistent with basic molecular genetics, would be
either via modification of already existing genetic information
(species differences in longevity reflecting differences in the
turning off of longevity-assurance systems during fetal development),
or through slight but significant changes in a number of interlocking
processes governing phenotypic expression. Either or both of these
mechanisms might explain the rapid evolution of life span within
species without necessitating the concurrent input of new genes.

Physiological data further supports the contention that DNA is a
primary target and that the rate of accumulation of various forms of

----
[*]This work was supported by National Cancer Institute Contract No.
Nol-CB-84226.

genetic damage may be a governing factor in longevity. When
different mammalian species are compared on a fraction of maximum
life span basis, most age-related changes observed appear to occur at
similar times (5). Likewise, the decline in "normal" physiological
and biochemical processes occurs at equivalent rates when maximum
life span within the placental mammals is normalized (6,7). The time
of onset of various degenerative diseases and loss of immune function
and wound-healing capacity also progress at similar rates in different mammalian species (8,9,7,4). These facts further emphasize a
commonality of target between species and differences in the rate of
loss of genomic fidelity.

The ability of an organism to maintain the stability of its unit
components determines its functional capacity. The higher the differentiated state of a system, the greater the amount of stability
required to maintain that state as a function of time. Stability can
be achieved by prevention, repair or redundancy. Instability occurs
when damage or noise is introduced into a system, where it remains
and may be expressed. In addition to external agents which produce
DNA damage, various internal processes also induce such damage. For
example, approximately 1,000 lesions occur per day per cell as a
result of apurinic sites induced at a 37°C body temperature. Thus,
while the number of internal and external DNA damaging events to
which animals are exposed is relatively constant, maximum achievable
life span among mammalian species is not. This suggests that if the
causal factor in aging is the expression or rate of accumulation of
DNA damage, then among different species there must exist different
degrees: 1) to which the DNA is protected from damaging agents and
2) for the removal of the damaged portions of DNA and of the expression of damaged regions of the genome. The net effect of the combination of these processes will be dependent on the absolute residual level of unrepaired DNA damage and on its expression.

PROCESSES RELATED TO THE CONSERVATION OF DNA STABILITY

Metabolite Induction and Removal

DNA damage arises partly as a result of the interaction of exogenously or endogenously generated free radicals and electrophilic
molecules with cellular DNA. Differences appear to exist with regard
to cell-mediated carcinogen activation among cultivated fibroblasts
derived from different species. An inverse correlation between
species life span and the capacity of cultured fibroblasts to activate the potent chemical carcinogen 7,12-dimethylbenz(a)anthracene
(DMBA) to its mutagenic form has been observed (10). Subsequent
studies by this group further confirmed this observation with several
independently isolated fibroblast strains from these same six
species, and also showed an excellent inverse correlation between
species life span and the rate and extent to which the metabolites of
the polycyclic aromatic hydrocarbon (PAH) DMBA bind to DNA (11). The

difference in extent of binding of DMBA to cellular DNA in these
species was over thirty-fold, with rat binding approximately 130
pmoles DMBA/mg DNA, rabbit 55 pmoles DMBA/mg DNA, and man less than
10 pmoles DMBA/mg DNA. It is not known whether other cell types or
tissues follow a similar pattern. Nor is it known whether a similar
life span correlation holds for metabolic activation and metabolite-
binding of other chemical carcinogens.

It has been proposed that the metabolites resulting from intracellular oxidation of DMBA are derived from epoxide intermediates,
and that these epoxides are the electrophilic species responsible for
the DNA-damaging properties of DMBA (12). These epoxides are formed
by microsomal oxidation of DMBA and benzo(a)pyrene (BP) as well as
other PAH (13). The major metabolic products of BP oxidations are
transdihydrodiols, phenols, and glutathione conjugates (13). For
PAH-containing exocylic methyl functions (e.g., DMBA), the situation
is considerably more complex, since these compounds form metabolites
from both ring oxidations and methyl hydroxylation (Fig. 1).
Cultured cells metabolize both DNA-damaging and non-DNA-damaging PAH
at roughly equal rates (14). However, human cells generally oxidize
PAH at a slower rate than rodent cells (15,16).

It has been established that the process of epoxide formation is
initiated by the action of the aryl hydrocarbon hydroxylase (AHH)
enzyme system found in the microsomal membrane (17). The AHH system
requires NADPH and oxygen, and contains the cytochromes P448 and P450
(18). AHH enzyme systems are present in the microsomes of most tissues that have been studied, but are generally found at the highest
concentration in hepatic cells (18). This general nature of the AHH
system may reflect its wide range of functions, including oxidation
of a wide variety of xenobiotic substances in both rodent (19) and
human (20) cells in vitro. Whitlock and Gelboin (21) have shown that
both RNA and protein synthesis are required for AHH induction. There
exists, however, evidence demonstrating induction of AHH by PAH in
the presence of inhibitors of protein synthesis (22). Similarly,
studies on the genetics of AHH inducibility have led to contradictory
results. Nebert at al. (23) have shown that the gene required for
AHH inducibility segregates as a simple autosomal dominant trait, and
that inducibility is an all-or-none phenomenon in all tissues of the
organism. Kouri et al. (24) also found that AHH inducibility in two
strains of mice, C57Bl/6 and DBA/6, behaved as a simple autosomal
trait, but only hepatic levels were measured. Weibel et al. (25), on
the other hand, observed that in some strains of mice the liver AHH
is not inducible via PAH, while the AHH levels in target tissues of
the same animal (i.e., lung, skin, small intestine and kidney) were
inducible. Additionally, studies comparing mice with a high (AKR)
vs. low (AF) incidence of leukemia for AHH induction via 3-methyl
cholanthrene (3MC) also indicate a genetic system more complicated
than a single Mendelian one (26).

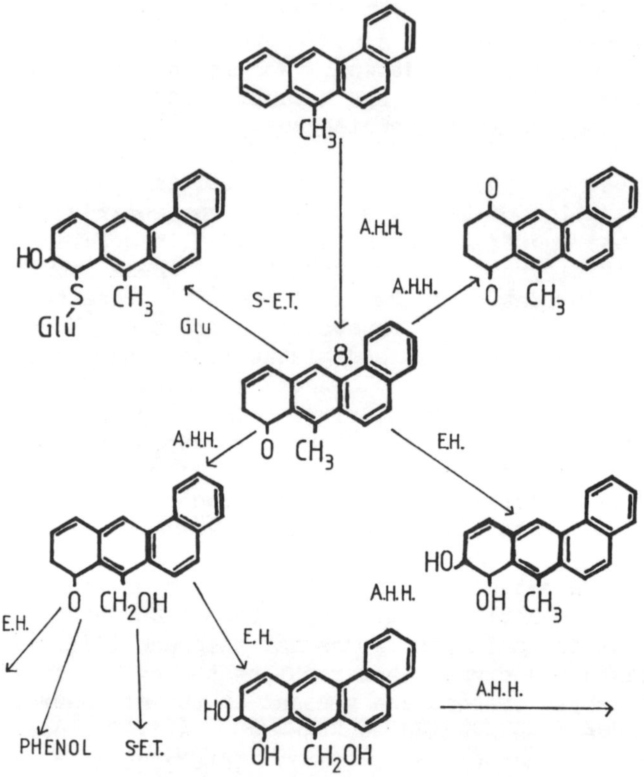

Fig. 1. Some examples of the possible metabolic pathways for
oxidation of 7-methylbenz(a)anthracene.

Kellerman et al. (20) have measured the 3MC induction in mitogen-
stimulated lymphocytes from man. They found the lymphocytes fell
into two to three groups (27): low (1.8-fold), medium (2.5-fold),
and high (5.6-fold). Their subsequent studies on families and
identical twins suggest that AHH inducibility in humans is under
genetic control. Similarly, aging rates in man also appear to be the
same in identical, but not fraternal, twins (28).

Since the capacity to perform metabolic activation correlates
well in an inverse fashion with species maximum achievable life span,
it would be interesting to determine if cells or animals treated with
PAH demonstrate any life span shortening effect minus tumor induction; whether non-DNA damaging analogs of these agents (i.e., DMBA
vs. 2F-DMBA) induce similar or different effects on life span; and if
blocking of AHH activation retards any life span shortening effects
observed. All of the experiments listed are feasible, since:

a) doses of carcinogens can be controlled so as to achieve anywhere
between 10 and 90 percent killing from carcinogen-induced tumors,
with the remaining fraction of survivors being monitored as to
variation in life span against controls; b) a series of DMBA analogs
with varying abilities to damage cellular DNA are available; and c)
inhibitors of AHH-catalyzed conversion of BP and DMBA to water-soluble derivatives are available.

Other factors affecting the extent of damage to cellular DNA by
DNA-damaging agents include the ability of other cellular components
to scavenge free radicals (e.g., vitamin E), break down nucleophilic
molecules (e.g., epoxide hydrase and superoxide dismutase), absorb
their deleterious interactions (e.g., attacks on membrane, protein,
and RNA rather than DNA), and modify their metabolism and rate of
removal. While the modes of action of certain of these phenomena are
well understood, their roles in aging are not. Ascribing any particular role for any of these events has an underlying pitfall: i.e.,
since several events exist, the modification of any single event
would be expected only to modify those facets of aging related to
that event or form of DNA damage, rather than all facets of aging.

The Induction of DNA Damage and Its Removal

Among the longevity-assurance genes, there are probably several
sets of genes responsible for both preservation of DNA damage and
control of the repair of such damage (29,4). For example, there are
at least four general categories of DNA repair: excision, strand
break, postreplication, and photoreactivation (30). Each of these
may have several subcategories. Of the various forms of DNA repair,
only large patch excision repair has been widely examined relative to
longevity (30).

Excision or prereplication repair of UV-induced damage has been
measured in a number of different species (31) by a number of
different techniques (32,33). Although these techniques measured
different parameters, they all seem to give similar estimates of
excision repair (29). These earlier studies tended to indicate that
human cells (34) and cow cells (35) were very efficient at dimer
excision (a direct measure of DNA damage and repair), while those
from the hamster (36) showed less excision repair than those from cow
or human, but more than cells from the mouse (36). A subsequent
study, attempting to minimize different variables between laboratories and cell strains, used primary cell cultures derived from the
same anatomical location of animals that had completed the same proportion of the species' maximal life span. This study showed an
excellent correlation between both the rate and extent of unscheduled
DNA synthesis induced by ultraviolet radiation, as measured by autoradiography, and the life span of seven species drawn from five
orders of mammals (29).

A subsequent study examined this correlation in a well-defined comparative system consisting of two Myomorph rodent species, Mus musculus and Peromycus leucopus, which are similar in size, organ weight, and gestation time, but which differ in life span by a factor of 2.5 (4). Agreement was observed between the life spans and the extend of UV-induced unscheduled DNA synthesis for primary fibroblast cell cultures derived from these two species. A determination of patch size (size of the repaired regions) following exposure of the cells to UV light agreed with the aforecited unscheduled DNA synthesis data, thereby confirming a genuine difference in excision repair between two species. These studies indicated that the previous results could not be accounted for by differences in the size of radio-labeled patches. Furthermore, no significant differences in either the amount of DNA per cell or in the rate and extent single-strand break repair following exposure of these cells to X-rays were observed between these two species (4).

A still more recent study using primate fibroblast cell cultures again supports the aforementioned correlation between unscheduled DNA synthesis, as determined by autoradiography, and species life span for UV-induced damage (37). In this study, eleven fibroblast cell cultures derived from punch biopsies of similar-aged primates were shipped blind and coded. These samples were exposed under identical conditions to identical fluences of ultraviolet light, and the extent of unscheduled DNA synthesis measured. The results were then exchanged for the code, and the data calculated. Again a direct correlation between extent of unscheduled DNA synthesis and species life span was observed, with longer-lived species being capable of approximately eight times more repair than shorter-lived species. Additionally, using the assay for endonuclease-sensitive sites, it now appears that UV-endo-sensitive sites are removed at approximately equal rates in all primate cell lines under low-salt conditions, and that in all cases additional sites can be demonstrated after treatment with high-salt. Experiments are now in progress to determine whether there exists species-dependent differences in chromatin structure in relation to the accessibility of damaged sites. Recently, studies which were performed under similar conditions on inbred rodent strains exhibiting approximately a three-fold difference in life span have suggested that this correlation holds between strains of the same species (38). Such studies have not yet been performed with any chemical agent. However, there do exist certain reports relevant to the discussion of this question. For example, as seen in Table 1, it has been observed that the hamster cell line BHK21/C13, which is excision positive for UV-induced cyclobutane-type pyrimidine dimers, is more proficient in removal of DNA adducts induced by benzo(a)pyrene from its DNA than the mouse cell line C57Bl over the same time period following exposure to the same concentration of BP (39). In these studies, the initial number of DN-BP adducts induced were approximately equal in each cell type. Additionally, Smith-Sonneborn (40) has recently used photoreactivation

Table 1.   Data on Removal of Chemical Carcinogens. These data
           are based on actual measurment of lost chemical adducts
           by chromatographic procedures, and do not reflect mere
           loss of specific activity from DNA.

Carcinogen	Cell-Type	Strain	Dimer Excision	Treatment Conc. (uM)	% Removal	Time of Removal	Reference
4NQO	E. Coli	H/r30	+	400	80	60 min.	Ikenaga et al., 1975
"	"	Hs30R	-	400	0	60 min.	"
"	mouse	A31-714	?	4	70	24 hr.	"
"	human	FL	+	4	60	24 hr.	"
"	human	XP	-	4	20	24 hr.	"
7BrMBA	hamster	V-79	+	0.1-0.2	50	30 hr.	Dipple and Roberts,1977
"	human	HeLa	+	0.1-0.2	50	30 hr.	"
"	human	lympho-cytes	+	1	15-17	12 hr.	"
"	human	lympho-cytes	+	5	15-19	6 hr.	"
"	human	lympho-cytes	-	5	1.4-2	6 hr.	"
"	E. Coli	WP2	+	38.5	70	30 min.	Venitt and Tarmy, 1972
"	E. Coli	WP2uvrA⁻	-	38.5	10	2 hr.	"
"	E. Coli	WP2(uvrA⁻)(exrA⁻)	-	38.5	0	2 hr.	"
BP	hamster	BHK21/C13	+	1.3	27.7	24 hr.	Cerutti et al., 1977
"	mouse	C57Bl	+	1.3	15.1	24 hr.	"

(the specific and direct monomerization of UV-induced cyclobutane-
type pyrimidine dimers) as an exquisite tool to demonstrate that the
life span shortening effects of UV-light in the clonal Paramecium
aging model system can be reversed. She speculates that, since the
treatment of UV-irradiated cells with photoreactivating light not
only overcomes the life span shortening effects of UV, but extends
life span significantly, this observation may result from the action
of a nondamage-specific repair recognition system in Paramecium which
is free to operate upon non-UV-induced damage in cellular DNA following photoreactivation. Interestingly, in single cell systems
there is precedent for such enzymes.

On the other hand, the Chinese hamster V-79 cell line appears to

be as repair-proficient for similar concentrations of 7-bromoethyl-
benz(a)anthracene-induced DNA damage as is the human cell line HeLa,
both removing approximately 50 percent of the total number of
DN-chemical complexes within 24 hours (41). Additionally, the rodent
cell line A31-714 appears to remove the DNA damage induced by
4-nitroquinoline-1-oxide (4NQO) at approximately the same rate and to
the same extent as human fetal lung cells in vitro (42). This latter
observation is especially interesting in light of the fact that 4NQO
is a classical UV-mimicking agent which produces DNA damage that is
not repaired in excision-defective strains of xeroderma pigmentosum
(42). Another possibly relevant observation is the study of
Ben-Ishai and Peleg (43), who showed that cell cultures taken from
mouse embryos between day 5 and day 19 of gestation have a high level
of UV-induced excision repair which subsequently is turned off just
prior to birth.

It is important to note that while these studies are intriguing,
they nevertheless represent studies performed with model agents.
They measure the repair of only a small number of the potential forms
of DNA damage as carried out by only a few of the various types of
excision repair over limited time frames, and use restricted method-
ologies under in vitro cell culture conditions. Any general extrapolation from these data to a process such as aging would be premature,
if not naive. Any alteration in the structure of DNA would be expected to lead to alteration in cellular function and the ability of a
system to respond to various external and internal stress factors.
Since there exist numerous forms of DNA damage and repair system, it
is a reasonable expectation that neither a single type of DNA damage
nor a lack of any individual type of repair would mimic the aging
process in all aspects. However, one would expect that individuals
exhibiting such defects would mimic, in some form or the other, certain facets of premature aging. Indeed, this seems to be the case
for selected human repair defective syndromes, such as xeroderma
pigmentosum, ataxia telangectasia, progeria, Down's syndrome,
Fanconi's anemia, etc. (44). Likewise, since no single agent induces
all forms of DNA damage uniformly and proportionately to what might
be expected to occur naturally, it would not be expected that any
single agent would bring forth uniformly and proportionately all
facets of aging. Again, this expectation is consistent with the
known facts (45).

Chromatin Structure and Its Possible Role in the Control of Genome Integrity

A number of studies on terminally differentiated and aging
post-mitotic cells (46-56) have shown that DNA in these cells
progressively accumulate strand breaks. Evidence has been presented
recently that in terminally differentiating postmitotic lens fibers,
single-strand breaks affect DNA in the region between nucleosomes,
and are converted to double-strand breaks giving rise to a multimeric

series of low M_w DNA fragments resembling those produced by Ca^{++}-dependent nuclease-catalyzed digestion of chromatin (57).

From earlier studies, it was hypothesized (51) that the progressive accumulation of damage in DNA in terminally differentiating and aging postmitotic cells is probably related to a defective DNA repair machinery. Considerable evidence now exists that in terminally differentiating and aging cells, excision-repair and strand-break rejoining does indeed become defective (54,58-67). Cellular DNA does not exist as a naked molecule, but rather in the form of a complex with histone and nonhistone protein (68). The DNA-histone complex forms a flexible string of closely packed beads of chromatin subunits, also called 'nubodies' or 'nucleosomes' (69,70), each containing a stretch of DNA (71,72) varying in length between species (73,74). These nucleosomes contain two molecules each of H2A, H2B, H3 and H4 (75,76) to form the "core particle" (77,78), which contains 165-212 base pairs of DNA, with 25-72 base pairs in the spacer or linker region outside the core particle (79,80). Histone H1 is associated with the spacer region (81-83).

It is generally assumed that the distribution of damaged sites in DNA produced by ionizing radiation or UV is random. While this may hold true for naked DNA, there is as yet no evidence on the validity of the above assumption for chromatin-associated DNA. Wilkins and Hart (84) found that a significant portion of pyrimidine dimers induced by UV is masked in nuclei and can be made fully accessible in vitro to UV-endonuclease by high-salt treatment, thereby showing for the first time preferential DNA repair. Treatment of mouse mammary cells with methyl methane-sulfonate and subsequent analysis of the site of damage and repair in chromatin suggest that either damaged sites are non-uniformly distributed, or that the repaired regions are distributed non-randomly relatively to the nucleosomes (85). In UV-irradiated human fibroblasts, the initial repair replication seems to occur preferentially in the linker region (86); nothing is known, however, concerning the frequency of occurrence of pyrimidine dimers in DNA associated with chromatin subunits. The above studies thus indicate that at least the accessibility of the damaged site in DNA is controlled by the chromatin organization, but say little about the precise structural parameter involved. A classical case demonstrating the complexity of this issue is found in V-79 cells, in which 85-90% of UV-induced dimers remain unexcised after six hours (87), although only 20% of the chromatin-DNA is associated with staphylococcal nuclease-resistant nucleosome core particles (Modak, D'Ambrosio, and Hart, unpublished data). Thus, any model conferring upon the chromatin subunits the role of controlling the accessibility of damaged sites to repair enzymes seems naive unless it takes into account histone-histone, histone-DNA, and nonhistone-DNA interactions. Perhaps the most overwhelming consideration is that DNA repair enzymes represent large complexes and must require at least a temporary weakening of the DNA-histone complex, if not its complete

disassociation or displacement in order to render accessible the
template DNA. Thus, while the existing data (85-87) emphasize the
importance of the chromatin organization, a direct extrapolation of
results on excision repair in purified DNA may be misleading at this
time. In any case, the template-active and repair-active fractions
of chromatin seem to be structurally distinct from the inactive
regions (84-86,88-91).

In attempts to investigate causes for the aging process, several
authors have analyzed the thermal melting behavior (92-96) and the
template activity for exogenous RNA polymerase (92,95,97,98) of
chromatin in aging tissues, but their results do not always agree.
Chromatin Tm increases as a function of age in bovine thymus and rat
liver (92,95). Similarly, it has been found that the chromatin
template activity for exogenous RNA polymerase decreases with age
(92,95,98). Complexity measurements suggest that the number of different types of RNA sequences expressed in mouse tissues decreases
with age (99). Taken together, these studies indicate that the
chromatin structure undergoes discrete changes during the aging process. Relevant to this, the DNA repeat size remains unchanged as a
function of time, although in old mice (28-33 months) a considerable
heterogeneity appears in the digestion products with staphylococcal
nuclease. Additionally, the proportion of staphylococcal nuclease-
sensitive fraction in mouse liver chromatin decreases from 50%
(1.75-18 months of age) to 38% at 28-33 months of age, so that the
actual proportion of DNA organized into chromatin subunits increases
from 70% at 18 months to 90% in very late age. Although these differences suggest that the histone:DNA ratio should increase, this has
not been found to be the case (98). Alternate explanations include
the possibility that there exists a free pool of histones in mouse
liver cells, or that at early and mid-ages half-nucleosome-like
structures similar to those suggested by Weintraub et al. (89) may
exist containing DNA which is fully sensitive to staphyloccocal
nuclease. In the latter case, the half-nucleosome pairs may
reassociate to form full nucleosomes, thus rendering resistance to
DNA from the staphylococcal nuclease. So far, it has not been possible to ascertain whether non-histone protein confers a nuclease-
resistant property upon chromatin-DNA, but this possibility cannot be
excluded at present. Non-histone proteins play an important role in
regulation of gene expression (68), but nothing is known of their
involvement in age-dependent genome inactivation.

Medvedev et al. (100,101) have recently found that histone H1 is
modifed in old cells. Two-dimensional electrophoretic analysis of
histones from mouse liver chromatin suggests that significant histone
modification may appear at 28-33 months of age. Histone modifications can be expected to affect the conformation of chromatin, e.g.,
an increased charge on H1 would result in condensation of the chromatin, while appearance of H4 with greater charge would tend to
increase histone:histone interactions, while at the same time

decreasing DNA:histone interactions. Thus, at present the evidence
is suggestive of significant changes in the chromatin structure as a
function of age. Detailed analyses are necessary, using a variety of
organ systems and comparative-evolutionary model systems, in order to
comprehend the molecular basis of changes in DNA:histone and
histone:histone interactions on one hand and increased concentration
of nucleosomes on the other. Such studies should shed light on the
possible cell cycle-, differentiation-, and age-specific modulation
of the stability and mobility of histone octamers along DNA in a
manner relevant to the understanding of the accessibility of
nucleosome-bound sites in DNA to the damaging agents and repair
enzyme on the one hand and to DNA and RNA polymerases on the other.

CONCLUSION

     Mammalian DNA in vivo can be damaged by normal body temperature
(102), X-rays, ultraviolet light, metabolites, free radicals, and
numerous chemical agents. Such damage, if not repaired, will lead to
alterations in various physiological functions. Accumulation of DNA
damage will result in accumulated changes in the information flow and
content of the genetic material. Four ways in which fidelity of
information flow can be maintained are: 1) prevention of the
induction of DNA damage; 2) repair of the resulting damage; 3)
redundancy of information content; and 4) repression of damaged
regions. Studies bearing on the first three of these indicate that:
1) fibroblasts derived from longer-lived species are less able to
metabolically activate certain chemical agents to their nucleophilic
forms than those derived from shorter-lived species; 2) fibroblasts
derived from longer-lived species generally are better able to excise
UV-induced DNA damage than those derived from shorter-lived species
and 3) redundancy of information content appears to play a minor role
in maintenence of DNA information flow. Little is presently known
about the role of chromatin in either the interference of DNA repair
processes or control of the expression of altered regions of the DNA.

     While a paucity of data exists regarding the role of DNA damage
in aging, it is a reasonable assumption that it will alter the flow
of information with a resultant decreased ability of the cell to
respond to either exogenously or endogenously generated stress.
Longevity assurance mechanisms which might serve to regulate the rate
of accumulation of such damage have been outlined above. Since: 1)
no human syndrome totally mimics the aging process, and yet many, if
not most, repair-defective syndromes exhibit certain facets of
premature aging, and 2) no known DNA-damaging agent brings forth in
time uniformly and proportionately all aspects of aging, but, for
those agents thus far studied, each appears to accelerate certain
aspects of aging, it therefore would appear that the total repair
capacity of a system for all forms of genetic damage must be studied
in order to strictly determine the role of DNA damage in the aging
process. Further, due to the complexity of the aging process and the

role of various cell-cell and tissue-tissue interactions, it would appear that these proceses would be best evaluated in vivo. Further, since each of these interlocking longevity assurance systems (each composed of multiple steps and sub-systems) is directly involved in maintaining the fidelity of the information content within the cell, then each must therefore be evaluated separately and in concert with one another in order to determine their overall importance in longevity.

REFERENCES

1. A. Comfort, in:"Ageing, The Biology of Senescence," Holt, Rinehart and Wilson, New York (1964).
2. W. Andrew, in:"The Fine Structure and Histochemical Changes in Ageing," Academic Press, New York (1968).
3. R. G. Cutler, Exp. Gerontol. 10:37 (1975).
4. G. A. Sacher and R. W. Hart, in:"Genetic Effects of Aging," D. Bergsma and D. Harrison, eds., Alan R. Liss, New York (1978).
5. P. Burch, in:"The Fine Structure and Histochemical Changes in Ageing," Academic Press, New York (1968).
6. C. Finch, in:"Animal Models for Biomedical Research IV", Nat. Acad. Sci. USA, Wash., D.C. (1971).
7. N. Shock, Ann. Rev. Physiol. 23:97 (1961).
8. A. Engel and R. Larsson, in:"Cancer and Aging," Norcliska Bakhandelns Forlag, Stockholm (1978).
9. T. Makinodan, E. Perkins, and M. Chen, Adv. Gerontol. Res. 3:171 (1971).
10. A. G. Schwartz, Exp. Cell Res. 94:445 (1975).
11. A. G. Schwartz and C. J. Moore, Exp. Cell Res. 109:448 (1977).
12. E. Boyland, Biochem. Soc. Symp. 5:40 (1950).
13. P. Sims and P. L. Grover, Adv. Cancer Res. 20:165 (1975).
14. M. E. Duncan and P. Brookes, Int. J. Cancer 4:813 (1970).
15. E. Huberman, J. K. Selkirk, and C. Heidelberger, Cancer Res. 31:2161 (1971).
16. M. E. Duncan and P. Brookes, Int. J. Cancer 9:349 (1972).
17. A. H. Conney, Science 178:576 (1972).
18. H. V. Gelboin, F. J. Weibel, and H. Kinoshita, in:"Chemical Carcinogenesis," P. O. P. T'so and J. A. DiPaolo, eds., Marcel Dekker, New York (1974).
19. D. W. Nebert and H. V. Gelboin, Arch. Biochem. Biophys. 134:76 (1969).
20. G. Kellerman, E. Cantrell, C. R. Shaw, Cancer Res. 33:1654 (1973).
21. J. P. Whitlock and H. V. Gelboin, J. Radiol. Chem. 249:2616 (1974).
22. J. P. Whitlock, and H. V. Gelboin, J. Biol. Chem. 248:6114 (1973).
23. D. W. Nebert, W. F. Benedict, J. E. Gielen, F. Oesch, and J. W. Daly, Mol. Pharmacol. 8:374 (1972).

24. R. E. Kouri, H. Ratrie, and C. E. Whitmore, J. Natl. Cancer Inst. 51:197 (1973).
25. F. J. Weibel, J. C. Leutz, and H. V. Belboin, Arch. Biochem. Biophys. 154:292 (1973).
26. K. Burki, A. G. Liebelt, and E. Bresnick, J. Natl. Cancer Inst. 50:369 (1973).
27. G. Kellerman, C. R. Shaw, M. Lugten-Kellerman, N. Engl. J. Med. 289:934 (1973).
28. A. Comfort, in:"Ageing, the Biology of Senescence," Holt, Rinehart and Wilson, New York (1964).
29. R. W. Hart, and R. B. Setlow, Proc. Natl. Acad. Sci. USA 71:2169 (1974).
30. D. E. Brash and R. W. Hart, J. Environ. Pathol. Toxicol. 2:79 (1978).
31. H. F. Stich and R. H. C. San, Proc. Soc. Exp. Biol. Med. 142:155 (1973).
32. J. E. Cleaver, in:"Methods in Cancer Research," vol. 9, H. Busch, ed., Academic Press, New York (1975).
33. R. W. Hart and J. E. Trosko, Interdisc. Top. Gerontol. 9:134 (1976).
34. J. E. Cleaver and J. E. Trosko, Photochem. Photobiol. 11:547 (1970).
35. J. E. Cleaver, Nature 270:451 (1977).
36. R. B. Setlow, J. D. Regan, and W. L. Carrier, Biophys. Soc. Abstr. 12:19a (1972).
37. K. Hall, C. Albrightson, and R. W. Hart, XIth Internat. Cong. Gerontol., Tokyo, Japan (1978).
38. V. Paffenholz, Mech. Ageing Dev. 7:131 (1978).
39. P. Cerutti, K. Shinohara, and J. Remsen, J. Toxicol. Environ. Health 2:1375 (1977).
40. J. Smith-Sonneborn, personal communications (1978).
41. A. Dipple and J. J. Roberts, Biochemistry 16:1499 (1977).
42. M. Ikenaga, Y. Ishii, M. Toda, T. Kakunaga, H. Takebe, and S. Kondo, in:"Molecular Mechanisms for Repair of DNA," P. C. Hanawalt and R. B. Setlow, eds., Plenum Press, New York (1975).
43. R. Ben-Ishai, and I. Peleg, in:"Molecular Mechanisms for Repair of DNA, P. C. Hanwalt and R. B. Setlow, Plenum Press, New York (1975).
44. R. W. Hart, S. D'Ambrosio, K. J. Ng, and S. P. Modak, Mech. Ageing Dev. 9:203 (1978).
45. R. W. Hart, K. Y. Hall, and F. B. Daniel, Photochem. Photobiol. 28:131 (1978).
46. S. P. Modak and F. J. Bollum, Exp. Cell Res. 62:421 (1970).
47. S. P. Modak and F. J. Bollum, Exp. Cell Res. 75:307 (1972).
48. S. P. Modak and G. B. Price, Exp. Cell Res. 65:289 (1971).
49. G. B. Price, S. P. Modak, and T. Makinodan, Science 190:917 (1971).
50. H. R. Massie, M. B. Baird, and R. J. Nicolosi, Arch. Biochem. Biophys. 153:736 (1972).

51. S. P. Modak, in:"Cell Differentiation," R. Harris, P. Allen, and
    D. Viza, eds., Munksgaard Publications, Copenhagen (1972).
52. S. P. Modak and H. Traurig, Cell Differentiation 1:351 (1972).
53. J. Piatigorsky, S. S. Rothschild, and L. M. Milstone, Dev. Biol.
    34:334 (1973).
54. P. Karran and M. G. Ormerod, Biochim. Biophys. Acta 299:54
    (1973).
55. K. J. Wheeler and J. T. Lett, Proc. Natl. Acad. Sci. USA 71:1962
    (1974).
56. M. F. Counis, E. Chaudun, and Y. Courtois, Dev. Biol. 57:47
    (1977).
57. D. W. Appleby and S. P. Modak, Proc. Natl. Acad. Sci. USA
    74:5579 (1977).
58. S. Goldstein, N. Engl. J. Med. 285:1120 (1971).
59. G. M. Hahn, D. King, and S. J. Yang, Nature 230:242 (1971).
60. F. E. Stockdale, Science 171:1145 (1971).
61. F. E. Stockdale and M. C. O'Neil, J. Cell Biol. 52:589 (1972).
62. R. W. Hart and R. B. Setlow, Mech. Ageing Dev. 5:67 (1976).
63. M. R. Mattern and P. Cerutti, Biochim. Biophys. Acta 395:48
    (1975).
65. G. E. Milo and R. W. Hart, Arch. Biochem. Biophys. 176:324
    (1976).
66. A. C. Chen, S. K. C. Ng, and I. G. Walker, J. Cell Biol. 70:685
    (1976).
67. J. Treton, S. P. Modak, and Y. Courtois, manuscript in
    preparation (1978).
68. A. Ruiz-Carillo, L. J. Wangh, and V. G. Allfrey, Science 190:117
    (1975).
69. A. Olins and D. E. Olins, Science 183:330 (1974).
70. P. Oudet, M. Gross-Bellard, and P. Chambon, Cell 4:281 (1975).
71. D. R. Hewish and L. A. Burgoyne, Biochem. Biophys. Res. Comm.
    52:504 (1973).
72. M. Noll, Nature 251:249 (1974).
74. E. M. Bradbury, in:"The Organization of Expression of Ekaryotic
    Genome," E. M. Bradbury and K. Javaherian, eds., Academic
    Press, New York (1977).
75. R. D. Kornberg, Science 184:868 (1974).
76. R. D. Kornberg and J. O. Thomas, Science 184:865 (1974).
77. B. Sollner-Webb and G. Felsenfeld, Biochemistry 14:2915 (1975).
78. R. Axel, H. Cedar, and G. Felsenfeld, Proc. Natl. Acad. Sci. USA
    70:2921 (1975).
79. J. O. Thomas, in:"The Organization and Expression of Eukaryotic
    Genome," E. M. Bradbury and K. Javaherian, eds. Academic
    Press, New York (1977).
80. N. R. Morris, Cell 9:627 (1976).
81. B. R. Shaw, T. M. Herman, R. T. Kovacic, G. S. Beaudreau, and K.
    E. van Holde, Proc. Natl. Acad. Sci. USA 73:505 (1976).
82. A. J. Varshavsky, V. V. Bakayev, and G. P. Georgiev, Nucleic
    Acids Res. 3:477 (1976).
83. J. P. Whitlock and R. T. Simpson, Biochemistry 15:3307 (1976).

84. R. J. Wilkins and R. W. Hart, Nature 247:35 (1976).
85. W. J. Bodell, Nucleic Acids Res. 4:2619 (1977).
88. W. Andrew, in:"The Fine Structure and Histochemical Changes in Ageing," Academic Press, New York (1968).
89. H. Weintraub, A. Worcel, and B. Alberts, Cell 9:409 (1978).
90. A. Garel and R. Axel, Proc. Natl. Acad. Sci. USA 73:3966 (1976).
91. H. Weintraub and M. Groudine, Science 193:848 (1976).
92. M. J. Pythilla and F. G. Sherman, Biochem. Biophys. Res. Comm. 31:340 (1968).
93. D. I. Kurtz and F. M. Sinex, Biochim. Biophys. Acta 145:840 (1967).
94. H. P. von Hahn, Gerontologia 16:116 (1970).
95. S. M. Zhelabovskaya and G. D. Berdyshev, Exp. Gerontol. 7:313 (1972).
96. D. I. Kurtz, A. P. Russel, and F. M. Sinex, Mech. Ageing Dev. 3:37 (1974).
97. H. Y. Samis and V. J. Wulff, Exp. Gerontol. 4:111 (1969).
98. B. T. Hill, Gerontologia 22:111 (1976).
99. R. G. Cutler, Proc. Natl. Acad. Sci. USA 72:4664 (1975).
100. Zh. A. Medvedev, M. N. Medvedeva, and L. I. Huschtscha Gerontology 23:334 (1977).
101. Zh. A. Medvedev, M. N. Medvedeva, and L. Robson, Gerontology 24:286 (1978).
102. T. Lindahl and S. Ljungquist, in:"Molecular Mechanisms for Repair of DNA," P. C. Hanawalt and R. B. Setlow, eds., Plenum Press, New York (1975).

EVIDENCE AGAINST SOMATIC MUTATION AS A

MECHANISM OF CLONAL SENESCENCE

George M. Martin, Holger Hoehn and Eileen M. Bryant

Division of Genetic Pathology
Center for Inherited Diseases
and Institute on Aging
University of Washington
Seattle, Washington 98195

SUMMARY

In order to carry out complementation tests of the somatic cell mutational theory of clonal senescence, methods were developed for the isolation of proliferating hybrid and parental tetraploid human cells which would not depend upon biochemical selection. Crosses between short-lived strains resulted in short-lived offspring and crosses between long-lived parents tended to be long-lived, in experiments involving skin fibroblast-like cells. Crosses between strains of contrasting longevities gave growth potentials approximately intermediate to those of the parentals.

Crosses were also carried out between euploid fibroblast-like cells and two other distinctive euploid cell types ("E," or epitheloid and "AF," or aminiotic fluid cells, both derived from second trimester aminotic fluid) (Hoehn et al., 1974), and both having replicative life spans which are much more limited than the fibroblast-like skin cell ("F" cells). Compared to F x F tetraploids, F x AF and F x E hybrids had lesser growth rates, but were superior to those of parental AF and E cells.

The results are interpreted as evidence in favor of a programmed mechanism for clonal senescence and against somatic cell mutation, at least for the case of mutations involving single copy DNA.

INTRODUCTION

It has been well established that normal diploid human somatic cells have limited replicative life spans in culture (for reviews, see 1,2). There is controversy concerning the probable mechanisms of such in vitro clonal senescence. Some investigators favor a genetic program related to cell differentiation, while others emphasize protein synthesis error catastrophe theories and somatic cell mutation (1,2).

We thought it useful to carry our complementation tests of the somatic cell mutation theory in hybrids synthesized between different strains. We reasoned that if such mutations were in fact random, predominantly recessive and involved (among other types of DNA) single copy DNA, crosses between strains with different prior in vivo and in vitro histories would be likely to demonstrate significant enhancements of their growth potentials because of the mutual complementation of defective genes significant for mitotic cell cycle function. The results failed to show evidence of such complementation.

This paper summarizes research which has been presented in more detail elsewhere (3,4).

METHODS

The papers by Hoehn et al. (3) and Bryant et al. (4) should be consulted for methodological details. The cell strains were derived from various human donors, via skin biopsy or from second trimester amniotic fluid. In the determination of replicative life spans, cultures were teminated when counts were equal or less than the input inoculum of 5×10^4 cells (weekly passages in 25 cm^2 plastic flasks). Cell fusions were carried out with a modification of the polyethylene glycol-dimethysulfoxide technique of Norwood et al. (5). Putative tetraploid clones were harvested after dilute plating, on the basis of morphology. Tetraploidy was confirmed cytogenetically and by the use of flow microfluorescence. Hybrid tetraploids were distinguished from parental tetraploids by electrophoretic detection of a heterodimer of glucose-6-dehydrogenase (G6PD), the parental strains having been chosen on the basis of contrasting G6PD types (A and B).

RESULTS

The first point to make is that at least a proportion of parental and hybrid clones was chromosomally stable throughout their replicative life spans. Those clones which were mixoploid (diploid + tetraploid) could well have resulted from inter-clonal contamination. Such cytogenetic stability is in contrast to what is observed with the more conventional hybrids between parents, one of which is aneuploid.

Figure 1 summarizes the longevities of parental diploid (A), parental tetraploid (B) and hybrid tetraploid (C) colonies derived

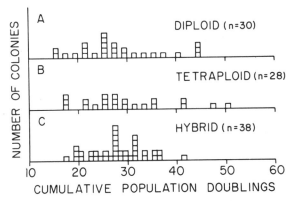

Fig. 1.   Comparison of clonal longevities: (A) parental diploids;
(B) tetraploids of single G6PD phenotype; (C) hybrid
tetraploids. Reproduced from Hoehn et al. (1978) with
permission of publisher.

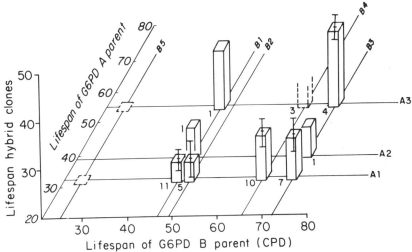

Fig. 2.   Life span of hybrid clones as a function of growth
potential of G6PD A and G6PD B parental mass cultures.
Each vertical tower represents mean (+ standard deviation)
life span of the number of hybrid isolates indicated by
arabic numerals at the base of each tower. The incomplete
tower (dashed outline) of cross A3 x B4 indicates loss of
isolates due to culture mishap. The flat squares with
dashed outline refer to attempts to obtain hybrids with an
extremely short-lived strain (B5) derived from a patient
with Werner syndrome (Bryant et al., 1978). Reproduced
from Hoehn et al. (1978) with permission of publisher.

from 12 experimental crosses between 7 different skin fibroblast strains. The histograms show that the modal value is quite comparable between the three sets of clones. There is no evidence of a complementation for enhanced replicative potential among the hybrids.

In Figure 2, a three-dimensional plot of the data of Figure 1 shows the results of crosses between cells from strains with contrasting life spans. It can be seen that crosses involving long-lived strains with short-lived strains give hybrids whose life spans fall approximately in between those of the parental lines. In contrast, crosses involving short-lived strains give short-lived hybrids, while crosses between long-lived strains give long-lived hybrids.

In Figure 3, the growth rates of groups of hybrid tetraploid fibroblast clones are compared with parental tetraploids. In keeping with the longevity data, the growth rates of the hybrids are intermediate to those of the parents.

"E" type cells rarely, if ever, can be cloned after trypsinization. Previous studies (6) have shown that such cultures grow for only about 10 cell doublings. For 9 F x E hybrids, the mean cumulative population doublings acheived were 20.5 + 2.3 (s.d.). Therefore, fusion of these epithelioid cells with fibroblast-like cells conferred upon the former the ability to be cloned and passaged, with resulting life spans intermediate between those of the parents.

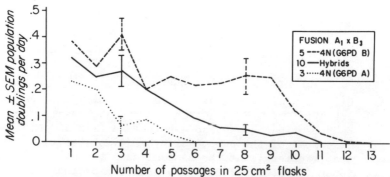

Fig. 3.   Mean growth rates of isolates obtained from crosses between hybrids and parental skin fibroblast cultures. The error bars represent standard errors at selected points. Reproduced from Hoehn et al. (1978) with permission of publisher.

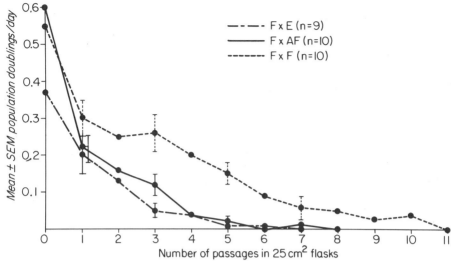

Fig. 4.   Growth histories of serially passaged hybrid isolates from
          F x E, F x AF, and a control F x F fusion. SEM, standard
          error of mean. Reproduced from Bryant et al. (1978) with
          permission of publisher.

The life spans of ten hybrid clones derived from crosses between
F and AF cells were also investigated. Once again, they gave results
(22.5 ± 7.6 cumulative population doublings) approximately intermediate between those of the two parents.

Figure 4 shows that the growth curves of the F x E and F x AF
hybrid tetraploids were consistently less than those of F x F tetraploids over a series of passages.

DISCUSSION

The first question that one must deal with in the interpretation
of the results is the extent to which the life spans of individual
clones from a mass culture reflect the life spans of the mass cultures. It is well established that there is a great deal of variation with respect to the growth potentials of such clones (7,8). In
the present experiments, however, the methods were such that only the
best growing clones could be studied, since only these provided
enough growth for the initial isolation and passaging. This automat-
ically eliminated a great deal of the variance. Furthermore, we
could experimentally demonstrate that a sample of 22 parental tetraploid clones from 5 strains showed a high correlation (r = 0.89) of
their replicative life spans with those of their respective parental
mass cultures (3).

Next, we might ask what kinds of mutations are likely to interfere with mitotic cell cycle function? In the case of the best studied eukaryotic model system, Saccharomyces cerevesiae, all such mutations so far analyzed genetically appear to be recessive (8). This may also be the case in mammalian cells (9). Therefore, complementation for random mutations at different sites within the genome should be observable in our system. No such complementation was detected.

One can also consider the possiblity that dominant mutations are of paramount importance in leading to clonal senescence. If this were the case, then tetraploid clones, with 4 genetic targets (of single copy DNA) per cell should have much shorter life spans than diploid clones, which have only 2 such targets per gene per cell. Figure 1 clearly shows that this is not the case.

It could be argued, however, that both dominant and recessive mutations play a role, thus obviating complementation. If this were the case, one would expect a greater statistical variance of longevities among hybrid clones, as occasionally, hybrids will be made in which there is a predominance of dominant mutations, giving very short life spans--or, alternatively, hybrids will be made in which there is a predominance of recessive mutations, giving complementation and enhanced life spans. (The effects of such dominant or recessive mutant alleles need not be lethal, but could act to slow the cell cycle, with the cumulative effects of many such mutations eventually leading to cessation of replication.) Although the total number of hybrids examined is limited, Figure 1 shows no such evidence of an increased variance of longevities; if anything, there is <u>less</u> variance among hybrids than among the tetraploid parentals.

Finally, one might argue that the mutations which are of importance are not those involving single copy DNA, but rather those that involve repetitive genes, such as those which code for ribosomal RNA and the various species of transfer RNA. DeMars (10) and Ohno (11) have reasoned that selection against mutations in single copy genes would lead to rapid elimination of the cells bearing such mutations, whereas mutations in reiterated genes could gradually accumulate, having the effect of a type of delayed dominance. DeMars and Ohno essentially invoke the Orgel hypothesis of protein synthesis error-catastrophe (12) to explain such delayed dominance. However, there are strong arguments why this may not be a valid general mechanism of clonal senescence (3).

In conclusion, we believe that the experiments we have cited count as strong evidence against somatic mutational theories of clonal senescene, certainly as it involves single copy DNA, although, as originally pointed out by Littlefield (13), one could not rule out a situation in which there were very large numbers of somatic mutations, such that complementation was not effective.

REFERENCES

1. G. M. Martin, Cellular aging--clonal senescence, Amer. J. Path. 89:484 (1977).

2. T. H. Norwood, Somatic cell genetics in the analysis of in vitro senescence, in:"Genetics of Aging," E. L. Schneider, ed., Plenum Press, New York (1978).

3. H. Hoehn, E. M. Bryant, and G. M. Martin, The replicative life spans of euploid hybrids derived from short-lived and long-lived human skin fibroblast cultures, Cytogenet. Cell Genet., 21:282 (1978).

4. E. M. Bryant, E. Crouch, P. Bornstein, G. M. Martin, P. Johnston, and H. Hoehn, Regulation of growth and gene activity in euploid hybrids between human neonatal fibroblasts and epithelioid amniotic fluid cells, Am. J. Hum. Genet., 30:392 (1978).

5. T. H. Norwood, C. J. Zeigler, and G. M. Martin, Dimethyl sulfoxide enhances polyethylene glycol mediated somatic cell fusion, Somat. Cell Genet. 2:263 (1976).

6   H. Hoehn, E. Bryant, L. Karp, and G. M. Martin, Cultivated cells from diagnostic amniocentesis in second trimester pregnancies. I. Clonal morphology and growth potential, Ped. Res. 8:746 (1974).

7. J. R. Smith and L. Hayflick, Variation in the life span of clones derived from human diploid cell strains, J. Cell Biol. 62:48 (1974).

8. L. H. Hartwell, Sequential function of gene products relative to DNA synthesis in the yeast cell cycle, J. Mol. Biol. 104:803 (1976).

9. R. M. Liskay and H. K. Meiss, Complementation between two temperature-sensitive mammalian cell mutants, each defective in G_1 phase of the cell cycle, Somat. Cell Genet. 3:343 (1977).

10. R. DeMars, Somatic cell mutations and cellular senescence, in: "Senescence Dominant or Recessive in Somatic Cell Crosses?" W. W. Nichols and D. G. Murphy, eds, Plenum Press, New York (1977).

11. S. Ohno and Y. Nagai, Genes in multiple copies as the primary cause of aging, in: "Genetic Effects on Aging, Birth Defects, Orig. Art. Series," Vol. XIV, Alan R. Liss, New York (1978).

12. L. E. Orgel, The maintenance of the accuracy of protein synthesis and its relevance to aging, Proc. Natl. Acad. Sci. USA 49:517 (1963).

13. J. W. Littlefield, Attempted hybridizations with senescent human fibroblasts, J. Cell Physiol. 82:129 (1973).

EPIDERMAL CARCINOGENESIS IN YOUNG

AND AGING ANIMALS

P. Ebbesen

Department of Tumor Virus Research
Institute of Medical Microbiology
22 Juliane Maries vej
DK-2100 Copenhagen, Denmark

Spontaneous epidermal carcinomas show an age (t) related incidence (I) conforming to the following expression:

$$I = ct^b$$

(c and b are constants) (1). As an explanation of these age incidence curves, the local multistep mutation hypothesis (2) is widely,
but not universally, accepted.

When it comes to epidermal carcinomas known to be elicited by
external factors in adult humans, most studies indicate that the risk
of cancer increases with the age of the first exposure (3-6), but
that there are important exceptions (6,7).

Experimental studies on epidermal carcinogenesis in young adult
and so-called old animals are numerous. However, in nearly all
cases, young animals are compared with what should be called middle-
aged animals--e.g., mice 14 months of age. About 80 per cent of a
cohort of untreated animals will still be alive at 14 months, and
this is comparable to a cohort of Danes of around 50 years of age.
When such young and middle-aged animals are treated with skin paint-
ings or irradiation, tumor incidence usually is unaffected by age (8).

However, if we turn to senescent animals, those left when 50 percent have died (comparable to a 70-year-old cohort of humans), very
little has been done in the way of studying epithelial carcinogenesis.

With mice, we have found senescent skin to be more susceptible to
chemical carcinogen than middle-aged or young skin. Work in progress

147

indicates the same to be the case when β-irradiation is used for tumor induction. By grafting skin from old donors to young recipients, we demonstrated that this increase in susceptiblity with advanced age also occurs when old skin is located on young syngeneic recipients. It therefore appears to be due to a local, autonomous aging process (9). This was further confirmed by the finding that skin of the same age grafted to young and old recipients remained equally susceptible (10).

What are the local, autonomous processes responsible for the increased susceptiblity of senescent skin? We do not know. One possibility is a spontaneous, stepwise alteration of normal cells, creating so-called variant cells which might need only a little further pushing to become malignant cells. This assumption would be in line with present knowledge about the persistent effect of carcinogen-initiators (11), and with the multistep hypothesis for spontaneous cancer development. There is, furthermore, in vivo evidence for the existence of such variant cells (12-14), and for variant cells being very susceptible to carcinogens (15). The apparent reversibility of in vivo malignancy, in certain cases (16,17), makes one wonder whether there exists a dynamic equilibrium between normal and cancer-like cells which shifts towards the abnormal, carcinogen-sensitive cells with aging, rather than a series of mutational events.

An alternative, or additional, explanation for the enhanced susceptiblity to carcinogen of senescent skin is some change in the intercellular regulatory mechanisms postulated to exist by Weiss and Kavanau (18).

We studied the effect on skin of young mice of a 30-50,000 MW extract of skin from old and young mice. Our finding was that while extract of young skin when injected intraperitoneally into young mice strongly inhibited mitosis of skin epithelial cells, extract of old skin, whether from an old mouse or a skin graft from an old donor on a young recipient, had hardly any inhibitory effect on young mice (19). In recently completed experiments, we found, furthermore, that the epithelial cells of middle-aged skin also react to intraperitoneal injection of extract from young skin with mitotic arrest. In contrast, senescent skin grafted on middle-aged recipients reacted with enhancement of the mitotic rate. And what was more surprising, this proliferative response to the extracts was also seen in the skin of middle-aged mice when the animals were carrying syngeneic grafts from senescent donors. Thus, extract of a young skin is likely to contain both a mitogen inhibitor and a mitogen stimulator; which one is dominating may depend on the age of the skin on which the test has been made (20). It may be pertinent to this that tumor cells growing in vivo (21) and in vitro (22) may lack mitotic inhibitor, and that injection of skin extract into carcinogen-treated skin may inhibit tumor development (23).

Summing up: 1) there is an enhanced susceptibility to carcinogen in senescent mouse skin which we believe should cause deliberations about safety regulations for humans; 2) both accumulation of variant cell and/or change in a local mitosis regulatory system should serve as working hypothesis for further studies.

REFERENCES

1. J. A. H. Lee, P. G. Chin, W. A. Kukull, R. S. Tompkins, and A. F. Wetherall, J. Natl. Cancer Inst. 57:753 (1976).
2. C. A. Nordling, Brit. J. Cancer 7:68 (1953)
3. R. A. M. Case, M. E. Hosker, D. B. McDonald, and J. T. Pearson, Brit. J. Industr. Med. 11:75 (1954).
4. R. E. W. Fisher, in:"Twelfth International Congress on Occupational Health," V. Kirjapaino, ed., Helsinski (1958).
5. J. F. Know, S. Holmes, R. Doll, and I. D. Hill, Brit. J. Industr. Med 25:293 (1968).
6. R. Doll, L. Morgan, and F. E. Speizer, Brit. J. Cancer 24:623 (1970).
7. D. H. McGregor, C. E. Land, K. Chorik, S. Tovokn, P. I. Liv, T. Wakabayashi, and G. W. Beebe, J. Natl. Cancer Inst 59:799 (1977).
8. R. Peto, F. J. C. Roe, P. N. Lee, L. Levy, and J. Clack, Brit. J. Cancer 32:411 (1975).
9. P. Ebbesen, Science 183:217 (1974).
10. P. Ebbesen, J. Natl. Cancer Inst. 58:1057 (1977).
11. I. Berenblum and P. Shubik, Brit. J. Cancer 3:383 (1949).
12. R. T. Prehn, Adv. Cancer Res. 23:203 (1976).
13. T.-W. Tao and M. M. Burger, Nature 270:437 (1977).
14. N. Haran-Ghera, J. Natl. Cancer Inst. 60:707 (1978).
15. P. M. Naha and M. Ashworth, Brit. J. Cancer 30:448 (1974).
16. G. B. Pierce, Amer. J. Pathol. 77:103 (1974).
17. M. C. Revilla, M. T. Gonzalez, M. Z. Balderas, and G. Romero, Nature 272:454 (1978).
18. P. Weiss and J. L. Kavanau, J. Gen Physiol. 41:1 (1957).
19. L. Olsson and P. Ebbesen, Exp. Gerontol. 12:59 (1977).
20. P. Ebbesen, L. Olsson, and C. Due, Exp. Gerontol. 13:365 (1978).
21. W. S. Bullough and J. U. R. Deol, Brit. J. Derm. 92:417 (1975).
22. P. Ebbesen and L. Olsson, in:"Antiviral Mechanisms in the Control of Neoplasia," P. Chandra, ed., NATO Advanced Study Center, Corfu, March 5-11, 1978.
23. S. A. Winkel and S. L. Smith, Nature 260:48 (1976).

TRANSLATIONAL ACTIVITY AND FIDELITY OF PURIFIED

RIBOSOMES FROM AGING MOUSE LIVERS

Nozumi Mori, Den'ichi Mizuno, and Sataro Goto

Faculty of Pharmaceutical Sciences
University of Tokyo
Hongo, Bunko-ku, Tokyo, Japan

INTRODUCTION

Since early years of modern molecular biology, it has been suggested that there must be some functional changes in the flow of
genetic information which are almost universal to any type of cells,
and hence very likely to be a general cause of functional deterioration during the aging of animals (1,2). In fact, various aspects of
transcription and translation have been studied in relation to both
the aging of tissues in vivo and cells in culture (3,4).

Production and accumulation of defective proteins during aging
appears to be of a rather general nature, and post-translational
modifications have been suggested to be a major cause of protein
alterations (5,6). In studies on viral infections, Pithe et al. (7)
could not find the production of defective viral proteins by senescent fibroblasts in culture. However, it is not certain whether the
frequency of translational error changes in tissues of old animals
where post mitotic cells predominate.

We have previously reported that 18S ribosome RNA accumulates,
relative to 28S ribosmal RNA, in the cytoplasm of some tissues during
the aging of mice (8). This observation was confirmed by an experiment in which a greater accumulation of free small subunits was present in the cytoplasm, relative to that of large subunits (9). These
observations raised the question as to whether or not there are any
functional changes in ribosomes in aging tissues.

Table 1.   Requirements for the Incorporation of Phenylalanine and
            Leucine in the Translation in Vitro (Mori et al., 1979).

Omission	^{14}C-Phenylalanine incorporated		^{3}H-Leucine incorprated	
	cpm	%control	cpm	%control
None	1245	100	5591	100
Ribosome	79	6	739	13
Factors	28	2	764	14
Poly(U)	63	5	1149	21
t-RNA	151	12	1327	24
Mg(CH$_3$COO)$_2$	45	4	723	13
Energy mixture	35	3	608	11

RESULTS AND DISCUSSION

Translational Activity of Purified Ribosomes

It is generally accepted that protein synthesis in vivo declines
with age in amimals. Since Mainwaring (10) reported an age-associated decrease in the activity of translation in a cell-free system
derived from mouse livers of various ages, several reports have
appeared in which translational activity of microsomes or polysomes
of tissues during aging have been shown to decline (11,12). However,
the components of protein synthetic machinery that are responsible
for this decrease in activity have not been identified in these
studies.

We therefore examined whether the ribosome itself is responsible
for the decrease (9). Ribosomes from mouse livers of various ages
were purified by treatment with puromycin and a high salt medium.
This type of purification has not been done in previous studies by
other investigators (10,11,12). In each such experiment, ribosomes
were prepared from each of three young and three old mice in parallel
to minimize the possibility of artifacts being introduced by the
preparation process. Ribosomes thus obtained were shown to be free
from mRNA, peptidyl tRNA and factors necessary for translation, as
shown in Table 1. Translational activity for these purified ribosomes was determined for poly(U)-dependent incorporation of phenylalanine, in the presence of aminoacyl tRNA synthetases and translational factors obtained from rabbit reticulocyte ribosomes as well as
tRNAs prepared from young mouse livers. As shown in Table 2, translational efficiency of the ribosomes was usually lower in older animals, confirming reports by other investigators who have used more
crude ribosome preparations (10,11,12). It should be noted that
variation in this activity in old animals is much greater than that
in young animals. This may indicate that variation at the translational level is a reflection of the variation of physiological age
among old individuals. Since, in our study, components other than

purified ribosomes were common in all assays, we may conclude that the decline in the activity of protein synthesis as animals age could be explained at least in part by the decreased activity of the ribosome itself. However, other components, such as tRNA, aminoacyl tRNA synthetases and translational factors, may also be responsible for the decline.

Coding Fidelity of Purified Ribosomes

The extent of mis-translation (i.e., mis-charging and mis-coding) may be increased by alterations in aminoacyl tRNA synthetases, tRNA, ribosomes and/or translational factors. Among these possibilities, we have examined whether there is any change in the level of mis-coding due to ribsomes during aging. As shown in Table 1, poly(U)-dependent incorporation of radioactive leucine, in the presence of sufficient amounts of non-radioactive phenylalanine, was dependent on components essential to translation. It was thus demonstrated that leucine was mis-incorporated into polypeptides, using a protein synthetic apparatus dependent on poly(U) that does not code for leucine. The level of mis-coding was defined as the molar ratio of leucine to phenylalanine incorporated in the standard assay system. Results of two sets of experiment are shown in Table 2. These data indicate that mis-coding was on the order of 10^{-3} under standard experimental conditions. We next examined the coding fidelity at various concentrations of magnesium ion, which is known to affect the activity and fidelity of translation in vitro (13,14). The incorporation of phenylalanine and leucine occurred at different optimal concentrations of the ion, and were independent of age. Thus, the level of coding fidelity of old ribosomes was essentially the same as that of young ribosomes. These findings do not necessarily exclude the possibility that changes occur in the fidelity of coding with age, because the fidelity in vivo should be much higher than that observed in the in vitro experiment where synthetic polymers were employed as a template. This point should be examined in more detail, using mRNA, which has natural initiation and termination codons.

The error frequency in translation during aging observed in vitro by other investigators (15,16), as well as by us, is summarized in Table 3. In all cases, the error was measured as the frequency of mis-incorporation of leucine in place of phenylalanine in a system for poly(U)-directed polypeptide synthesis. The results are not consistent with each other in either the level of error or the magnitude of the change with age. This could be due to differences in the assay system used, which may be critical for the fidelity of translation in vitro.

CONCLUSION

Functional alterations of purified ribosomes from mouse liver

Table 2. Summary of the Efficiency and the Coding Fidelity of Translation in Vitro of Mouse Liver Ribosomes as Determined by Poly(U) Dependent Assay System.

Amount of amino acid incorporated is expressed as pmoles per A260 unit of ribosome per 40 min. Infidelity level is the molar ratio of leucine to phenylalanine incorporated. av. ± S.D.: average ± standard deviation. (Mori et al., 1979)

	age of mouse	phenylalanine incorporated	av. ± S.D.	leucine incorporated	infidelity level ($\times 10^3$)	av. ± S.D.
Exp.1	Young 2 mon.	9.8		0.108	11.9	
	2 mon.	13.5	11.6 ± 1.9	0.124	9.3	9.8 ± 1.9
	2 mon.	11.5		0.093	8.1	
	Old 21 mon.	6.4		0.411	62.5	
	22 mon.	10.2	6.8 ± 3.3	0.096	9.4	18.5 ± 21.6
	22 mon.	3.7		0.037	9.9	
Exp.2	Young 2 mon.	14.8		0.087	5.8	
	2 mon.	15.6	14.3 ± 1.6	0.096	6.1	5.7 ± 0.4
	2 mon.	12.5		0.066	5.3	
	Old 15 mon.	8.5		0.026	3.1	
	19 mon.	11.1	11.9 ± 3.9	0.037	3.3	4.9 ± 1.4
	19 mon.	16.1		0.100	6.3	

Table 3. Fidelity of Translation <u>in vitro</u> as Determined by Poly (U)
Dependent Phenylalanine or Leucine Incorporation.
The level of error is shown as molar ratio of leucine to
phenylalanine incorporated (x 10^{-3}).

animal and tissue (age)	system	level of error	reference
mouse liver (2 mon. vs. 31 mon.)	microsome chick embryo factors E.coli amino acyl tRNA 4 mM Mg++	100 vs. 70	Kurtz,1975
rat liver (3 mon. vs. 12 mon.)	ribosome corresponding pH 5 fraction 10 mM Mg++	0.2 vs. 0.6	Mariotti and Ruscitto,1977
mouse liver (2 mon. vs. 22 mon.)	ribosome mouse tRNA rabbit reticulo-cyte factors 10 mM Mg++	7 vs. 6	Mori et al,1979

were examined in relation to the age of the experimental animals.
This study suggests that an age-associated decline in protein synthetic activity can be ascribed, at least in part, to the ribosome
itself. The coding fidelity of ribosomes does not change with age in
our poly(U)-dependent assay system.

Obviously, additional studies are required, using natural mRNA as
a template, to further define age-associated alterations of components in each step of translation.

REFERENCES

1. Z. A. Medvedev, Ageing at the molecular level, <u>in</u>:"Biolgical
    Aspects of Ageing," N. W. Shock, ed., Columbia University
    Press, New York (1962).
2. L. E. Orgel, The maintencance of the accuracy of protein syn-
    thesis and its relevance to ageing, <u>Proc. Nat. Acad. Sci.
    U.S.A.</u> 49:517 (1963).
3. R. G. Cutler, <u>in</u>:"Interdisciplinary Topics in Gerontology," H.
    P. von Hahn, ed., Vol. 9 and 10, S. Karger, Basel (1976).
4. F. M. Sinex, The molecular genetics of aging, <u>in</u>:"Handbook of
    the Biology of Aging," C. E. Finch and L. Hayflick, eds., Van
    Nostrand Reinhold Co., New York (1977).
5. D. Gershon, Current status of age altered enzymes: Alternative
    mechanisms, <u>Mech. Ageing Dev.</u> 9:189 (1979).
6. M Rothstein, The formation of altered enzymes in aging animals,
    <u>Mech. Ageing Dev.</u> 9:197 (1979).

7. J. Pitha, E. Stork, and E. Wimmer, Protein synthesis during
    aging of human cells in culture, Exp. Cell Res. 94:310 (1975).
8. N. Mori, D. Mizuno, and S. Goto, Increase in the ratio of 18S
    RNA to 28S RNA in the cytoplasm of mouse tissues during
    ageing, Mech. Ageing Dev. 8:285 (1978).
9. N. Mori, D. Mizuno, and S. Goto, Conservation of ribosomal
    fidelity during ageing, Mech. Ageing Dev. 10:379 (1979).
10. W. I. P. Mainwaring, The effect of age on protein synthesis in
    mouse liver, Biochem. J. 113:869 (1969).
11. G. W. Britton and F. G. Sherman, Altered regulation of protein
    synthesis during aging as determined by in vitro ribosomal
    assays, Exp. Gerontol. 10:67 (1975).
12. D. K. Layman, G. A. Ricca, and A. Richardson, The effect of age
    on protein synthesis and ribosome aggregation to messenger
    RNA in rat liver, Arch. Biochem. Biophys. 173:246 (1976).
13. J. M. Gilbert and W. F. Anderson, Cell-free hemoglobin
    synthesis. II. Characterization of the transfer ribonucleic
    acid-dependent assay system. J. Biol. Chem. 245:2342 (1970).
14. M. R. Capecchi, Polarity in vitro, J. Mol. Biol. 30:213 (1967).
15. D. I. Kurtz, The effect of ageing on in vitro fidelity of
    translation in mouse liver, Biochim Biophys. Acta 407:479
    (1975).
16. D. Mariotti and R. Ruscitto, Age-related changes of accuracy and
    efficiency of protein synthesis machinery in rat, Biochim.
    Biophys. Acta 475:96 (1977).

INTERACTION OF HORMONES WITH RECEPTORS AND

ALTERATIONS OF THESE PROCESSES WITH AGE

George Roth

Gerontology Research Center
Baltimore, Maryland

INTRODUCTION

We have been studying alterations in hormone action during the aging process. If one looks in the literature at studies of hormonal responses during aging, it becomes readily apparent that many responses at both the physiological and biochemical levels have been observed to change (for reviews, see refs. 1 and 2). In many cases, the changes are in a negative direction: decreased responsiveness or decreased sensitivity to various hormones. In some cases, however, there is no change; and in a few situations there may actually be increases in sensitivity. However, the large majority of changes for many different hormones, target cells, and tissues are post-maturational reductions in responsivenss.

In order to better understand the mechanisms involved in such changes, we are using the knowledge gained by endocrinologists, biochemists, and molecular biologists, who have elucidated the mechanisms of the hormone action at the cellular or molecular levels, independent of aging. These are rather complex processes, with many molecular events occurring between the time that the hormone reaches the cell and the time that the final biological effect is elicited. We can make some generalizations, however, especially in the case of the initial event--attachment of hormones to specific cellular receptors. These receptors can be located on the cell surface, as is the case of the catecholamines, glucagon, or insulin. Alternatively, receptors can be located inside the cell, as is the case with the steroid and thyroid hormones. Subsequent to this initial interaction, many other biochemical events occur. There are age changes in many of these intercellular events, but for the purposes of this

157

paper, I am going to limit discussion to the interactions of hormones
with receptors, and to how these processes change during aging.

HISTORICAL BACKGROUND

     I want to briefly review some of the studies of hormone receptors
during the aging process. I have grouped these studies of changes in
hormone receptors during aging into four categories. The first of
these are those studies that show hormone receptor concentrations
which decrease during senescence (Table 1). (References to all the
cases cited in Tables 1-4 can be found in reference 2). In essentially all the studies mentioned here, the changes in receptors that
occur are in the apparent concentration of quantity of the receptors,
rather than in the binding affinity or in the tightness of the fit.
Those hormone receptors which are present in old cells and tissues
are just as capable of binding the hormone as are those present in
the young tissues.

     The first group of hormones listed here (in Table 1) are the
steroids. Studies have taken place using many tissues. Also shown
are some correlations between biological responsiveness and changes
in receptor concentrations that have been carried out in some of
these tissues. The reader will notice some apparent conflicts,
contradictions or discrepancies in Tables 1-4. This is typical of
aging research in general. Possible reasons for these particular
disagreements have been discussed elsewhere (2). Changes have also
been reported for some hormone receptors that are located on the cell
surface, such as those for insulin, the adrenergic agents, acetyl-
choline, gonadotropin, and dopamine.

     In the case of some hormone receptor changes which occur during
senescence, changes are progressive over the entire life span. It is
interesting to note that if one compares the relative decreases in
different species with different maximal or different mean life spans
(for example, in two rat strains, in the rabbit or in the human) that
the relative uptake or binding loss is, in many cases, fairly com-
parably expressed as a function of the percentage of the life span
completed (Fig. 1). So, this may indicate that there is some genetic
specificity and that the changes that occur are not simply thermodynamic, but do have something to do with the life span of the
species.

     Some receptors have been reported to change only during early
adulthood or else have not been examined during the latter phase of
the life span (Table 2). Again, many different tissues, species, and
hormones have been studied.

     Table 3 shows some receptor studies in which no changes have been
reported. A few of these are similar to some of the systems in which
changes have been reported. As mentioned above, possible reasons for

Table 1. Decreases in Hormone Receptor Concentrations
During Senescence

Hormone Receptor	Tissue or Cell	Species	Concomitantly Reduced Biological Response
Corticosteroid)	Splenic lymphocytes	Rat	Inhibition of uridine uptake
	Cerebral Cortex	Rat	
	Cortical Neurons	Rat	
	Skeletal Muscle	Rat	
	Adipose Tissue	Rat	
	Adipocytes	Rat	Inhibition of glucose oxidation
	Liver	Human	
	Skin Fibroblasts (WI-38)	Human	Prolongation of in vitro life span
Androgen)	Liver	Rat	Induction of α2μ globulin
	Ventral Prostate	Rat	Maintainance of cell content
	Lateral Prostate	Rat	
	Hypothalamus	Rat	
	Pituitary	Rat	
	Testes	Rat	
Estrogen)	Uterus	Rat	Induction of phospho-fructokinase
	Uterus	Mouse	
	Brain	Rat	Induction of acetylcholin-esterase
Insulin)	Skin Fibroblasts	Human	Stimulation of glucose uptake
β-adrenergic)	Lymphocytes	Human	
	Adipocytes	Rat	Lipolysis
	Cerebellum	Rat	
	Corpus Striatum	Rat	
Acetylcholine)	Cerebral Cortex	Rat	
	Cerebellar Cortex	Rat	
Gonadotropin)	Testes	Rat	
Dopamine)	Corpus Striatum	Rat	Induction of turning behavior
Low Density Lipoprotein)	Lung Fibroblasts (WI-38)	Human	

these discrepancies have been discussed elsewhere. Table 4 shows
some actual increases in receptor levels during senescence. Thus, a
whole spectrum of observations exists: decreases during the entire
life span, decreases early in the life span, no change, and actual
increases.

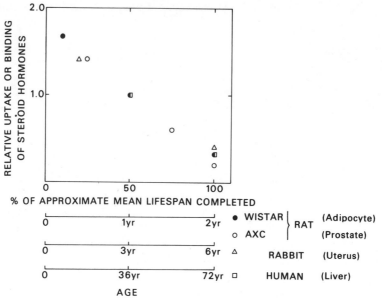

Fig. 1.   Representative age changes in steroid hormone uptake or
          binding in different species. Receptor concentrations or
          uptake rates for steroid hormones were compared in differ-
          ent genotypes. Values obtained for the 50% point of mean
          life span were arbitrarily classified as 1.0. Data are
          adapted from studies cited in ref. 2.

     At this point, I would like to focus on one or two studies in
which we have been involved. One of them deals with the membrane-
associated hormone receptors and the other with intercellular
receptors. Many investigators have reported that the ability of
adenylate cyclases in various brain regions to respond to dopamine
changes with increasing age (see ref. 1). The maximal response seems
to be progressively reduced with increasing age in most studies.
Several species have now been examined with respect to dopaminergic
stimulation of adenylate cyclase in the corpus striatum. These
include mice, rats and rabbits.

METHODS AND RESULTS

     In collaboration with our behavioral group at the Gerontology
Research Center, we examined the concentration of dopaminergic receptors in the corpus striatum region of the brain, as well as some
dopaminergic behavioral modifications (3). We used ^{3}H-haloperidol as
the ligand for receptor binding studies. At the time the work was
done (several years ago), many groups were using this compound, which
is a potent dopaminergic antagonist. More recently, spiroperidol, a
much more specific ligand, has been employed. The data were analyzed

Table 2. Decreases in Hormone Receptor Concentrations During
         Early Adulthood

Hormone Receptor	Tissue or Cell	Species	Concomitantly Reduced Biological Response
Corticosteroid)	Liver	Rat	
	Thymus	Rat	
Androgen)	Cerebral Cortex	Rat	
Insulin)	Liver	Rat	
β-andrenergic	Erythrocyte	Rat	Stimulation of adenylate cyclase
	Pineal	Rat	
Glucagon)	Adipocyte	Rat	Stimulation of lipolysis
Prolactin)	Prostate	Rat	
	Seminal Vesicles	Rat	
Thyroid)	Cerebral Hemisphesis	Rat	

Table 3. Unaltered Hormone Receptor Concentrations During Adulthood

Hormone Receptor	Tissue or Cell	Species
Corticosteroid)	Liver	Rat
	Liver	Mouse
	Cerebral Cortex	Mouse
	Hypothalamus	Mouse
	Hippocampus	Mouse
Androgen)	Anterior Prostate	Rat
	Dorsal Prostate	Rat
	Seminal Vesicles	Rat
	Prostate	Dog
Insulin)	Liver	Mouse
	Heart	Mouse
β-adrenergic)	Cerebral Cortex	Rat
Low Density Lipoprotein)	Skin Fibroblasts	Human
Growth Hormone)	Liver	Mouse

Table 4. Increases in Hormone Receptor Concentrations During
         Senescence

Hormone Receptor	Tissue or Cell	Species
Androgen)	Seminal Vesicles	Rat
Estrogen)	Seminal Vesicles	Rat
Insulin)	Skin Fibroblasts	Human
Epidermal Growth Factor)	Lung Fibroblasts (WI-38)	Human

by the method of Scatchard (4), plotting the bound over free hormone
concentration as a function of the bound concentration (Fig. 2).
These were experiments in which crude membrane preparations were
incubated with various concentrations of ^{3}H-ligand. Non-specific
binding was determined by competition with excess unlabeled dopamine. From such analysis, one can see that the concentration of
receptors (as taken from the intercept on the abscissa) is reduced
about 35% between 6 months to 25 months of age. Wistar rats from the
Gerontology Research Center were used in these experiments. The
slopes of the two lines are not significantly different, indicating
no change in binding affinity. When data were obtained from six
experiments using these two age groups, no change in binding efficiency, but a significant 40% reduction in the concentration of the
receptors, was detected. This is roughly comparable to the reduction
in the ability of dopamine to stimulate adenylate cyclase. More
recently, confirming data have been obtained from the laboratory of
Finch using mice (5) and Makman using rabbits (6). Both groups have
employed the newer tritiated dopaminergic antagonist, spiroperidol.

Under these conditions, one observes much less non-specific
binding, and is able to generate more precise data. Data from all
three laboratories are basically in agreement that this particular
receptor is lost with age. The loss is probably closely related to
the loss in ability to stimulate adenylate cyclase, as reported by
many investigators

Now, I would like to deal with the system on which we are
spending more of our time. This is the rat epididymal fat pad
adipocyte and the effect of glucocorticoid hormones, which work
through intracellular receptor systems. Two rat strains have been
employed, the CD Sprague-Dawley from Charles River Breeding

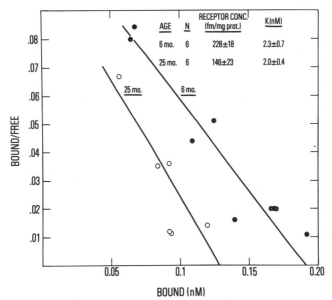

Fig. 2. Scatchard analysis of ^{3}H-haloperidol specific binding to
crude membranes of rat corpus striatum. Binding studies
were performed as described in ref. 3. Statistics from 6
individual experiments are pictured in the inset.

Laboratories, as well as our own Wistar strain. Two strains are
utilized, since they exhibit different patterns of adipocyte size
increase (7). In the Sprague-Dawley rat, the epididymal fat pad
adipocytes continue to increase in size throughout the life span,
whereas in Gerontology Research Center Wistar rats, hypertrophy
ceases after roughly 4-6 months of age; and one can compare the
mature and senescent animals without having to worry about the
effects of cell size superimposed on the effects of cell age.

Another reason we chose the epididymal fat pad adipocyte system
is that it is a relatively static postmitotic cell system. Cell numbers remain relatively constant throughout the life, so one can be
reasonably confident of dealing with the same population of cells in
the senescent animals as in the young animals. We don't have to
worry about complex shifts in cell populations, so we can be relatively confident that the change we are looking at is restricted to this
particular cell type, rather than including the loss of a small population of hormone responsive cells. We have examined glucocorticoid
receptor levels by the method of Scatchard (4) in cells of three age
groups (Fig. 3). As with the dopamine receptors mentioned above,
there is no change in the slope, therefore, no change in the binding
affinity. However, there is a progressive reduction with increasing
age in the apparent concentration of receptor sites.

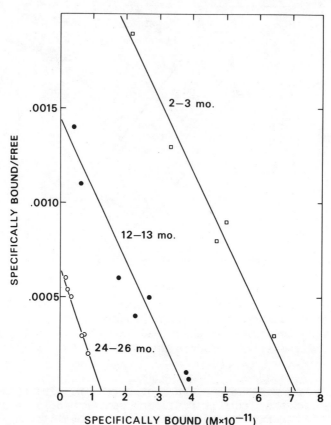

Fig. 3.   Scatchard analyses of specific glucocorticoid binding in
adipocyte cytosols.   Cytosols of adipocytes from 2-3 mo.
(□), 12-13 mo. (●), and 24-26 mo. (○).   Wistar rats were
prepared, and specific dexamethasone binding was assessed
as described in ref. 7.

    We are also interested--in fact, more interested--in the action
of the hormone and how it changes with age. Thus, we have examined
one particular response of adipocytes to glucocorticoid hormones, the
ability of glucocorticoids to inhibit the rate of glucose utilization
by these cells. Dexamethasone is the synthetic glucocorticoid that
we used for this effect. We measured the ability of this synthetic
corticoid to inhibit glucose oxidation in fat cells from the three
age groups. Again, as with the dopamine-sensitive adenylate cyclase
data shown above, progressive reduction with increasing age in
glucocorticoid responsiveness is also observed (Fig. 4).

    Figure 5 shows some statistics with respect to the reduction in
binding sites for glucocorticoid hormone receptors in the three age

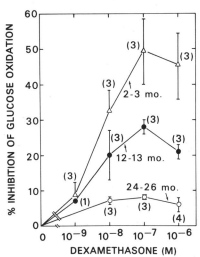

Fig. 4.   Effect of dexamethasone concentration on inhibition of
          glucose oxidation in young, mature, and senescent rat
          adipocytes. Dexamethasone inbibition of glucose oxidation
          in Wistar rat adipocytes was determined as in ref. 7.
          Values are the mean ± standard errors for the number
          of experiments in parentheses.

groups and the reductions in the ability of the hormone to inhibit
glucose utilization. There is a fairly close relationship between
the two. In fact, it has been demonstrated that if the receptors are
blocked with other types of steroids, they are inactive with respect
to this particular response. No dexamethasone effect can be
observed. So, there appears to be very close, if not causal, relationship between the receptor and the response loss.

DISCUSSION

     Now, I would like to digress a bit, using the same system to
discuss what we feel is the change in the cell membrane which may in
part contribute to some of the change in responsiveness to glucocorticoid. For a number of reasons, we were enticed to look a little
bit more closely at the changes that occur between young adulthood
and maturity, although this is not the true senescence phase of the
life span. In looking at the literature, we realized that many
people felt that the effect of glucocorticoid hormones on glucose
metabolism was secondary to inhibition of the glucose transport
system within the cell membrane. In other words, people felt that
any inhibition of glucose oxidation was simply the consequence of the
reduced entry of glucose into the cell in the presence of dexamethasone. Indeed, if one looks at the effect of dexamethasone on both

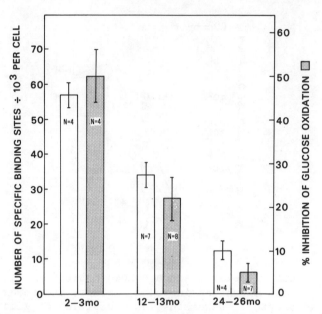

Fig. 5.   Effect of age on glucocorticoid receptor concentration and
          inhibition of glucose oxidation in rat adipocytes. Data as
          for Figs. 3 and 4 were compiled for the number of
          experiments shown inside the bars. Values are the means
          ± standard errors.

glucose transport and metabolism in cells from the young 2-3 month
old animals, there is essentially no difference in the response
curves. However, if one looks at the mature animals, one still can
get a pretty good effect on inhibition of glucose by dexamethasone,
but there is no effect on glucose transport (Fig. 6). This suggests
that the two processes may be dissociable, at least under conditions
of increased age or increased cell size. In the senescent animals,
there is a statistically significant dexamethasone effect on glucose
oxidation, but again, no effect on the transport system (8).

     The possibility exists that this apparant decrease in the abil-
ity of dexamethasone to effect transport has something to do with the
metabolism of glucose. We therefore used two other glucose analogs,
2-deoxyglucose and 3-0 methyl glucose, both of which are either mini-
mally metabolized or not metabolized at all, and repeated our experiments. Again we found large inhibition of sugar transport in the
young animals, but essentially no effect at all in the mature or senescent animals.

     We can also express our data in terms of molecules of glucose
which are either taken into the cell or metabolized. These basal

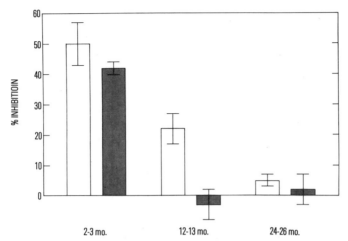

Fig. 6. Effect of age on the ability of dexamethasone to inhibit
         glucose transport and metabolism. Effects of dexamethasone
         on adipocyte glucose transport and metabolism were deter-
         mined as described in ref. 8. Values are the means ±
         standard errors for 3-8 separate experiments for each
         group. Open bars, glucose oxidation; shaded bars, glucose
         transport.

levels of glucose uptake are essentially unchanged with age, so that
when we express our values as percentages, we might equally well
express them in terms of absolute molecules of sugar transported or
metabolized. Thus, the effect that we observed is not due to some
intrinsic change in the basal rate of transport of metabolism.

     Since in the mature animals, there did not appear to be any
effect of dexamethasone on glucose transport, we examined the glucose
phosphorylation system. In the 2-3 month old animals, there is a
very good correlation between the inhibition of glucose oxidation and
the inhibition of glucose phosphorylation. This, of course, is due
to the fact that transport is inhibited. However, in the mature 12
to 13 month old animals, where there is no effect at all of dexamethasone on glucose transport, we do observe that the effect on glucose
phosphorylation is comparable to the amount of inhibition of glucose
oxidation. Thus, there appears to be some sort of compensatory
mechanism whereby the phosphorylation step is independently effected
by dexamethasone. We don't know the mechanism here, but this does
appear to account for the fact that one can still inhibit glucose
oxidation without inhibiting transport in these older cells.

     We think that the insensitivity to dexamethasone that we see is
the consequence of the generalized refractoriness of the membrane
with increasing age or increasing cell size. Other agents which can

Table 5. Effects of Insulin, Vitamin K_5, and H_2O_2 on Glucose
Uptake by Young and Mature Adipocytes

Addition	Glucose Uptake (% of Control)	
	Young Cells	Mature Cells
None	100	100
Insulin, 500 μU/ml	467 ± 51	132 ± 19
Vitamin K_5, 10 μg/ml	559 ± 62	94 ± 1
H_2O_2, 0.3 mM	222 ± 4	98 ± 1

Adipocytes were prepared and glucose uptake was measured as described in
reference 8. Values are the means $\pm$ standard errors for three experiments.

moderate glucose transport are also less effective in older animals
(Table 5). Insulin, vitamin K-5, and hydrogen peroxide, all of which
stimulate the glucose transport system, show this decreased sensitivity.

We are now interested in possible molecular mechanisms that
might be involved in these changes, such as reduced rates of glucocorticoid receptor synthesis, increased rates of receptor degradation, malformation or blocking of aged receptors, and possible neuro-
endocrine-systemic mechanisms that may be involved.

SUMMARY

A variety of hormone receptor concentrations appear to decrease
during aging. Such reductions seem to be closely, if not causally,
related to reduced responsiveness. The receptors appear to be lost
from target cells during aging. The simple loss of target cells from
target tissues is not a sufficient explanation for decreased hormone
concentrations, since we can observe these changes in static cell
populations. Currently, we are attempting to elucidate the molecular
and neuroendocrine mechanisms that are involved in these changes, and
we would like to apply some of the mechanisms of hormone receptor
control to these problems of altered responsiveness.

REFERENCES

1. G. S. Roth, Mech. Ageing Dev. 9:497 (1979).
2. G. S. Roth, Fed. Proc. (in press).

3. J. A. Joseph, R. E. Berger, B. T. Engel, and G. S. Roth, _J. Gerontol._ 33:643 (1978).
4. G. Scatchard, _Ann. N.Y. Acad. Sci._ 51:660 (1949).
5. C. E. Finch (personal communication).
6. M. H. Makman, H. S. Alin, L. J. Thal, N. Sharpless, B. Dvorkin, S. G. Horowitz, and M. Rosenfeld, _Fed. Proc._ (in press).
7. G. S. Roth and J. N. Livingston, _Endocrinology_ 99:831 (1976).
8. G. S. Roth and J. N. Livingston, _Endocrinology_ (in press).

CELLS, SIGNALS, AND RECEPTORS: THE ROLE

OF PHYSIOLOGICAL AUTOANTIBODIES

IN MAINTAINING HOMEOSTASIS

Marguerite M.B. Kay

Laboratory of Molecular and Clinical Immunology
Geriatric Research, Education and Clinical Center
(691/11G)
V.A. Wadsworth Medical Center
Los Angeles, California   90073, USA

INTRODUCTION

Macrophages can distinguish mature "self" from senescent "self" cells. This is reflected by their ability to phagocytize cells which have reached the end of their functional lifespan, while sparing the mature cells. For example, mononuclear phagocytes of the liver and spleen remove syngeneic lymphocytes as well as antibody-coated red blood cells (RBC) (1,2,3). Erythrophagocytosis also occurs in lymph nodes (4). Studies on the fate of aged RBC indicate that they are eliminated intracellularly by mononuclear phagocytes rather than by osmotic lysis both in vitro and in situ (5 6,7,8,9). In this way, mononuclear phagocytes may perform an essential homeostatic role by permitting the more efficient mature cells to carry out their vital functions without hindrance from the less efficient senescent cells, or by preventing pathological reactions which could arise as a consequence of senescent cells dying and decaying within the organism.

The mechanism by which macrophages make such a fine distinction between mature and senescent cells has fascinated and eluded biologists for years. This paper summarizes my investigations into the mechanisms by which macrophages may make this distinction.

Initially, I hypothesized that Ig in normal human serum attaches to the surface of senescent RBC until a critical level is reached which results in phagocytosis (3,10). Human RBC were utilized as a

model system because mononuclear phagocytes routinely phagocytize RBC
at the end of their 120-day lifespan and because they are an ideal
experimental system in many respects. Large numbers of RBC are
readily available, and senescent cells can be easily separated from
mature cells. RBC membranes have been extensively characterized
biochemically and they have a smooth regular surface which does not
"cap" or ingest labels.

MATERIALS AND METHODS

    Isolation of Ig from old RBC. Blood was obtained from 41 healthy
individuals. Young RBC were removed, and the remaining RBC were
washed 3 times with 50 volumes of phosphate buffered saline (PBS), pH
7.4. Ig was eluted from 50-250 ml of packed RBC by the method of
Kochwa and Rosenfield (11), as methods of elution which did not
result in dissociation of antigen-antibody bonds (e.g., temperature
and glycine-NaOH buffer, pH 8), did not result in Ig elution in our
hands. Preliminary experiments indicated that Ig could be eluted
from old, but not young, RBC. The RBC eluate from 31 individuals was
assessed without further purification. Antibody from the RBC eluates
of each of 10 individuals was isolated with an anti-Fab immunoabsorbent column. Fab was obtained from normal human IgG by papain
digestion and column chromatography (12,13, An Chaun Wang, personal
communication). Purity was determined by immunodiffusion (ID),
immunoelectrophoresis (IEP), and polyacrylamide gel electrophoresis
(PAGE). Antisera to Fab was obtained by immunizing a goat with eight
weekly injections of 1 mg of pure Fab, as determined by ID and IEP.
After 10 weeks, the goat was bled and the immune serum incubated with
an immunoabsorbent that was made by binding Fab covalently to Sepharose 4B through a 13 atom spacer (aminohexyl derivative of Sepharose
4B; 14). After thorough washing, the beads were poured into a 7.5 ml
glass column (Bio Rad) and the antibodies specific for Fab were
eluted with 0.1 M glycine-HCl, pH 2.3. The eluted antibody, determined with a recording spectrophotometer, was neutralized with 1 N
NaOH, concentrated, and dialysed against PBS, pH 7.4. The anti-Fab
antibodies obtained by this procedure were specific for Fab and
reacted with pure IgA and IgM as well as IgG, as determined by ID and
IEP. Conversely, specific anti-IgA, IgG, and IgM reagents reacted
only with the specific Ig class. Anti-Fab specific antibodies were
coupled to aminohexyl Sepharose 4B and used to isolate Ig from RBC
eluates. The Ig was eluted from the anti-Fab column in the same
manner as described for anti-Fab antibodies, then concentrated with
an Amicon Diaflow with PM 10 filter. The quantity of IgG eluted per
ml of packed RBC was 270 $\pm$ 60 ng (mean $\pm$ std. error), as determined
by radial immunodiffusion with Ultra Low Level Diffu-gen plates, lot
#55822, Oxford Laboratories, Foster City, Calif.

    Mononuclear phagocytes. Mononuclear cells from human peripheral
blood were isolated on "Lymphoprep" and washed three times with
Medium 199. The percentage of mononuclear phagocytes was determined

by spreading an aliquot of mononuclear cells on a slide, or by making
a cytocentrifuge preparation of mononuclear cells and staining with
May-Gruenwald-Giemsa or with esterase (15), and performing differential cell counts with a 64X or 100X oil immersion objective (Zeiss).
The number of mononuclear phagocytes was calculated by multiplying
the total number of mononuclear cells times the percentage of mononuclear phagocytes. Polymorphonuclear leukocyte contamination was
less than 1%. Mononuclear cells were diluted with bicarbonate buffered Medium 199 with Methicillin/Gentamycin (100 µg/ml) and gluta-
mine so that the concentration of mononuclear phagocytes was 6-10 x
10^5/ml, and 1 ml was pipetted into each tube. After a 1 hr incubation at 37°C in an atmosphere of humidified air containing 5% CO_2,
nonadherent cells were removed by vigorous washing.

Phagocytosis assay. The phagocytosis assay utilized for these
studies measured phagocytosis rather than attachment, osmotic lysis,
or adhesion of RBC to glass tubes. Light microscopy and transmission
electron microscopy of cultures after 30 mins and 3 hrs demonstrated
that RBC in various stages of degradation were present inside mononuclear phagocytes with some phagocytes having as many as 20 RBC
inside them (16). Scanning electron microscopy of the cultures after
3 hrs demonstrated that only RBC which were partially engulfed were
visible on the surface (16). When young RBC were added to 20 tubes
containing mononuclear phagocytes, 100% of the RBC were recovered 3
hrs later. When RBC stored without Ig were added to 16 tubes containing mononuclear phagocytes, 98--100% of the RBC were recovered 3
hrs later. Negative controls were utilized throughout the study.
These included young RBC, RBC aged in vitro and incubated in medium
without serum or in Ig depleted serum, neuraminidase treated RBC
incubated in culture medium, and young RBC incubated in allogeneic Ig
eluted from senescent cells. These cells were not phagocytized, as
indicated by the recovery rates noted above. Mononuclear phagocyte
viability at the end of culture was 98-100% as determined by trypan
blue dye exclusion.

Young and senescent RBC. RBC from freshly drawn blood were
depleted of white cells and reticulocytes, then separated into young,
middle-aged and old (senescent) populations by their differences in
density (17). At the end of the density separation, young RBC are at
the top of the gradient and the old RBC are at the bottom, as determined by the distribution of recently synthesized   Fe-labeled RBC
(18).

Stored RBC. Freshly isolated young RBC were washed 3 times with
50 volumes of Medium 199, resuspended at a concentration of 10% in
Medium 199 without serum, to avoid IgG binding, or alpha minimum
essential medium (AMEM) with 10% fetal calf serum (FCS), and transferred to tissue culture flasks. RBC were stored for 2-4 wks at 4°C.

Not all of the RBC populations were needed for the purpose of these experiments. Those in excess of the required numbers remained in storage for a total of five months. When these cells were subsequently examined, it was found that all old RBC and approximately half of the middle-aged RBC had lysed. The young RBC populations, however, were essentially free of lysed cells. This reaffirms that the method of cell separation employed in the present experiment is successful and that different cell populations have different membrane properties. It suggests that storage of RBC in vitro may be a reasonable parallel model for aging in vivo, because young RBC survive at least 150 days, and that old RBC have the potential for lysis if stored, without macrophages, for an extended period of time. It is possible that the mechanism by which membrane lesions are generated during storage in vitro may not be the same as that by which lesions are generated in vivo as cells age. However, the lesions themselves may be identical.

Incubation of RBC with Ig eluted from senescent cells. Stored RBC were washed and resuspended to a concentration of $1.5-2.0 \times 10^9$ RBC per ml. Twenty micrograms of Ig were added to 1 ml of the cell suspension, which was incubated at 37°C for 30-60 mins in a shaking water bath. The RBC were then washed three times with medium and incubated with mononuclear phagocytes. Approximately 10-15 RBC were added per phagocyte and the volume was adjusted to 0.24-0.40 ml per tube. Following incubation for three hours at 37°C, the percent of phagocytized RBC was calculated as described previously (3). This culture method supports a maximum of $\simeq 50\%$ phagocytosis.

The maximum percent phagocytosis obtainable appears to be limited by depletion of nutrients in the media. Addition of new medium at the end of 3 hrs results in additional phagocytosis of RBC: $46 \pm 11\%$ of the RBC were phagocytized during 6 hrs when new media was not added, whereas $61 \pm 2\%$ were phagocytized when new media was added after the first 3 hr incubation. If old RBC are added to cultures that have been incubated without RBC for the first 3 hrs, without changing media, there is no significant phagocytosis (only $8 \pm 7\%$ of the RBC were phagocytized). Finally, an additional $40 \pm 3\%$ of the old RBC, harvested from cultures after a 3 hr incubation, are phagocytized when added to new cultures with fresh media.

Neuraminidase treated RBC. Freshly isolated young RBC were washed 3 times with 50 volumes of Medium 199; incubated with 3.35 units of Vibrio cholerae neuraminidase (Behring Diagnostics, which was tested and found to be lipase and protease free) per 10^{10} RBC at 37°C in PBS, pH 6.8, for 30-60 min; and washed again. They were incubated in Medium 199 containing 20 µg of either autologous or allogeneic Ig eluted from senescent cells, washed 3 times, and incubated with autologous mononuclear phagocytes.

Scanning Immunoelectron Microscopy. Aliquots of the RBC used in

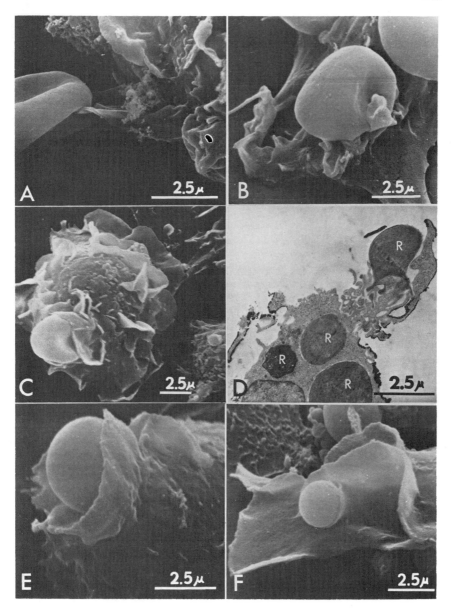

Fig. 1.   Scanning electron micrographs of stages in the phagocyto-
          sis of senescent RBC by macrophages. D is a transmission
          electron micrograph showing RBC (indicated by "R") inside
          of a macrophage. From (63).

phagocytosis experiments were incubated in the IgG fraction of goat
antihuman IgG for 30 min at 37°C, washed, incubated in rabbit

anti-goat IgG conjugated to ferritin for 30 min at 4°C, washed, and
prepared for scanning electron microscopy (3,10,19,20,21). Preparations were viewed with an Hitachi HFS-2 field emission, scanning
electron microscope with 3 nm resolution. Between 200 and 300 cells
were viewed in each preparation at magnifications from 20,000 to
100,000. Scanning time per preparation was 18-36 hrs.

RESULTS

    Kinetics of Phagocytosis of RBC. Freshly drawn RBC were separa-
ted into young and old populations by density and were washed and
stored in vitro and then incubated with macrophages. Samples were
removed for analysis at various intervals up to 6 hr (Fig. 1). The
results indicate that the percent phagocytosis is greatest during the
first hour of incubation, and 90% of the phagocytosis occurring
during a 6 hr incubation is complete by the end of 2 hr (Fig. 2).
These results are in agreement with those of Morita and Perkins (6),
who used absorbance of hemoglobin to determine the number of RBC
remaining at the end of a phagocytosis experiment. Based on the
results of these experiments, a 3 hr incubation time was selected for
subsequent studies.

    Requirement for Ig. Freshly drawn human RBC were incubated with
the IgG fraction of rabbit anti-human RBC antibody (Cappel Lab.) for
30 min at 37°C, washed three times with Medium 199, and added to
macrophages. Controls consisted of RBC incubated in Medium 199 or
Ig-depleted serum. Sixty-three percent (63%) of the RBC (standard
error of mean, 19%) treated with rabbit anti-human RBC reagent were
phagocytized, whereas only 3-7% phagocytosis was observed in the
controls. Rabbit IgG was demonstrated on the surface of the RBC with
SIEM (3). These results indicate that IgG can initiate phagocytosis

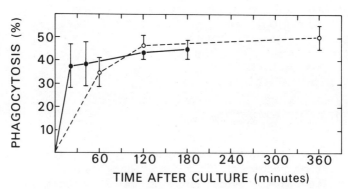

Fig. 2.   Kinetics of phagocytosis of RBC aged in situ (o) and
           stored RBC (●). Zero time samples were not taken in the
           experiment since preliminary studies consistently showed
           no phagocytosis at this time. Sample size per culture,
           4. Vertical bars indicate standard error. From (3).

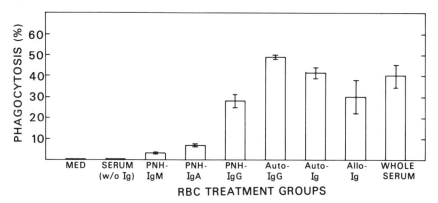

Fig. 3.   Phagocytosis of stored RBC. Stored RBC were washed and
           incubated in Medium 199, autologous Ig-depleted or agamma
           serum (serum w/o Ig), pooled normal human IgM, IgA, or IgG
           (PNH-Ig), autologous IgG (Auto-IgG), autologous Ig
           (Auto-Ig), allogeneic Ig (Allo-Ig), or autologous, fresh,
           whole serum. RBC were then washed and incubated with
           macrophages. Vertical bars indicate one standard error of
           the mean. From (3).

and might be required. However, the RBC were deliberately coated
with foreign IgG in the form of a specific antibody. Therefore, it
could not be determined from this procedure whether normal circulating Ig would attach to RBC. In order to test this, human RBC were
stored in vitro for 14 days at 4°C in Medium 199. They were then
incubated for 1 hr in Medium 199, autologous Ig, autologous IgG,
another individual's allogeneic Ig, or pooled, normal human
(PNH) IgG, PNH-IgM, PNH-IgA, washed, and incubated with the individual's macrophages. The results of these experiments (Fig. 3) demonstrated that (a) the percent phagocytosis of stored RBC ("0"-RBC)
incubated in IgM and IgA is only slightly more than that in medium
alone ($\leq 10\%$); (b) the percent phagocytosis of stored RBC incubated
in autologous IgG was essentially the same as that of stored RBC
incubated in either autologous whole serum or the Ig fraction
(42-49%); and (c) allogeneic Ig and PNH-IgG ($\geq 30\%$ phagocytosis) were
not as effective as autologous whole serum, Ig, or IgG in promoting
phagocytosis, although they had not been tested for blood group
compatibility. These results, which confirm the requirement for Ig,
indicate that normal circulating Ig can attach to RBC, and suggest
that the Ig that attaches is IgG. They further suggest that
macrophages discriminate not only between classes of Ig, but also
between their own and "foreign" Ig. These experiments support, but
do not prove, the initial working hypothesis which states that
immunoglobulins attach to the surface of aging RBC until a threshold
level is reached, at which time macrophages no longer recognize the
RBC as a "self" cell.

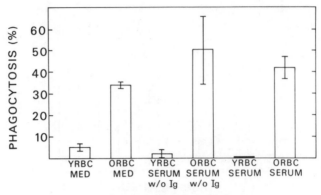

Fig. 4.   Phagocytosis of RBC aged in situ. Freshly drawn RBC were
           separated by density into young and old RBC populations,
           washed, resuspended in Medium 199 (Med), autologus agamma
           serum (serum w/o Ig), or autologous fresh, whole serum
           (serum), and incubated with autologous macrophages.
           Vertical bars indicate one standard error of the mean.
           From (3).

Demonstration of Phagocytosis of Aged RBC Bearing Autologous IgG
In Situ. In an attempt to test this hypothesis directly, and to
determine whether the Ig which attached in situ was IgG, the following experiments were performed.

     Freshly drawn human RBC were separated into young and old popula-
tions according to their different densities and washed three times
with Medium 199. Aliquots from each population were incubated with
scanning immunoelectron microscopy marker conjugates and prepared for
scanning electron microscopy. At the same time, each population was
incubated with macrophages in Medium 199, Ig-depleted serum, or whole
serum. A consistent difference in phagocytosis, greater than 30%,
was observed between young and old populations of RBC whether the
final incubations were performed in medium without serum, in autologous Ig-depleted serum, or whole serum containing Ig (Fig. 4). This
indicated that the Ig was attached in situ to the RBC, and that
phagocytic recognition was not inhibited by other serum components.
Scanning immunoelectron microscopy of the two populations revealed
that young RBC were essentially unlabeled, whereas senescent RBC were
heavily labeled with SV40 anti-human IgG, but not with T2 anti-human
IgA or with KLH anti-human IgM. The fact that only 30-40% of the
senescent RBC were ingested suggests that a threshold level of IgG
may be required.

     This tentative view is consistent with the observation, using
scanning immunoelectron microscopy, that the number of IgG molecules

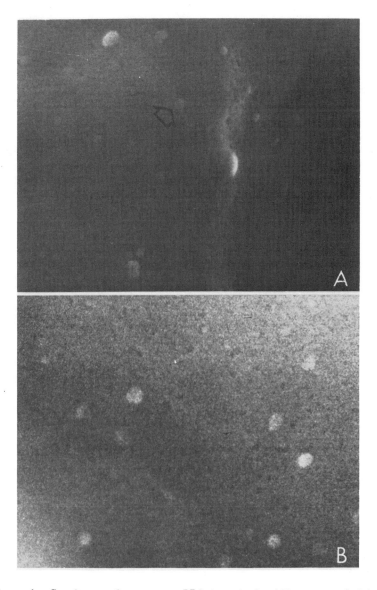

Fig. 5.   A. Surface of a young RBC treated with neuraminidase,
             incubated in IgG, washed, and incubated with
             ferritin-conjugated antihuman IgG. From (16).

          B. A higher magnification of ferritin-labeled RBC. From
             (16).

on senescent RBC varied between 20 to 50 per half cell. It is also
possible that the macrophages were engorged with RBC and had, therefore, ceased ingesting. However, this seems unlikely as the macro-
phage:RBC ratio was 1:10.

On the basis of these findings, it can be concluded that IgG
attaches in situ to senescent human RBC, making them vulnerable to
phagocytosis by macrophages.

Phagocytosis of Neuraminidase-Treated Young RBC. The preceding
experiments elucidate a mechanism by which macrophages recognize
"senescent-self" cells. The next obvious question is, "How does IgG
recognize senescent cells?" It is known that: (a) approximately 10%
of the RBC membrane is comprised of glycoproteins (22); (b) removal
of sialic acid from circulating glycoproteins results in their
removal (23,24,25); (c) transient autoimmune hemolytic anemias sometimes follow respiratory infection with viruses such as influenza
which contain neuraminidase, and that (d) "autoantibody" is generally
formed against molecular precursors of blood groups rather than
intact molecules. Therefore, it was hypothesized that autologous IgG
recognizes determinants which are exposed by removal of sialic acid
from membranes of RBC as they age. The following experiments were
performed in order to test this hypothesis.

Young RBC were incubated with neuraminidase, a microbial enzyme
which cleaves sialic acid groups from glycoproteins, washed, then
incubated in either Medium 199, autologous Ig, or autologous IgG,
washed again, and incubated with autologous macrophages. Results were
that: (a) neuraminidase-treated young RBC incubated in medium were
not phagocytized (0% phagocytosis), whereas those incubated with
either autologous Ig or IgG were ($\geq$ 45% phagocytosis); (b) IgG is as
effective as total Ig; and (c) the percent phagocytosis of neuraminidase-treated young RBC is approximately equal to that of in situ aged
senescent RBC.

Scanning immunoelectron microscopy, utilizing the tri-labeling
technique, demonstrated the presence of IgG on the surface of neuraminidase-treated young RBC (Fig. 5). These results suggest that
young RBC can be artificially aged by neuraminidase treatment and
that IgG binds to receptors exposed by removal of sialic acid (pre-
sumably carbohydrate moieties).

The results presented thus far suggest that macrophages can distinguish senescent from mature self RBC on the basis of selective
attachment of autologous IgG to the membrane of senescent RBC. The
presence of IgG on senescent cells is presumptive evidence that an
immunological receptor-IgG binding has occurred. However, such evidence by itself does not establish that the Ig is a homeostatic autoantibody directed against normal constituents of the cell membrane.
Definitive evidence for the role autoantibodies play in the selective

removal of senescent cells can be obtained by first dissociating the
antibodies from senescent cells and then by demonstrating their
specific immunologic reattachment to homologous senescent, but not to
mature cells, leading to destruction of only the senescent cells by
mononuclear phagocytes.

Identification and Characterization of Old RBC Ig. Ig was eluted
from RBC aged in situ. It was shown to be an IgG containing kappa
and lambda light chains by immunodiffusion and immunoelectrophoresis. Other Igs were not detected by immunodiffusion, immunoelectrophoresis, or polyacrylamide gel electrophoresis. Thus, the antibody
attached to senescent cells is an IgG which is polyclonal with respect to light chains.

IgG Binding and Specificity Experiments. In order to determine
whether the IgG eluted from old RBC aged in situ would reattach to
homologous cells, the IgG was incubated with autologous or allogeneic
young stored RBC. These RBC were then washed and incubated with
autologous mononuclear phagocytes. The percent phagocytosis, of
stored RBC incubated with autologous IgG and then with autologous
mononuclear phagocytes ($46 \pm 0\%$), was essentially the same as that of
RBC aged in situ ($50 \pm 4\%$). Mononuclear phagocytes phagocytized
autologous stored RBC incubated with autologous IgG ($27 \pm 0\%$ phagocytosis), as well as allogeneic stored RBC incubated with autologous
IgG ($56 \pm 4\%$ phagocytosis). However, they did not phagocytize allogeneic cells which had not been incubated with IgG (0% phagocytosis),
nor did they phagocytize young allogeneic cells which were incubated
with allogeneic IgG ($5 \pm 3\%$ phagocytosis). IgG was demonstrated on
the surface of stored RBC incubated with IgG eluted from autologous
or allogeneic cells with scanning immunoelectron microscopy. Absorption of the eluted IgG with stored RBC, but not with freshly isolated
young RBC, abolished its phagocytosis-inducing ability (Table 1).

These binding and specificity experiments indicate that: (a) IgG
is required for the phagocytosis of stored autologous and allogeneic
RBC; (b) non-specific binding of IgG does not play a major role in
these experiments because absorption of both pooled normal human IgG
and IgG eluted from senescent cells with stored RBC abolishes its
phagocytosis-inducing activity; (c) IgG eluted from senescent RBC is
reactive against stored, but not young, cells; and, (d) IgG eluted
from senescent RBC cannot discriminate between autologous and allogeneic cells. The last two findings suggest that the receptor site
appearing on the surface of cells aged in situ and that appearing on
stored cells is the same, or closely related, for all individuals.
Likewise, absorption of pooled normal human IgG with stored RBC
abolished its phagocytosis-inducing ability (Table 2).

To confirm these findings and to determine the nature of the membrane molecules that are altered during RBC aging in situ, young RBC
were treated with neuraminidase, the microbial enzyme that cleaves

Table 1. Phagocytosis of Stored RBC ("O" RBC) Incubated with IgG
          Eluted from Senescent Cells Before and After Absorption
          with Stored RBC or Freshly Isolated Young RBC (YRBC)

EXPT	QUANTITY*	PHAGOCYTOSIS (%) ± SEM[+]		
		Before Absorption	After Absorption with YRBC	After Absorption with "O" RBC
1	3	49 ± 2	43 ± 9	0
2	3	35 ± 1	34 ± 7	0
3	3	43 ± 11	46 ± 16	0

*Quantity (μg) of IgG added to 1.5 x 10^8 RBC in 1 ml of Medium 199.

[+]SEM, standard error of the mean of triplicate or quadruplicate cultures.

sialic acid groups from glycoproteins. Neuraminidase treated RBC
incubated in medium alone were not phagocytized (0% phagocytosis),
whereas those incubated in autologous and allogeneic IgG eluted from
old RBC aged in situ were phagocytized (% phagocytosis: 35 ± 2 and 46
± 6, respectively). IgG was observed with scanning immunoelectron
microscopy on the surface of neuraminidase-IgG treated RBC, but not
on RBC treated with neuraminidase alone.

The observation that the IgG eluted from RBC aged in situ recognizes the receptor exposed by removal of sialic acid groups suggests
that the receptor exposed as cells age naturally in situ may be the
same as, or analogous to, that exposed by the removal of sialic acid
in vitro. Membrane glycoproteins may be losing sialic acid as cells
age, thus exposing the molecular determinants to which IgG binds.
Another possibility is that the structural association between glycoproteins and integral membrane proteins may be disrupted during
aging, leading to exposure of cryptic antigens. In such a case, one
could speculate that neuraminidase acts, not by exposing new sugars,
but by changing glycoprotein-protein interactions through removal of
sialic acid.

To determine whether the Fab or Fc portion of IgG attaches to

Table 2.   Phagocytosis of Stored RBC Incubated with Pooled Human
           IgG Before or After Absorption of the IgG with Stored
           RBC*

EXPT	QUANTITY	PHAGOCYTOSIS (%)	
	of IgG (µg)[+]	Before Absorption	After Absorption
		(Mean ± SEM)[++]	
1	30	42 ± 17	0
2	30	32 ± 4	0
3	300	52 ± 2	0
4	300	28 ± 6	0

*IgG was absorbed over night at 4°C with RBC aged in vitro.

[+]The quantity of IgG (µg) was added to 2 x 10^8 RBC which were incubated

for 30 min at 24°C and then 30 min at 4°C, washed, and incubated with

autologous mononuclear phagocytes. The quantity of IgG (µg) was adjusted so

that it was the same both for absorbed and unabsorbed IgG, as determined by

radial immunodiffusion.

[++]Mean ± the standard error of the mean of quadruplicate cultures.

RBC, receptor blockade studies were performed. The results are summarized in Figure 6. Stored RBC were incubated for 30 minutes with
either pooled normal human IgG, its Fab or its Fc fragment. The RBC
were washed, and all three groups were incubated with IgG for another
30 mins. RBC were washed again and incubated with autologous mononuclear phagocytes (Fig. 6A). For the control cultures, stored RBC
were treated with IgG, Fab, or Fc before they were exposed to mononuclear phagocytes (Fig. 6B). Control results show that phagocytosis
was achieved by exposing the RBC to IgG. Treatment with Fab or Fc
did not promote phagocytosis. Experimental results show that
treatment of RBC with Fab prior to incubation with IgG reduced the

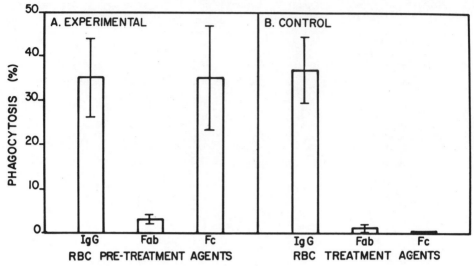

Fig. 6. A.   Susceptibility to phagocytosis of aged RBC as
             influenced by their pretreatment with either IgG, Fab
             or Fc before exposure to IgG. Stored RBC were
             incubated with either IgG, Fab. or Fc for 30 min,
             washed, and incubated with IgG for 30 min. The RBC
             were washed and incubated with mononuclear phagocytes
             for 3 hr.
        B.   Susceptibility to phagocytosis of aged RBC as
             influenced by their exposure to either IgG, Fab, or
             Fc. Stored RBC were incubated with either IgG, Fab or
             Fc for 30 min, washed and then incubated with
             mononuclear phagocytes for 3 hr. Bars indicate
             standard error of the mean; sample size, 6.

phagocytosis to essentially 0, whereas pretreatment with Fc did not
inhibit phagocytosis (Fig. 1A). Thus, these blockade studies demonstrate that IgG binds to old RBC via its Fab region. Binding of Fab
but not Fc was also demonstrated with scanning electron microscopy.
Binding of the IgG molecule to aged RBC via the Fab region is consistent with an immunological binding of IgG with a surface receptor.
The Fc portion of IgG would then be available to the macrophage Fc
receptor.

     These experiments suggest that the IgG eluted from senescent RBC
is an autoantibody, as it specifically reattaches to homologous RBC
via its Fab region and initiates their selective destruction by mononuclear phagocytes.

     Receptor Identification Studies. (The preliminary experiments
directed toward identifying the IgG-binding receptor on old RBC were

performed in collaboration with Dr. Hans Lutz, Department of Biochemistry, Swiss Federal Institute of Technology, Zurich, Switzerland.
Details of these experiments will be published elsewhere.)

There are several possible explanations for the mechanisms by
which appearance of a "new" receptor, such as the IgG-binding receptor, could occur with age. One possibility is the exposure of cryptic or hidden antigens that have existed as long as the cell has.
These antigens could be blocked, for example, by steric hindrance of
neighboring molecules. Alteration of the "shielding" molecules with
age, possibly through loss of one of their subunits, could result in
exposure of the receptor. Likewise, age-associated alterations in
membrane fluidity or in the interactions of molecules within the
membrane could result in exposure of cryptic antigens by allowing
molecular drift.

Another possible explanation is that subunits of surface molecules are lost with aging, thus exposing "new" antigenic determinants. In this case, the altered molecule, itself, would be the
receptor. Loss of a subunit could result in a change in the conformation of the protein. The receptor could be a sugar or amino acid
sequence behind the lost subunit, or it could result from a confor-
mational change in the molecule.

As an initial approach to this issue, we decided to isolate molecules that were potential receptor candidates. Based on data derived
from previous studies (3,26), which indicated that neuraminidase
treatment can increase IgG binding and phagocytosis of RBC, we sus-
pected that the receptor was a sialoglycoprotein or sialopeptide.
For this reason, we prepared glycophorin enriched vesicles (27). The
vesicles contain the sialoglycoproteins (PAS_1-PAS_4), a sialoglycoprotein that appears in the tracking dye region on polyacrylamide gel
electrophoresis, and trace contaminants of other minor proteins that
are not sialoglycoproteins (27). We used vesicles rather than soluble antigen for four reasons. First, it was necessary to determine
whether the receptor was indeed a sialoglycoprotein before proceeding
to isolate and purify it. Second, we were concerned with the possibility that membrane glycoproteins would aggregate when isolated or
when manipulated in an aqueous environment. Third, it is easier to
work with vesicles than with soluble antigens. Finally, other membrane components, such as protein component 3 or lipids, can be added
to the vesicles, enabling us to investigate the effect of these components on the receptor and IgG binding.

Isolation of potential receptors away from other membrane components allows differentiation between binding through exposure of
cryptic antigens and binding through alteration of the receptor
itself. If the appearance of an IgG-binding receptor on senescent
cells were due to exposure of a cryptic antigen, then the receptor
from young and old cells should bind IgG equally when isolated. On

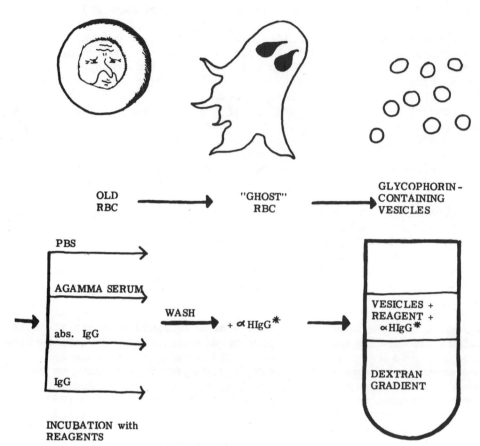

OLD RBC → "GHOST" RBC → GLYCOPHORIN-CONTAINING VESICLES

PBS

AGAMMA SERUM

WASH → + α HIgG*

abs. IgG

IgG

VESICLES + REAGENT + α HIgG*

DEXTRAN GRADIENT

INCUBATION with REAGENTS

Fig. 7.   Design of receptor identification experiments. Serum and
           buffy coat were removed from one unit of freshly obtained
           human blood. Cells were then resuspended in Medium 199
           and placed in tissue culture flasks at 4°C if they were
           to be stored, or were separated into young and old popula-
           tions and processed on the same day. For vesicle prepara-
           tion, cells were washed 4 times with PBS and lysed with
           hypotonic PBS (27). RBC ghosts were incubated in 10mM
           sodium acetate, washed with 0.1 mM ETDA, then 0.5 M NaCl,
           followed by 5 mM phosphate buffer, pH 7.4. The RBC ghosts
           were extracted with Triton X-100 (0.15%). After centrifu-
           gation, extracted supernates were washed with Bio Beads SM
           2 overnight at 4°C, resulting in vesicle formation (for
           details, see ref. 27). The vesicles were then incubated
           with PBS, agamma serum, autolgous IgG (10.5 mg), IgG or
           absorbed with stored RBC, for 1 hr at 4°C. After 2
           washes with PBS, vesicles were incubated with ^{125}I labeled

the other hand, if the receptor were a membrane molecule that has been altered by a deletion or addition, then the receptor from senescent cells should bind more IgG than the receptor from young cells.

Binding of IgG to Glycophorin-Containing Vesicles Prepared from Stored RBC. The experiments were performed with vesicles prepared from stored RBC as described in Figure 7. After equilibrium centrifugation (Fig. 8), vesicles incubated with PBS or agamma serum remained in the upper half of the gradient and the ^{125}I labeled anti-human IgG remained in the upper third of the gradient. Vesicles incubated with autologous IgG pelleted on the bottom of the tube along with bound anti-human IgG.

The amount of anti-human IgG bound to the vesicles was estimated from the amount of free anti-IgG (786 cpm per μg) on the gradient, after correcting for recovery of anti-IgG as determined by cpm, because of technical difficulties. Approximately 284 ng of anti-IgG was bound per μg protein to vesicles incubated with human IgG, while approximately 28 ng was bound to vesicles incubated with Ig-depleted serum. The amount of IgG bound is probably the same as the amount of anti-human IgG bound (3). However, it could be twice as much, since IgG has two binding sites. These results suggest that the IgG binding receptor on stored RBC copurifies with sialoglycoproteins.

Binding of IgG to Glycoprotein Containing Vesicles Prepared from RBC Aged in Situ. Vesicles were prepared from young, middle-aged, and old RBC populations. They were incubated with Ig reagents as described in Fig. 4. The results, which are summarized in Table 3, show that more ^{125}I labeled anti-human IgG or Protein A binds to vesicles from the senescent cell fraction than to vesicles from the middle-aged RBC fraction. The least label is bound to vesicles from the young RBC population. Increasing the amount of protein component 3 by increasing the amount of Triton X-100 used for extractions enhanced total IgG binding to vesicles from both young and old fraction cells, but not the difference in the amount of IgG bound between the fractions.

---

specific antibodies of goat anti-human IgG (anti-H IgG) prepared by the affinity chromatography and labeled by the lactoperoxidase method for 1 hr at 4°C. The mixture was then layered on a dextran gradient (ρ 1.005, 1.008, 1.012, 1.016, 1.020, and 1.025). Gradients were centrifuged for 8 hours in a SW27 rotor in a Beckman LS-50 preparative centrifuge at 25,000 rpm. Fractions were monitored during collection with a recording spectrophotometer. Radioactivity of the fractions was measured with a Searle gamma counter, and protein was determined by the method of Lowry.

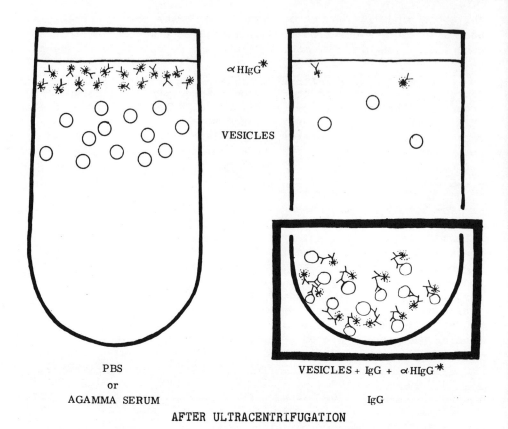

PBS
or
AGAMMA SERUM

VESICLES + IgG + αHIgG *

IgG

AFTER ULTRACENTRIFUGATION

Fig. 8.   Binding of IgG to glycoprotein-containing vesicles
           prepared from stored RBC. Vesicles were incubated with Ig
           reagents as described in Figure 4. After centrifugation
           on a dextran gradient, ^{125}I-labeled anti-human IgG that
           was not bound to vesicles was in the upper third of the
           gradient, and vesicles that were not labeled were in the
           upper half of the gradient. Labeled vesicles were on the
           bottom of the gradient. No radioactivity was detected in
           the bottom of the control gradient (incubated with PBS or
           agamma serum and then anti-human IgG). Fifty-nine percent
           of the radioactivity recovered from the gradient
           containing vesicles incubated with IgG was in the pellet.

Binding of ^{125}I labeled anti-human IgG or Protein A to vesicles
from the young population could be due to technical problems, such as
trapping of the label between vesicles during pelleting of the
vesicles, influx of the label into the vesicles during incubation
with subsequent resealing of the vesicles, sub-optimal separation of
RBC populations, or damage to young RBC during the preparative

Table 3. Binding of [125]I Labeled Anti-Human IgG or Protein A
          to Glycophorin-Containing Vesicles Isolated from Young,
          Middle-Aged, or Senescent RBC Populations Pre-Incubated
          with Autologous or Allogeneic IgG[1]

		IgG Binding[2]		
		(ng Protein A or anti-human		
Expt.		IgG bound per μg sialic acid)		
No	IgG Source	Cell Fraction		
		Young	Middle-aged	Old
1	autologous	50	70	90
		(0)	(20)	(40)
2	allogeneic	14	21	39
		(0)	(7)	(25)
3	allogeneic	9	21	26
		(0)	(12)	(17)

[1]Vesicles were incubated with autologous or allogeneic IgG,
washed, and incubated with ^{125}I labeled anti-human IgG (Expt 1)
or Protein A (Expt 2 and 3).
[2]Numbers in parentheses indicate relative anti-human IgG or
Protein A binding when the amount bound to vesicles from the
young cell fraction is subtracted from that bound to the middle-
aged and old fraction. This calculation was performed because
total binding of label to vesicles from young RBC incubated with
IgG was not significantly different from that of old RBC that
were incubated with IgG that had been absorbed before use with
RBC ghosts.

procedure. On the other hand, such binding could indicate the presence of a small number of the IgG binding receptor molecules in the
membranes of young cells.

As an independent method of assessing binding of IgG to vesicles,

Table 4.   Phagocytosis-Inducing Ability of IgG Absorbed with
           Glycophorin-Containing Vesicles (GCV) from Young,
           Middle-Aged, or Senescent Cell Fractions

				Phagocytosis (%)[3]		
				Mean ± SEM		
	Quantity (ug)			Source of Vesicles		
Expt	of IgG per	Vesicle Components[2]		Used for Absorption		
No	50 µg GCV[1]	protein	lipids	YG	MA	OLD
1	250	+	–	36±3	ND	5±5
2a	125	+	–	55±6	38±9	0
2b	125	+	+	42±3	34±7	0
2c	125	–	+	32±3	38±5	ND

[1]IgG was absorbed with vesicles from young (YG), middle-aged (MA), or senescent (OLD) cell fractions for 24-48 hrs at 4°C. Vesicles were removed by centrifugation and the supernate was incubated with approximately 150 x 10^6 stored RBC for 1 hr at 4°C. RBC were washed and incubated with macrophages.

[2]Vesicle components: a plus (+) indicates that the component was present; a minus (–) indicates that it was not.

[3]SEM, one standard error of the mean. The percent phagocytosis of RBC incubated with IgG that was not also absorbed was 41±3% for Expt 1 and 32±2% for Expt 2.

the phagocytosis inducing ability of IgG absorbed with vesicles from young, middle-aged, and old cell fractions was examined. The results, which are summarized in Table 4, show that absorption of IgG with vesicles prepared from senescent cells abolished the phagocytosis inducing ability of IgG, whereas absorption with vesicles prepared from young cells did not. Addition of lipids to the vesicles

did not significantly alter the results. Absorption of IgG with
lipids alone did not alter its phagocytosis-inducing ability. The
phagocytosis-inducing ability of IgG eluted from senescent cells
could be absorbed with vesicles prepared from senescent cells.

The results of the preceding experiments indicate that the IgG
binding receptor on senescent RBC copurifies with the sialoglycoproteins and is not a lipid. The receptor is not merely a cryptic antigen, but is a "new" antigen that appears on RBC membranes as they age
because there is a significant difference in IgG binding between vesicles isolated from young and old cells, as determined by two independent assays. If the receptor were merely a cryptic antigen, then
isolation of the receptor in vesicles, without the other "shielding"
molecules, should result in equal binding of the IgG, regardless of
the cell fraction from which it was prepared. This was not the
case. Furthermore, addition of lipids to the vesicles does not alter
IgG binding.

DISCUSSION

The results presented herein confirm the earlier studies from
this laboratory (3,10,20) by demonstrating that macrophages distinguish between senescent and mature RBC on the basis of selective IgG
attachment, and firmly establishing the existence of autoantibodies
with intrinsic physiologic and homeostatic functions. The IgG that
binds to senescent RBC in situ and stored RBC in vitro is an autoantibody, as it specifically attaches to old cells via the Fab
region, thus initiating their selective destruction by macrophages.
The IgG autoantibody is directed against an altered membrane protein
or sialoglycoprotein, not a cryptic antigen. It is interesting to
speculate that the IgG binding antigen may be a fragment of a higher
molecule weight membrane molecule that is produced through the action
of endogenous proteases or results from a change in activity of a
membrane bound enzyme(s) which maintains membrane integrity.

The IgG autoantibody protects RBC from lysis for the first 10-15
days of storage in vitro in serum (Kay, unpublished). It also
induces phagocytosis of senescent RBC by macrophages. As a result,
senescent cells are removed from the circulation instead of lysing
(4,5,6,8). Thus, the membranes and hemoglobin of the approximately
1.93×10^{11} (Footnote *) senescent cells that are removed daily are
enzymatically degraded by macrophages rather than being released into
the circulation by lysis. Lysis of RBC could be detrimental to an
individual's survival. For example, individuals with elevated plasma

---

*The number of senescent cells removed per day is calculated as
follows: 5.1×10^9 RBC/ml blood divided by 120 days = 4×10^7
senescent RBC per ml at the end of their life span. This is
multiplied by the blood volume (69 ml/Kg times 70 Kg = 4830 ml).

iron levels, as are seen with overt hemolytic anemia or destruction
of ferritin-containing liver cells (e.g., viral hepatitis), are
extremely susceptible to even a small innoculum of invading pathogens
(29). Iron enhances the virulence of bacteria and can neutralize the
microbiostatic action of serum (for review of the subject, see 28).

The IgG described herein is a physiologic autoantibody, as it
contributes to the maintenance of homeostasis by permitting the more
efficient mature cells to carry out their vital functions without
hindrance from the less efficient senescent cells, or from pathological reactions which could arise as a consequence of senescent
cells dying or decaying within the organism. Thus, the existence of
homeostatic autoantibodies has been demonstrated experimentally
probably for the first time. Since these autoantibodies are part of
the normal immune mechanism for removing cells, the B cell clones
producing these antibodies cannot be "forbidden" (29), nor need the
presence of these autoantibodies be attributed to an age-related
decrease in suppressor cell function (30,31).

Some authors have attributed macrophage removal of senescent
cells to a reduction in net negative surface charge with aging of RBC
(32,33). However, recent reports indicate that there are no differences between young and senescent RBC in net surface charge densities, as determined by several different methods (34,35).

Other investigators have attributed removal of senescent RBC to
direct interaction between desialylated RBC and macrophages that is
not mediated by IgG (36). This assumption is based on the observation that neuraminidase treated rat RBC bind to Kupffer cells and to
unseparated spleen cells (36). There are several problems with this
assumption. First, it has been shown that attachment of a cell or
particle to a specific receptor on a macrophage is not sufficient to
trigger phagocytosis (37,38). The following examples clearly demonstrate that attachment does not lead to phagocytosis.

Complement coated RBC are bound to the macrophage membrane but
are not ingested. When IgG coated pneumococci are added to the
macrophage preparations which have already bound complement coated
RBC, the macrophages ingest an average of 15-20 pneumococci, but not
the attached RBC (38). Thus, the response of the macrophage membrane
to a phagocytic stimulus is highly selective.

In addition, the distribution of IgG molecules on the potential
particle is of great importance to a macrophage. For example, macrophages will ingest B lymphocytes if they are diffusely coated with
antibodies against lymphocyte surface antigens which do not cap.
Capped lymphocytes treated with IgG anti-immunoglobulin are bound but
not ingested. Surprisingly, macrophages will clean capped immunoglobulins from the surface of lymphocytes without apparently damaging
them.

Evidence from many different laboratories has shown that IgG is required for phagocytosis of RBC. Jancik and Schauer (39) have shown that the phagocytosis of desialylated erythrocytes in vitro requires serum factors and that circulating erythrocytes are coated with IgG following desialylation. Durocher (40) has shown that immunoglobulins bind to desialylated rat RBC. In contrast to the studies on removal of desialylated serum glycoproteins (23,24,25), galactose oxidase treatment of desialylated RBC does not improve their survival nor does it reduce immunoglobulin binding (40). Cellular deformability does not seem to contribute to destruction of RBC (40).

Steer (41) has shown that infusion of desialylated chromium labeled lymphocytes into rabbits results in rapid uptake of these cells by the liver. However, incubation of desialylated lymphocytes with Fab fragments prior to infusion results in a marked decrease in hepatic uptake. This is consistent with the finding reported here and elsewhere (26) that the Fab portion of IgG binds to RBC, leaving the Fc portion free to interact with the Fc receptor on macrophages.

There is still some controversy regarding sialic acid content of aged RBC. Some authors report that senescent RBC have slightly lower levels of sialic acid (35), while others found identical levels of sialic acid in glycophorin of both young and senescent RBC (43). It is possible that sialic acid is lost from sialoglycoproteins besides glycophorin.

It has been suggested that the autoantibody described here and in previous studies from my laboratory may simply be the T-agglutinin which binds to an exposed β-galactose residue on desialylated RBC. However, the T-agglutinin belongs to the IgM class. The antibody which binds to senescent RBC is IgG, as determined by four different methods. Furthermore, IgM antibodies have not been observed on senescent RBC (3). A recent investigation using two mouse strains, one with and one without serum T agglutinin, demonstrated that T-agglutinin does not participate in the removal of desialylated RBC (44).

The concept of self-tolerance is a basic tenet of immunology. Ehrlich used the term, "horror autotoxicus" to describe autoimune disease which was felt to result from a breakdown in internal regulation that prevented reactions against "self." The demonstrated existence of physiologic autoantibodies requires a revision of this view. Besides the physiologic autoantibody described herein, for which a homeostatic function has been demonstrated and a mechanism of action has, in part, been elucidated (Fig. 9), autoantibodies are being found with increasing frequency in normal, healthy individuals (45-48). Essentially 100% of the young healthy individuals tested in this laboratory have low levels of antibodies to thyroglobulin (Kay, unpublished). Injection of the polyclonal activator, lipopolysaccharide (LPS), into mice results in production of IgM antibodies which are specific for mouse IgG (48). Immunogen injection has the same effect. Plaque-forming cells producing IgM anti-IgG autoantibody have been demonstrated (48). Autoantibodies against mouse RBC treated with bromelain have been described, and plaque forming cells producing autoantibody against bromelain treated mouse RBC have been demonstrated (49,50). The function or significance of cells capable of responding to bromelain treated RBC is unclear at this time because bromelain hydrolyzes proteins, peptides, amides and esters of amino acids and peptides, and because bromelain treatment represents a non-physiologic situation. The implication of such studies is that mice have a high proportion ($\geq$ 50%) of cells that recognize endogenous antigens. The problem with these studies is that bromelain may generate many "new" antigens by altering many molecules. Further, alteration of a self recognition antigen, such as one of the H-2 antigens, could result in recognition of the molecule as "non-self" or "altered self" (51), just as addition of a single sugar (α-N-acetyl-galactosamine) to a glycosphingolipid produced by adenocarcinoma of the stomach and colon leads to a "non-self" antigen passing as a "self" antigen (52).

In 1964, Swartzendruber (53) described removal of plasma cells by macrophages in the spleen of mice between 3 and 6 days after primary immunization, as determined by electron microscopy. Phagocytosis of plasma cells was most extensive on day 6. Jerne et al. (54), utilizing a plaque assay, reported a 90% decrease in the number of antibody-producing cells in the mouse spleen between 4 and 7 days after primary immunization with the same antigen. Schooley (55), using autoradiography, estimated the mean-life of a plasma cell at 8-12 hr after the last division in a stimulated lymph node. In addition, the phagocytosis of plasma cells observed by Swartzendruber correlates with the log phase of antibody appearance in the circulation (56). In view of the preceding, it is tempting to speculate that a clone(s) of plasma cells, and thus, antibody production to a specific immunogen, is terminated at the log phase of antibody appearance in situ by phagocytic macrophages. It is possible that an autoantibody similar to the one described herein is responsible for initiating the phagocytosis of terminally differentiated plasma cells. Antiidiotypic antibody directed toward the Fab or Fc region might be responsible for initiating phagocytosis.

One of the implications of such speculation is that multiple myeloma might result from a defect in macrophages or a regulatory autoantibody allowing plasma cells to function autonomously. Freed of their normal mechanism of destruction, plasma cells could then accumulate and the plasmacytosis of multiple myeloma would result.

It is possible that autoantibodies may also function as a regulatory mechanism for initiating and/or terminating metabolic processes. This is suggested by studies into the pathophysiology of certain disease processes. For example, thyroid-stimulating immunoglobulin

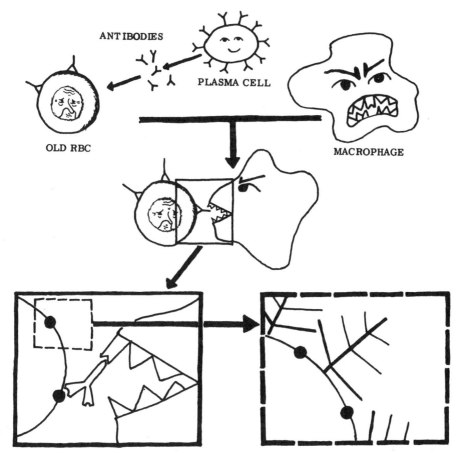

Fig. 9.   Summary of our knowledge of the autoantibody that
           initiates removal of senescent red cells.   Autologous
           plasma cells produce IgG antibodies against receptors on
           red cells.   The Fab region of the IgG autoantibody binds
           to receptors and autologous macrophages recognize and bind
           to the Fc region of the IgG autoantibody and phagocytize
           the red cell.   This is depicted in the diagram on the
           lower left.   The diagram on the lower right is a schematic
           diagram of the receptor on the RBC, which is represented
           as a branched glycoprotein.   The circles represent
           adjacent membrane proteins.

(TSI) is an IgG autoantibody that binds to the thyroid follicular
cell's receptor or a component thereof.   TSI stimulates cyclic adeno-
sine monophosphate and endocytosis of colloid droplets, displaces
thyroid stimulating hormone from membrane sites and results in excessive levels of circulating thyroid hormone (58).   The existence of an
autoantibody that can initiate the activities of an endocrine gland,

even though it is associated with a disease, suggests the possibility
that other autoantibodies may exist which act as initiators of homeostatic processes. Less dramatic examples of immunoglobulins initiating metabolic processes are the "capping" that is observed following
binding of anti-immunoglobulin reagents to lymphocyte membranes and
the DNA synthesis initiated by culturing lymphocytes with anti-immunoglobulin (19,59,60).

It is interesting that greater than 90% of the immunoglobulin
molecules in human serum are of the IgG class. IgG has the longest
half-life and the highest rate of synthesis of any immunoglobulin
class (61). A calculation of the amount of IgG in a human being
reveals that each of us has approximately a quarter of a kilogram.
This is rather excessive unless IgG serves physiologic functions
other than opsonization of occasional bacteria. One of these
physiologic functions is the removal of senescent cells. Others
remain to be elucidated.

ACKNOWLEDGEMENTS

This is publication number 020 from the Laboratory of Molecular
and Clinical Immunology and publication number 032 from GRECC,
Wadsworth Hospital Center, Los Angeles, California 90073. This work
was supported by NIH Grant HL 22671. This work was performed, in
part, in a building belonging to the Research Service of Wadsworth VA
Hospital. I am grateful to Dr. Lynn Baker for drawing Figures 4, 5,
and 6 for me.

REFERENCES

1. M. A. Klauser, L. J. Hirsch, P. F. Leblond, J. K. Chamberlain,
    M. R. Klemperer, and G. B. Segel, Contrasting splenic
    mechanisms in the blood clearance of red blood cells and
    colloidal particles, Blood 46:965 (1975).
2. V. Silobcic, B. Vitale, M. Susnjic, V. Tomazic, and I. Basic,
    Acute graft-versus-host reaction in mice. 3. Organ
    distribution of injected 51 chromium labeled lymphocytes, Exp.
    Hemat. 4:103 (1976).
3. M.M.B. Kay, Mechanism of removal of senescent cells by human
    macrophages in situ, Proc. Natl. Acad. Sci. USA 72:3521 (1975).
4. F. Smith, Erythrophagocytosis in human lymph-glands, J. Path.
    Bact. 78:383 (1958).
5. C. R. Jenkin and K. Karthigasu, Elimination hepatiques des
    erythrocytes age et alteres chez le rat, Compt. Rend. Soc.
    Biol. 161:1006 (1967).
6. T. Morita, and E. H. Perkins, A simple quantitative method to
    assess the in vitro engulfing and degradative potentials of
    mouse peritoneal phagocytic cells. J. Reticuloendothel. Soc.
    2:406 (1965).

7. A. E. Stuart, and R. A. Cumming, A biological test for injury to the human red cell, Vox Sang. 13:270 (1967).

8. D. S. Nelson, Macrophages in auto-immunity, the disposal of effete cells and chronic inflammation, in:"Macrophages and Immunity," Amer. Elsevier Pub. Co., New York (1969).

9. D. Gemsa, C. H. Woo, H. H. Fudenberg, and R. Schmid, Erythrocyte catabolism by macrophages in vitro. The effect of hydrocortisone on erythrophagocytosis and on the indication of heme oxygenase, J. Clin. Lab. Invest. 52:812 (1973).

10. M. M. B. Kay, Mechanism of macrophage recognition of senescent red cells, Gerontologist 14(5):33 (1974).

11. S. Kochwa and R. Rosenfield, Immunochemical studies of the Rh system. I. Isolation and characterization of antibodies, J. Immunol. 92:682 (1964).

12. A. Nisonoff, F. C. Wissler, L. N. Lipman, and D. L. Woernley, Separation of univalent fragments from the bivalent rabbit antibody molecule by reduction of disufide bonds, Arch. Biochem. Biophys. 89:230 (1960).

13. J. J. Cebra, D. Guval, H. I. Silman, and E. Katchalski, A two-stage cleavage of rabbit y-globulin by a water-insoluble papain preparation followed by cysteine, J. Biol. Chem. 236:1720 (1961).

14. C. L. Cambiasco, A. Goffinet, J.-P. Vaerman, and J. F. Feremans, Glutaraldehyde-activated aminohexyl-derivative of Sepharose 4B as a new versatile immunoabsorbent, Immunochemistry 12:272 (1975).

15. J. Mueller, R. G. del Brun, H. Buerki, H.-U. Keller, M. W. Hess, and H. Cottier, Non-specific acid esterase activity: A criterion for differentiation in mouse lymph nodes, Eur. J. Immunol. 5:270 (1975).

16. M. M. B. Kay, Kupffer cells: Homeostatic functions during aging, in:"Liver and Ageing," D. Platt, ed., F.K. Schattauer Verlag, Stuttgart (1977).

17. J. R. Murphy, Influence of temperature and method of centrifugation on the separation of erythrocytes, J. Lab. Clin. Med. 82:334 (1973).

18. E. R. Borun, M. G. Figueroa, and I. M. Perry, The distribution of Fe^{59}-tagged human erythrocytes in centrifuged specimens as a function of cell age, J. Clin. Invest. 36:676 (1957).

19. M. M. B. Kay, Multiple labeling technique used for kinetic studies of activated human B lymphocytes, Nature 245:425 (1975).

20. M. M. B. Kay, Multiple labeling technique for scanning immuno-electron microscopy, in:"Principles and Techniques of Scanning Electron Microscopy," M.A. Hayat, ed., Van Nostrand and Reinhold Co., New York, (1978).

21. M. M. B. Kay, High resolution scanning electron microscopy and its application to research on immunity and aging, in:"Immunity and Aging," T. Makinodan and E. Yunis, eds., Plenum Press, New York (1978).

22. T. Steck, The organization of proteins in the human red blood cell membrane, J. Cell Biol. 62:1 (1974).

23. C. J. A. van den Hamer, G. Morell, I. H. Scheinberg, J. Hickman, and G. Ashwell, Physical and chemical studies on ceruloplasmin. IX. The role of glactosyl residues in the clearance of ceruloplasmin from the circulation. J. Biol. Chem. 245:4397 (1970).

24. A. G. Morell, G. Gregoriadis, I. H. Scheinberg, J. Hickman, and G. Ashwell, The role of sialic acid in determining the survival of glycoproteins in the circulation, J. Biol. Chem. 246:1461 (1971).

25. W. E. Pricer Jr. and G. Ashwell, The binding of desialylated glycoproteins by plasma membranes of rat liver, J. Biol. Chem. 246:4825 (1971).

26. M. M. B. Kay, Role of physiologic autoantibodies in the removal of senescent human red cells, J. Supra. Mol. Stuct. 9:555 (1978).

27. H. U. Lutz, A. von Daniken, G. Semenza, and T. H. Bachi, Glycophorin-enriched vesicles obtained by a selective extraction of human erythrocyte membranes with a non-ionic detergent, Biochim. Biophys. Acta., in press.

28. E. D. Weinberg, Iron and susceptibility to infectious disease, Science 148:952 (1974).

29. F. M. Burnet, "Immunological Surveillance," Pergammon Press, Oxford, England (1970).

30. H. H. Fudenberg, Genetically determined immune deficiency as the predisposing cause of "autoimmunity" and lyphoid neoplasia, Amer. J. Med. 51:295 (1971).

31. M. E. Gershwin and A. D. Steinberg, Suppression of autoimmune hemolytic anemia in New Zealand (NZB) mice by syngeneic young thymocytes, Clin. Immunol. Immunopath. 4:38 (1975).

32. Y. Marikovsky, D. Danon, and A. Katchalsky, Agglutination by polylysine of young and old red blood cells, Biochim. Biophys. Acta 124:154 (1966).

33. E. Skutelsky, Y. Marikovsky, and D. Danon, Immunoferritin analysis of membrane antigen density: A. Young and old human blood cells. B. Developing erythroid cells and extruded erythroid nuclei, Eur. J. Immunol. 4:512 (1974).

34. G. V. F. Seaman, R. J. Knox, F. J. Nordt, and D. H. Regan, Red cell aging. I. Surface charge density and sialic acid content of density-fractionated human erythrocytes, Blood 50:1001 (1977).

35. S. J. Luner, D. Szklarek, R. J. Knox, G. V. H. Seaman, J. Y. Josefowicz, and B. R. Ware, Red cell charge is not a function of cell age, Nature 269:719 (1977).

36. D. Aminoff, W. F. V. Bruegge, W. C. Bell, K. Sarpolis, and R. Williams, Role of sialic acid in survival of erythrocytes in the circulation: Interaction of neuraminidase-treated and untreated erythrocytes with spleen and liver and the cellular level, Proc. Natl. Acad. Sci. USA 74:1521 (1977).

37. A. F. LoBuglio, R. S. Cotran, and J. H. Jandl, Red cells coated with immmunoglobulin G: Binding and sphereing by mononuclear cells in man, Science 158:1582 (1967).

38. J. Michl and S. C. Silverstein, Role of macrophage receptors in the ingestion phase of phagocytosis, in:"Birth Defects: Original Article Series," 14 (2), R.A. Lerner and D. Bergsma, eds., The National Foundation--March of Dimes, White Plains, New York (1978).

39. J. M. Janicik, R. Schauer, K. H. Andres, and M. von During, Sequestration of neuraminidase-treated erythrocytes. Studies on its topographic, morphologic and immunologic aspects, Cell. Tiss. Res. 186:209 (1978).

40. J. R. Durocher, J. Supramol. Struct. Suppl. 2:199 (1978).

41. C. J. Steer, Kupffer cells and glycoproteins: Does a recognition phenomenon exist? Bull. Kupffer Cell Fdn. I:26 (1978).

42. A. Baxter and J. G. Beeley Surface carbohydrates of aged erythrocytes, Biochem. Biophys. Res. Commun. 83:466 (1978).

43. H. U. Lutz and J. Fehr, Total sialic acid content in glycophorin remains unchanged during senescence of human red cells, submitted.

44. G. Perret, D. Bladier, L. Gattegno, and P. Cornillot, The role of T-agglutinin in the disappearance of erythrocytes artificially aged by desialylation, Mech. Ageing Dev., in press.

45. W. J. Martin and S. E. Martin, Thymus reactive IgM autoantibodies in normal mouse sera, Nature 254:716 (1975).

46. J. C. Roder, D. A. Bell, and S. K. Singhal, Regulation of the autoimmune plaque-forming cell response to single-strand DNA (sDNA) in vitro, J. Immunol. 121:38 (1978).

47. D. W. Dresser and A. M. Popham, Induction of IgM anti-(bovine)-IgG response in mice by bacterial lipopolysaccharide, Nature 264:552 (1976).

48. D. W. Dresser, Most IgM-producing cells in the mouse secrete auto-antibodies (rheumatoid factor), Nature 274:480 (1978).

49. A. E. Bussard, M.-A. Vinit, and J. M. Pages, Immunochemical characterization of the autoantibodies produced by mouse peritoneal cells in culture, Immunochemistry 14:1 (1977).

50. E. J. Stelle and A. J. Cunningham, High proportion of IgG producing cells making autoantibody in normal mice, Nature 274:483 (1978).

51. G. M. Shearer, Cell-mediated cytotoxicity to trinitrophenyl-modi-fied syngeneic lymphocytes, Eur. J. Immunol. 4:527 (1974).

52. P. Levine, Self-nonself concept for cancer and diseases previously known as "autoimmune" diseases, Proc. Natl. Acad. Sci. USA 75:5697 (1978).

53. D. C. Swartzenbruber, Phagocytized plasma cells in mouse spleen observed by light and electron microscopy, Blood 24:432 (1964).

54. N. K. Jerne, A. A. Nordin, and C. Henry, The agar plaque technique for recognizing antibody-producing cells, in:"Cell-Bound Antibodies," D.B. Amos and H. Koprowski, eds.,

Wistar Press, Philadelphia (1963).

55. J. C. Schooley, Autoradiographic observations of plasma cell
    formation, J. Immunol. 86:331 (1961).

56. C. G. Congdon and T. Makinodan, Splenic white pulp after antigen
    injection: Relation of time of serum antibody production,
    Am. J. Path. 39:697 (1961).

58. D. H. Solomon, The nature of Graves' hyperthyroidism,
    in:"Autoimmune thyroid diseases--Graves' and Hashimoto's,"
    J. Brown, moderator, Ann. Intern. Med. 88:379 (1978).

59. M. C. Raff, Two distinct populations of peripheral lymphocytes in
    mice distinguishable by immunofluorescence, Immunology 19:637
    (1970).

60. D. J. Scribner, H. L. Weiner, and J. W. Moorhead, Anti-immuno-
    globulin stimulation of murine lymphocytes. V. Age-related
    decline in Fc receptor-mediated immunoregulation, J. Immunol.
    121:377 (1978).

61. H. N. Eisen, "Immunology," Harper and Row Publishers, Inc.,
    Hagerstown, Md (1974).

62. M. M. B. Kay, Hodgkin's Disease: A war between T lymphocytes and
    transformed macrophages? in:"Lymphocytes and Macrophages in
    Cancer Patients, Vol. 1, Recent Results in Cancer Research,"
    G. Mathe, I. Florentn, and M.-C. Simmler, eds., Springer-
    Verlag, New York (1976).

CHANGES IN SYNAPTIC STRUCTURE AFFECTING

NEURAL TRANSMISSION IN THE SENESCENT BRAIN

William Bondareff

Department of Anatomy and
Institute of Psychiatry
Northwestern University Medical School
Chicago, Illinois, USA

INTRODUCTION

Neural transmission involves electrochemical interactions between two neurons along a region of interneuronal contact known as a synapse. In vertebrate nervous systems these interactions are mediated by transmitter substances, which react with receptor sites on synaptic membranes affecting their permeability to various ions. Synaptic membranes are modified segments of neuronal plasma membranes, and their properties vary in different types of synapses.

Among synapses found in mammalian brains, axodendritic synapses are probably most numerous. They involve the axonal plasma membrane of one neuron and the dendritic plasma membrane of another. They consist of three parts: an axonal terminal or presynaptic component; a dendritic or postsynaptic component; and a modified segment of the extracellular space, the synaptic cleft. The interaction between presynaptic and postsynaptic components, which facilitates both initial contact in early embryogenesis and functional interactions later, appears to depend in part upon the presence of complex macromolecules. These include glycoproteins and glycolipids, which are structural components of the pre- and post-synaptic membranes. It is believed that the side chains and terminal groups of these plasma membrane-associated macromolecules extend into the synaptic cleft, where they may interact with one another and with other macromolecules, perhaps proteoglycans.

A relationship between synaptic structure and function is indicated by the fact that interneuronal transmission in the fetus is heralded by the appearance of synapses with adult-like structure.

The return of function after deafferentation in young and adult
animals is similarly associated with the appearance of synapses, and
the character of the returning function appears to depend upon the
accuracy with which synaptic connections are remade with previously
deafferentated neurons (1). As a relationship between synaptic
structure and function exists in immature and mature animals, it
seems reasonable to anticipate that a similar relationship exists in
senescence and that senescent changes in neuronal function can be
associated with changes in synaptic structure and distribution.
Age-related changes in the structure/function relationship of
synapses are, however, not well known. They have been the subject of
recent studies (2,3), and their discussion here is predicated upon
the observation that synaptic loss typically occurs in the brain of
the senescent rat, and is not necessarily dependent upon an antecedent loss of neurons (4), although neuronal loss in senescence is
well known (5).

MATERIALS AND METHODS

Axo-dendritic synapses of the dentate gyrus molecular layer were
compared in hippocampi of young adult and senescent male Fischer-344
rats. The hippocampus was chosen for study because of its presumed
relationship to memory and learning functions, and the dentate gyrus
because its anatomy is well known. The animals, bred under pathogen-
free conditions, were commercially available from the Charles River
Breeding Laboratories (Wilmington, Massachusetts). Their natural
history and pathology has been characterized (6). The 50% mean survival age is 29 months; the maximal survival age appears to be about
36 months; and the incidence of pathological changes in the brain is
small. Rats of the Fischer-344 strain of 24 and 3 months of age,
therefore, seemed well suited for studies of aging.

RESULTS

Attention was focused on the axo-dendritic synapses of a specific
part of the dentate gyrus portion of the hippocampus (see refs.
14,19). The postsynaptic component of these synapses appears to consist primarily of dendrites of dentate gyrus granule cells, but the
presynaptic component is less well-defined. Synapses were first
counted in an electron microscope study of the middle third of the
molecular layer (4). When compared with synaptic counts of the same
region of 3-month-old rats, a 27% decrease in the number of synapses
per unit of square area of neuropil was found in the 24-month-old
animals (Fig. 1). Unfortunately, it was difficult to determine
whether this loss of synapses reflected an antecedent age-related
insult to the pre- or post-synaptic neurons involved in the synapses. There was, however, no age-related change in the number of
postsynaptic granule cell bodies (nor in synaptic size, nor in tissue
volume), and it appeared, therefore, to depend upon changes to the
presynaptic component (7). This conclusion was supported by a later

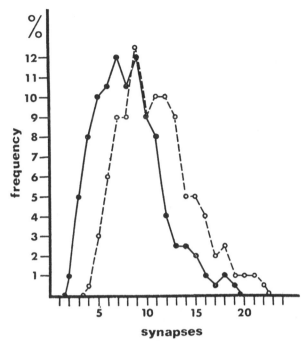

Fig. 1.   Frequency distribution of synapses in a unit of square
          area of the dentate gyrus molecular layer of 3-month-old
          (broken line) and 25-month-old (solid line) rats. A shift
          to the left in 25-month-old rats indicates a smaller
          percentage of unit areas in which a given number of
          synapses were counted due to a 27% decrease in the number
          of synapses (see reference 4).

electron microscope study (8) in which an almost identical loss of
synapses was found in the supragranular portion of the molecular
layer, where presynaptic elements have been shown to be different
from those found in the middle third portion. Again, no decrease in
the number of postsynaptic granule cell bodies could be demonstrated.

    A loss of axo-dendritic synapses has also been found in the
visual area of the cerebral cortex of the senescent Fischer-344 rat
(9) and the cerebellar cortex (10). In the latter, a 33% decrement
in the axo-dendritic synapses of 25-month-old Fischer-344 rats was
found to involve axo-spinous synapses selectively. The number of
these synapses, between parallel fibers (axons) and Purkinje cell
dendritic spines, seemed to decline in senescence, while those
between climbing fibers and dendritic shafts were spared.

    Lest the misinterpretation be given that synaptic loss in the
senescent hippocampus involves only axo-dendritic synapses and that

there is some property of the axo-dendritic synapse which makes it
uniquely susceptible to the aging process, it should be noted that
axo-somatic synapses may be lost also. These synapses were counted
in an electron microscope study of perikarya of dentate gyrus granule
cells which accumulate lipofuscin pigment, but appear otherwise
normal in 25-month-old Fischer-344 rats. Their number, as compared
with that of 3- to 4-month-old young adults, appeared to be constant. There was, nevertheless, a 15% decrease in synapses per
length of plasma membrane surface, which amounted to a 22% decrease
in the percentage of the granule cell surface covered by synapses in
senescent animals.

DISCUSSION

   The time course of these age-related losses of synapses is not
known; nor are the neurobiological processes by means of which they
occur. Among the many possible factors which may contribute to synaptic loss and effect a decline in neural transmission in senescence,
the following are of particular interest.

Age-Related Change in Neuron-Neuroglial Relationships

   Although our studies of the dentate gyrus have been extensive, no
indication of synaptic degeneration or of phagocytosis has ever been
encountered. Assuming that products of cell degeneration are generally removed by phagocytosis, this suggests that the loss of synapses
found at 24 months must have occurred some time earlier, so as to
allow sufficient time for the products of degeneration to be removed
by phagocytosis and the debris-laden phagocytes to be cleared from
the tissue. Such a process might be anticipated if synaptic loss
were part of a continuous process of synaptic rebuilding, as was suggested earlier (11). If, during adulthood, synapses were being
formed and deformed, the rate of deformation would increase with age
such that, as senescence were approached, more synapses would be lost
than formed. The number of microglial cells, which are the principal
phagocytes of the central nervous system, might increase with age, as
has been found in cerebral cortex (12). There is no evidence that
the number of microcytes increases in the senescent dentate gyrus,
and no evidence that microcytes laden with phagocytized remains of
synapses are cleared from the dentate gyrus prior to the 24th month.
There is, however, evidence that a process of remodelling occurs in
the dentate gyrus as a function of age.

   Although there appears to be no change in the number of microglial cells in the hippocampus of the senescent rat, there is evidence of an increase in the number of astrocytes (13). An electron
microscope study of the supragranular region selected for morphometric analysis of synapses (14) did not demonstrate any change in the
number of astrocytic cell bodies, but did show a 45% increase in the
volume fraction of astrocytic processes (Table 1). As no change in

Table 1. Number and Volume Fraction of Astroglial Process
          Profiles in the Supragranular Zone of the Dentate Gyri
          of Young Adult (3 months of age) and Senescent (25
          months of age) Rats (14)

	Volume Fraction	
	3 Months	25 Months
Mean ± S.E.M. per animal	0.114 ± 0.006	0.184 ± 0.008
	0.083 ± 0.006	0.141 ± 0.008
	0.098 ± 0.007	0.120 ± 0.007
	0.094 ± 0.007	0.136 ± 0.007
	0.082 ± 0.007	0.097 ± 0.007
Mean ± S.E.M. per group	0.094 ± 0.006	0.136 ± 0.014
Percent of 3-month-old group		144.7
Significance level		P < 0.01

the dimensions of the whole dentate gyrus could be demonstrated,
there would appear to be a redistribution of its parts in the senescent rat.

Injury of Postsynaptic Neurons

Although a voluminous literature might lead to the assumption
that synaptic loss is associated with an antecedent loss of neurons
in the dentate gyrus, available data indicate no such loss. The
data, however, are conflicting. On the one hand, counts of granule
cells in senescent Fischer-344 rats have failed to demonstrate any
significant age-related decrease (7,8). On the other hand, a whit-
tling away of the dendritic trees of neurons appears to be a fairly
generalized characteristic of aging, and has been described in several areas of the brain (9,15-18).

Decreases in both the volume fraction and surface area of dendrites, coincident with the age-related changes in synapses and
astrocytes described above, have been demonstrated by morphometric
analysis of the supragranular portion of the dentate gyrus and shown
to reflect an absolute loss of dendrites (19). That these decreases
are disproportionate (Table 2) probably indicates the selective loss

Table 2.   Volume Fraction and Surface Area of Dendritic Shafts in
           3-Month-Old and 25-Month-Old Rats (19)

	Volume Fraction		Surface Area	
	3 Months	25 Months	3 Months	25 Months
Mean ± S.E.M. per Animal	0.407 ± 0.016	0.346 ± 0.012	2.13 ± 0.07	1.31 ± 0.08
	0.421 ± 0.011	0.406 ± 0.015	1.90 ± 0.06	1.63 ± 0.06
	0.422 ± 0.015	0.395 ± 0.012	1.77 ± 0.07	1.46 ± 0.06
	0.365 ± 0.013	0.329 ± 0.011	1.78 ± 0.08	1.21 ± 0.04
	0.451 ± 0.015	0.333 ± 0.015	1.91 ± 0.07	1.29 ± 0.06
Mean ± S.E.M. per group	0.413 ± 0.014	0.362 ± 0.016	1.90 ± 0.06	1.38 ± 0.07
% of 3-month-old group		87.6		72.6
Significance		$P < 0.05$		$P < 0.001$

of smaller diameter, distal dendritic branches in the dentate gyrus,
as might have been predicted from the findings of others (see above)
in other parts of the brain. The mechanism of this loss is unknown
and its relationship to synaptic loss in the dentate gyrus is
unknown. However, it does not appear to be prerequisite for synaptic
loss, because the loss of synapses is the same whether it is determined relative to the square area of neuropil or to a unit length of
dendrites found in the senescent dentate gyrus (8) (Table 3).

Injury of Presynaptic Neurons

     There has been no systematic enumeration of neurons presynaptic
to synapses found in the dentate gyrus. There is evidence, however,
that neurons of the septal nucleus, which contribute presynaptic
cholinergic afferents to synapses in the supragranular region of the
dentate gyrus, take up and incorporate ^{3}H-fucose into glycoproteins
similarly in animals 24 and 3 months of age (20). Yet, the intraneuronal transport of fucose-labeled glycoproteins through axons of
the septohippocampal pathway was shown to be slowed in 25-month-old
Fischer-344 rats. This was shown by labeling the medial septal
nucleus of young adult and senescent rats with ^{3}H-fucose and comparing the times of arrival of ^{3}H-fucose labeled glycoproteins in the
hippocampus as a function of age (20). The arrival times differed
significantly, reflecting a 30% reduction in the rate of axonal
transport of glycoproteins to synapses remaining in the dentate gyrus
of senescent rats (Fig. 2). Since glycoproteins are components of
presynaptic membranes, such an age-related decrement in the amount

Table 3. Number of Synapses Involving Dendritic Shafts and Spines in the Supragranular Zone of the Dentate Gyrus of Young Adult (3-month-old) and Senescent (25-month-old) Rats (19)

	Per Tissue Square Area (66 sq. μm)				Per Dendrite Unit Length (10 μm)			
	Shafts		Spines		Shafts		Spines	
	3 Months	25 Months	3 Months	25 Months	3 Months	25 Months	3 Months	25 Months
Mean ± S.E.M. per Animal	2.6 ± 0.2	1.6 ± 0.1	17.0 ± 0.5	13.1 ± 0.4	6.3 ± 0.9 (n = 248)	4.7 ± 0.9 (n = 195)	4.2 ± 0.6	3.5 ± 0.6
	3.5 ± 0.2	1.0 ± 0.1	14.2 ± 0.6	13.6 ± 0.4	8.4 ± 1.3 (n = 253)	3.1 ± 0.6 (n = 239)	3.7 ± 0.8	3.6 ± 0.6
	2.4 ± 0.2	2.0 ± 0.2	14.6 ± 0.5	11.2 ± 0.4	7.2 ± 1.1 (n = 265)	3.2 ± 0.6 (n = 230)	7.7 ± 1.4	3.7 ± 0.6
	2.1 ± 0.2	2.3 ± 0.2	14.7 ± 0.4	9.7 ± 0.5	6.2 ± 0.8 (n = 300)	5.4 ± 1.0 (n = 225)	7.4 ± 0.9	3.5 ± 0.7
	2.5 ± 0.2	1.7 ± 0.1	13.6 ± 0.6	8.2 ± 0.4	7.0 ± 1.0 (n = 320)	4.2 ± 0.9 (n = 211)	6.0 ± 1.1	3.3 ± 0.7
Mean ± S.E.M. per Group	2.6 ± 0.2	1.7 ± 0.2	14.8 ± 0.6	11.2 ± 1.0	6.8 ± 0.2	4.1 ± 0.4	5.8 ± 0.8	3.5 ± 0.1
Per Cent of 3-month-old group		65.4		75.7		60.4		60.3
Significance Level	P < 0.02		P < 0.02		P < 0.001		P < 0.05	

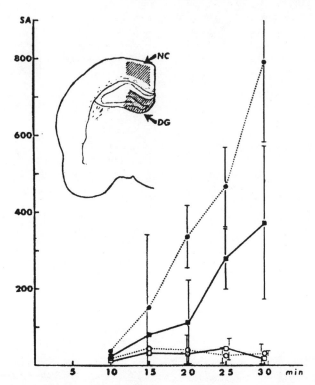

Fig. 2. Specific activities of the TCA-PTA-insoluble fractions of
the dentate gyrus (closed symbols) and neocortex (open symbols) at various time intervals after ^{3}H-fucose injection
into the medial septal nucleus of young adult (dotted line)
and senescent (solid line) rats. The dentate gyrus (DG)
with its hilus and the neocortex (NC) overlying the hippocampal formation were excised from a 1 mm thick coronal
brain section through the most rostral part of the dentate
gyrus (left upper corner). Each point on the graphs represents the mean specific activity obtained for a group of 5
rats, and 95% confidence intervals of the means are indicated by bars. Time after the end of ^{3}H-fucose injection is
plotted on the abscissa against specific activities of the
corresponding fraction on the ordinate (see reference 20).

and/or rate of glycoproteins transported to axonal terminals can be
expected to indicate a failure of presynaptic neurons to maintain the
integrity of their synaptic membranes in senescence.

Change in the Extraneuronal Microenvironment

The formation and maintenance of synaptic structure depends upon
adequate neuronal metabolism. Neuronal metabolism, in turn, depends

upon a physiological relationship between neurons, blood vessels sup-
plying them, and the extracellular space through which neuronal-vas-
cular exchanges occur. Although little is known about the vascular
compartment of aging Fischer-344 rats, it has been shown that the
blood-brain barrier, at least that to ^{14}C-sucrose, is intact at 28
months (21). It has been shown that the depth of penetration of
ruthenium red from the free ventricular surface into the substance of
the dentate gyrus decreases in the 25-month-old Fischer-344 rat (22),
indicating a change in charge density of intercellular polyanions in
the extracellular spaces of senescent brain. The nature of this
change is unknown, but it correlates directly with the 50% reduction
in volume of the extracellular space which was described in the rat
cerebral cortex by Bondareff and Narotzky (23).

This description of structure/function relationships in the senescent brain has focused on the rearrangement of structural components and the presumed relationship between this rearrangement and
faulty intraneuronal transport of glycoproteins. That the latter
might be more than merely temporarily related to structural alterations of synaptic membranes is suggested by two peculiarities of
neurons in senescent rats. First, a change in Concanavalin A binding patterns of neurons isolated from the lateral vestibular nuclei
of 24-month-old rats was demonstrated by fluorescence microscopy
(24). Second, a decrease in the sensitivity of cationized ferritin
binding capacity of synaptosomes isolated from the brains of senescent rats was demonstrated to neuraminidase (25). Both suggest age-
related changes in glycoprotein composition and are compatible with
structural changes in presynaptic membranes. It is unknown how such
changes might be related to functional impairment or to the
rearrangement of structural components in the dentate gyrus of senescent rats.

REFERENCES

1. A. Globus, Brain morphology as a function of presynaptic morphology and activity, in:"The Developmental Neuropsychology of
   Sensory Deprivation," H. Reisen, ed., Academic Press, New
   York (1975).
2. W. T. Greenough, R. W. West and T. J. DeVoogd, Subsynaptic plate
   perforations: Changes with age and experience in the rat,
   Science 202:1096 (1979).
3. P. W. Landfield and G. Lynch, Impaired monosynaptic potentiation
   in in vitro hippocampal slices from aged, memory-deficient
   rats, J. Gerontol. 32:523 (1977).
4. W. Bondareff and Y. Geinisman, Loss of synapses in the dentate
   gyrus of the senescent rat, Am. J. Anat. 145:129 (1976).
5. W. Bondareff, The neural basis of aging, in:"Handbook of the
   Psychology of Aging," J. E. Birren and K. W. Schaie, eds.,
   Van Nostrand Reinhold, New York (1976).

6. G. L. Coleman, S. W. Barthold, G. W. Osbaldiston, S. J. Foster, and A. M. Jones, Pathological changes during aging in barrier-reared Fischer-344 male rats, J. Gerontol. 32:258 (1977).

7. Y. Geinisman and W. Bondareff, Decrease in the number of synapses in the senescent brain: A quantitative electron microscopic analysis of the dentate gyrus molecular layer in the rat, Mech. Ageing Dev. 5:11 (1976).

8. Y. Geinisman, W. Bondareff, and J. T. Dodge, Partial deafferentation of neurons in the dentate gyrus of the senesent rat, Br. Res. 134:541 (1977).

9. M. L. Feldman, Aging changes in the morphology of cortical dendrites, in:"Neurobiology of Aging," R. D. Terry and S. Gershon, eds., Raven Press, New York (1976).

10. R. Glick, and W. Bondareff, Synapses in the cerebellar cortex of the senescent rat, J. Gerontol. (in press).

11. C. Sotelo and S. L. Palay, Altered axons and axon terminals in the lateral vestibular nucleus of the rat, Lab. Invest. 25:653 (1971).

12. D. W. Vaughan and A. Peters, Neuroglia cells in the cerebral cortex of rats from young adulthood to old age, J. Neurocyt. 3:405 (1974).

13. P. W. Landfield, G. Rose, L. Sandles, T. C. Wohlstadtes, and G. Lynch, Patterns of astroglial hypertrophy and neuronal degeneration in the hippocampus of aged, memory-deficient rats, J. Gerontol. 32:3 (1977).

14. Y. Geinisman, W. Bondareff, and J. T. Dodge, Hypertrophy of astroglial processes in the dentate gyrus of the senescent rat, Am. J. Anat. 153:3 (1978).

15. D. W. Vaughan, Age-related deterioration of pyramidal cell basal dendrites in the rat auditory cortex, J. Comp. Neur. 171:501 (1977).

16. J. W. Hinds and N.A. NcNelly, Aging of the rat olfactory bulb: Growth and atrophy of constituent layers and changes in size and number of mitral cells, J. Comp. Neur. 171:345 (1977).

17. M. E. Scheibel, R. D. Lindsay, U. Tomiyasu and A. B. Scheibel, Progressive dendritic changes in aging human cortex, Expt. Neurol. 47:392 (1975).

18. M. E. Scheibel, R. D. Lindsay, U. Tomiyasu and A. B. Scheibel, Progressive dendritic changes in aging human limbic system, Ep. Neurol. 53:420 (1976).

19. Y. Geinisman, W. Bondareff, and J. T. Dodge, Dendritic atrophy in the dentate gyrus of the senescent rat, Am. J. Anat. 152:321 (1978).

20. Y. Geinisman, Y. Bondareff, and A. Telser, Transport of ^{3}H-fucose labeled glycoproteins in the septo-hippocampal pathway of young adult and senescent rats, Br. Res. 125:182 (1977).

21. S. I. Rapoport, K. Ohno, and K. D. Pettigrew, Society for Neuroscience Abstracts (1978).

22. W. Bondareff and S. Lin-Liu, Age-related change in the neuronal
     microenvironment: Penetration of ruthenium red into
     extracellular space of brain in young adult and senescent
     rats, Am. J. Anat. 148:57 (1977).
23. W. Bondareff and R. Narotzky, Age changes in the neuronal
     microenvironment, Science 176:1135 (1972).
24. K. D. Bennett and W. Bondareff, Age-related differences in
     binding of Concanavalin A to plasma membranes of isolated
     neurons, Am. J. Anat. 150:175 (1977).
25. S. Lin-Liu and W. Bondareff (unpublished).

ROLE OF THE IMMUNE SYSTEM IN AGING[*]

Takashi Makinodan

Geriatric Research, Education and Clinical Center (GRECC)
Wadsworth Medical Center
Los Angeles, CA 90073
and the Department of Medicine, UCLA
Los Angeles, CA 90024

INTRODUCTION

Since the turn of the century, there has been a continuum of medical breakthroughs controlling life-shortening diseases. As a consequence, more people are now living longer than they were at the turn of the century. Unfortunately, life extension means chronic disorders to many of the elderly. This has created a trememdous socio-economic burden throughout the world. Thus, during the past decade, there has been a growing emphasis in biomedical research towards control of age-related chronic disorders, in order to enable the elderly to extend their healthy years of life.

To this end, various physiologic systems are being investigated, with the major emphasis on those with systemic homeostatic functions. Among them is the immune system. It is an attractive model system for the following reasons: (a) loss of immunologic vigor is one of the characteristics of perhaps all aging mammals; (b) the decline in normal functions of the immune system seems to trigger infectious, neoplastic, autoimmune and immune complex diseases; (c) the pattern of rise and fall in activity of the immune system with age is inversely related to the death rate; (d) our understanding of the immune system's differentiation process at the cellular, molecular and genetic levels is more comprehensive than that of perhaps

[*]This is publication no. 026 from GRECC, VA Wadsworth Medical Center, which has been supported in part by The Medical Research Service of VA and the Department of Energy (Grant no. ET 76-S-03-0034 P.A. 264).

213

any other system, and therefore it appears to be amenable to successful manipulation; and (e) circumvention of the declining function of
the immune system may minimize the severity of diseases of the elderly.

My task is to present an overview of the two major issues con-
fronting us on aging and immunity or immunologic aging. One is at
the cellular level and the other at the organismic level. At the
cellular level, it concerns the nature of decline in normal immunologic vigor with age. At the organismic level, it concerns the causal
nature of the inverse relationship between immunologic aging and
increase in susceptibility to various diseases. These discussions
will be preceded by a brief discussion of age-related changes in
immune functions.

LOSS OF IMMUNOLOGIC VIGOR WITH AGE--IMMUNOLOGIC AGING

The immune system protects the body in a highly specific manner
against foreign invasion by viruses, bacteria, fungi and protozoans,
and against one's own somatic cells which have been damaged or under-
gone transformation into cancer cells. Obviously, any factor or
event that can decrease the normal surveillance activity of the
immune system will permit growth of invasive antigens (e.g., bacteria
and cancer cells) which can, in turn, disrupt various physiological
functions of the body. Hence, it should be apparent that the immune
system plays a major role in the preservation of life.

The bone marrow, thymus, spleen and lymph nodes comprise the
major organs of the mammalian immune system. The bone marrow and
thymus are generally referred to as the primary or central organs of
the immune system because they become lymphocytic first in embryogenesis, and thereafter serve as the source of precursor cells. The
spleen and lymph nodes, on the other hand, are referred to as secondary or peripheral organs. It is in these peripheral organs that
immunity is initiated. The cells of the immune system can be subdi-
vided into (a) stem cells, (b) thymus-derived T lymphocytes, (c) bone
marrow-derived B lymphocytes, which upon antigen stimulation give
rise to plasma cells, and (d) macrophages. In a typical immune response, the latter three cell types communicate with each other in a
highly specific manner, and undergo proliferation and maturation
(i.e., clonal differentiation).

In general, immunologic activity increases rapidly after birth to
a peak level at sexual maturity followed by a gradual decline. The
onset and rate of decline, however, will vary with the type of immune
response and the species. The decline with age appears to be characteristic of aging mammals, as it has been observed not only in
humans (1), but also in all experimental mammals examined (2-7).
Therefore, it has been commonly referred to as "immunologic aging."

Moreover, as with immunodeficient children (8) and immunosuppressed
adults (9), the decline is associated with an increase in the incidence of infectious, autoimmune, immune complex, and cancerous diseases (1,10). Thus, there are two major issues in Immunogerontology. At the cellular level, it concerns the nature of cellular and
humoral changes responsible for immunologic aging. At the organismic
level, it concerns the causal nature of the inverse relationship
between immunologic aging and the increase in susceptibility to immunologically involved diseases of aging (infections, autoimmune and
immune complex diseases, cancer, amyloidosis, etc.).

FACTORS RESPONSIBLE FOR IMMUNOLOGIC AGING

The immunologic network is highly complex and multifaceted, so
the multifactorial etiology of immunologic aging should not be a sur-
prise (1,10-14). At the tissue level, changes in both the environment and the immune cells have been shown to be responsible.

Very little is known of the nature of the responsible factor(s)
in the cellular environment, but the findings indicate that two types
of factors are involved: deleterious substances of molecular and
viral natures, and essential substances of nutritional and hormonal
natures. Support for the first possibility came initially from the
cell-impermeable diffusion chamber studies by Price and Makinodan
(15), who showed that young mouse cells can be inhibited in their
immunologic performance when exposed to in vivo plasma fluid factors
of old mice. More recently, Rivnay et al. (16) found that the lipid
microviscosity is 20% higher in the plasma membrane of lymphocytes of
old than that of young mice, due mainly to the age-related elevation
of the cholesterol/phospholipid ratio. Elevation in lipid microviscosity could be a major contributory factor in the kinetic sluggish-
ness of old cells, as it can decrease the rate of protein diffusion.
Support for the second possibility comes from the observation of Bach
et al. (17), who found that secretion of thymic factors essential for
T cell maturation decreases with age in parallel with thymic involution, and of Bilder and Denkla (18), who found that hypophysectomy
plus hormonal replacement therapy had a pronounced immunorestorative
effect on old but not young rats.

There are 3 possible types of cellular changes which can cause
immunologic aging: (a) an absolute decrease in the number of antigen-responsive cells through cell death caused possibly by autoimmune
cells or by the Hayflick phenomenon (19), (b) functional alteration
of immune cells caused by genetic and epigenetic events, and (c) a
relative decrease in the number of antigen-responsive cells as a
result of interference by specific and nonspecific factors. Studies
over the past decade show that all 3 types of change do indeed occur
with age. Perhaps the least dramatic and consistent is the decrease
in number of antigen-responsive cells, which varies with population

sampling, ranging from no change with age to only a modest decrease
(10). Changes intrinsic to immune cells include findings such as:

a) Decrease with age in the number of surface theta receptor
   antigens of mouse splenic T cells (20), which differentiate into stem cells, T cells, B cells and macrophages.
b) Increase with age in the frequency of aneuploidy in circulating human T cells (21).
c) Decrease with age in the number of nuclear actinomycin
   binding sites in circulating human lymphocytes (22).
d) Decrease with age in nuclear histone acetylation of circulating human lymphocytes (23).
e) Decrease with age in the ability of mouse bone marrow
   stem cells to repair ionizing radiation-induced DNA
   damage (24).
f) Decrease with age in the Fc receptor-mediated immunoregulation of mouse splenic B cells (25).
g) Decrease with age in the ratio of cyclic AMP/cyclic GMP
   levels of unstimulated and stimulated mouse spleen cells
   (26).

Changes caused by alteration in the regulatory factors with age
include such findings as:

a) The inability of precursor cells of old mice to interact
   with each other as efficiently as those of young mice in
   response to antigenic stimulation (15,27,28).
b) An increase with age in the number of suppressor T and B
   cells (28-30).
c) A decrease with age in the number of suppressor T cells
   in short-lived autoimmune-susceptible mice and in humans
   (31-33).
d) An increase with age in the number of helper T cells in
   humans (33).
e) A decrease with age in the ability of carrier-primed
   mouse T cells to enhance B cells in their antibody
   response (34).
f) A parabolic pattern of change with age in the avidity of
   antibody (35).

RELATIONSHIP BETWEEN IMMUNOLOGIC AGING AND DISEASES OF AGING

An issue that has not been resolved satisfactorily is whether the
decline to a threshold level predisposes an individual to disease, or
whether disease compromises normal immunologic activities. Circumstantial evidence tends to favor the former possibility.

One appproach toward resolving this issue is to perturb the
immune system of adult individuals before their normal activities

decline, and then to assess the immunologic, pathologic, and actuarial changes kinetically. The system can be perturbed by altering
either the onset of the decline and/or the rate of decline. Another
approach is to perturb the immune system of old individuals whose
normal immune functions are already reduced, and then assess the
immunologic, pathologic and actuarial changes kinetically. The system can be perturbed by further reductive, by preventive, or by restorative means. Although all three approaches should be attempted to
resolve this complex triangular relationship of aging, decreased
immune function and increased incidence of disease, the latter two
approaches are preferred. They would lend themselves more effectively
to the study of both cellular and molecular mechanisms responsible
for the decline in normal immunologic activities with age. For these
reasons the discussion will be limited to these latter approaches.

Intervention by Preventive Methods

Internal Body Temperature Control. Liu and Walford demonstrated
that the life span of an annual fish can be extended by subjecting it
to mild hypothermia during the last half of its life (36). The immunologic implication of this observation is intriguing. However, further studies are required to understand the significance of the life
extending effect of hypothermia on the relationship between immunity
and disease.

Tissue Ablation. In controlling a disease that can disrupt normal immune functions and shorten the life span, one approach is to
remove the tissue from which a disease originates or that promotes it
(provided the tissue is not essential). This approach was first
employed successfully by Furth over 30 years ago (37). He thymectomized a short-lived, thymoma-susceptible AKR strain of mice at young
adulthood. The incidence of leukemia decreased drastically; as a
consequence, the mice lived significantly longer. This approach was
also used successfully by us in long-lived hybrid mice (38). We
found that the survival time of mice splenectomized at about 100
weeks of age can be nearly doubled over that of sham-splenectomized
mice. Splenectomy was performed at about 100 weeks because previous
studies had shown that many old mice were dying at about 2 years of
age of reticulum cell sarcoma originating in the spleen (39).

Although this method is not practical in humans, it could be used
in experimental animals to resolve the types of diseases emerging
late in life that can compromise general and specific immune functions.

Genetic Manipulation. Genetic manipulation has been performed in
both long-lived and short-lived strains of mice In studies with
long-lived mice, it was reasoned that aging is influenced genetically
by only a limited number of regulatory genes, that the immune system

plays a major role in aging (40), and that a "super-regulatory gene complex system" of the immune system (41), i.e., the H-2 region of chromosome 17 in the mouse and the HLA region of chromosome 6 in the human, is the major histocompatibility complex (MHC) system. Inbred congenic strains of mice differing only at the H-2 region were therefore assessed for their age-related immune functions, age-specific diseases and life spans (42,43). Variation in these parameters between congenic mice within a given inbred strain was as great as that observed between different inbred strains of mice. One would have expected a greater uniformity in life span, immunologically associated disease pattern, and immunologic activities between congenic sets of mice within an inbred strain than between inbred strains, if the MHC system in the mouse did not exert a significant influence upon aging, age-related immunologic abnormalities and life span. It can be argued, therefore, that the MHC system plays a major role in age-associated immunologic abnormalities and life span in mice.

The focus with short-lived mice has been on susceptibility to autoimmune and immune complex manifestations (44). These studies showed that more than one gene is involved in susceptibility to autoimmune and immune complex diseases. An example is reflected in a comparison of life spans of different inbred mouse strains and their hybrids; e.g., the mean life span of autoimmune-susceptible NZB, NZW, (NZB x NZW)F_1, (NZB x CBA)F_1 and nonautoimmune-susceptible CBA mice were 12, 21, 12, 29, and 28 months, respectively.

Genetic manipulation is not practical in humans, but it can be used to dissociate the relative roles that genetic and environmental factors play in aging. To this end, Greenberg and Yunis have been studying the influence of HLA haplotype on immune responsiveness and life span in aging humans (45).

Dietary Manipulation. About 45 years ago, McCay et al. (46) first discovered that the life span of rats can be extended significantly by restricting their caloric intake during growth. Recently a more exhaustive study was carried out, also in rats, by Ross and Bras (47,48) that confirmed and extended the classical work. They found that early caloric restriction decelerates the aging rate, as judged by age-related biochemical and pathological changes. Walford et al. (49) subsequently demonstrated that the immune systems of long-lived mice subjected to a calorically restricted but nutritionally supplemented diet, mature slowly and manifest age-associated changes belatedly. Fernandes et al. (50,51) showed that a diet high in fat and relatively low in protein, which favors reproduction in experimental rodents, significantly increased cell-mediated autoimmune manifestations and shortened the life expectancy of short-lived, autoimmune-susceptible mice. In contrast, a diet low in fat, which is less favorable for reproduction, decreased autoimmune manifestations and prolonged the life expectancy of these mice. Further, they showed that the life span of these short-lived autoimmune-susceptible mice can be dramatically extended by restricting their caloric intake (52).

Intervention by Restorative Methods

Tissue Ablation. As mentioned earlier, the tissue ablation approach, has been used as a preventive method. It has also been recently used very effectively by Bilder and Denckla in an attempt to restore normal immune functions (18). Denckla hypothesized that hypothyroidism in old individuals could be caused by a substance(s) secreted by the pituitary that competes with thyroid hormones for the same target cell receptors, including those of the immune system, and that secretion of the substance begins shortly after sexual maturity (53). He reasoned that if this were correct, hypophysectomy of aging individuals supplemented with standard hormone replacement therapy should have a beneficial effect. Accordingly, old and young rats were hypophysectomized and subjected to hormone replacement therapy. The results showed that hypophysectomy had a pronounced immunorestorative effect on old rats, but had no effect on young rats.

This method is not practical in humans. However, hypophysectomized old rats could be used to resolve the problem of the relationship between the immune system's "aging clock" and its extrinsic "pacemaker." Moreover, if the pituitary substance can be purified, a specific antiserum reagent could be prepared and used clinically. It appears, then, that this type of tissue ablation study has both basic and clinical importance.

Cell Grafting. Grafting of thymus, spleen, lymph nodes and bone marrow has been attempted individually or in combinations in genetically compatible old recipients with varying success in terms of immunologic restoration and extension of life span.

Fabris et al. demonstratrated most impressively that the life span of short-lived, growth-hormone deficient, hypopituitary dwarf mice can be extended as much as 3- to 4-fold by injecting large doses of lymph node cells (54). A comparable life-prolonging effect was obtained by injecting growth hormone and thyroxin into dwarf mice with intact thymi, but not into dwarf mice whose thymi had been removed beforehand. These results indicate that the pituitary "turns on" the immune system through the thymus, and the T cells "turn on" the endocrine system through the pituitary. Injection of young spleen or thymus cells into old, autoimmune-susceptible, short-lived mice has had less spectacular results. The appearance of certain types of auto-antibodies (55) was delayed, but not prevented permanently, and the life-prolonging effect was minimal (56). Similarly, multiple thymus grafts did extend their life expectancy, but only by 1 month (57). Furthermore, the age-associated pathological changes were unaltered by these treatments (58).

The first attempts to graft young thymus or bone marrow cells into old nonautoimmune-susceptible, long-lived mice were also not too encouraging, as the life span was not extended appreciably, nor was the immune response elevated (59,60). Subsequent studies on the mechanism of decline with age in normal immune functions suggested to us the reason that these earlier cell grafting attempts were not successful. These studies revealed that the loss of immunologic vigor is due in part to changes in the T cell population (61), in part to the reduced rate at which stem cells can self-generate and generate progeny cells (62), and in part to the inability of involuted thymus to transform precursor cells to T cells efficiently (63). Therefore, we exposed long lived old mice to low dose radiation to destroy most of their immune cells and grafted into them both newborn thymus and young adult bone marrow stem cells. This treatment restored their immune functions to levels approaching those of adult mice (64) for at least six months after graft treatment in mice with a normal mean life span of 27 months (an equivalent to 0.22 of a mean mouse life span, or about 15 human years). Current immunorestorative studies by cell grafting should resolve what influence, if any, grafting will have on the frequency and severity of diseases of the aged and whether cell grafting can alter the life expectancy of short-lived and long-lived mice.

Studies by Perkins et al. (65) on susceptibility to infection have also generated encouraging data. These showed that old mice can be made to resist lethal doses of virulent Salmonella typhimurium by injecting them before exposure with spleen cells from young genetically compatible mice which had been immunized with the vaccine. Their findings also indicated that sensitized spleen cells can persist in the recipients for a long time after injection, and that spleen cells can be stored cryogenically for an extended period of time without loss of immunologic activity. This means that the method of Perkins et al. (65) may have a practical application in random bred species.

Chemical Therapy. Only a few chemical agents have been shown to possess immunorestorative activity. These include thymic hormones, certain free radical inhibitors (antioxidants), double-stranded polynucleotide, and mercaptoethanol.

It seems obvious that thymic hormones will be used to prevent immunologic aging or restore immunologic vigor, since the loss of the latter has been clearly shown to be associated with the failure of thymus to continue synthesizing T cell maturation hormones (17,63). Surprisingly, however, there has been no systematic study on their effectiveness in preventing immunologic aging, and studies on their use as immunorestorative agents have been few--but nevertheless encouraging. Friedman et al. (66) found that thymus humoral factor (THF), prepared by N. Trainin, can enhance the T cell dependent graft-vs-host activity in vitro of spleen cells from old but not

young mice. This would indicate that THF is not acting as a non-
specific adjuvant agent. Otherwise, THF also would have enhanced the
activity of young spleen cells. Less encouraging are the preliminary
findings of Bach (67). Using T cell-dependent lymphocyte-mediated
cytotoxicity (LMC) as the assay, she found that circulating thymic
factor (TF) treatment in vivo is effective in preventing the accelerated decline in LMC activity of adult thymectomized mice, but
ineffective in normal young and middle-aged (75-86 weeks old) mice.
It would appear that TF may be promoting the emergence of suppressor
cells in these normal mice. Whether or not it would be effective in
old mice, as demonstrated by Friedman et al. (66), remains to be
proven.

Weksler et al. (68) were able to partially restore the antibody-
forming capacity of old spleen cells by exposing them to another
preparation of thymic hormones, thymopoietin. In contrast, Martinez
et al. (69) failed to demonstrate the effectiveness of thymopoietin,
ubiquitin and synthetic serum thymic factor, prepared by G. Goldstein, in restoring T cell mitogenic response and resistance to tumor
cells. The test mice were thymectomized either neonatally or at 1
month of age, and then subjected to treatment with one of the hormones. Unfortunately, no attempt was made to assess the effectiveness of a mixture of these hormones. According to A. Goldstein (70),
T cell maturation requires many steps, and several different types of
thymic hormones are necessary for the generation of mature functional
T cells.

A. Goldstein et al. (70) using still another preparation of thymic hormone, thymosin, have found that repeated injections of the
hormone can alleviate many of the symptoms in mice and humans manifesting immunodeficiency diseases. In addition, repeated injection
of thymosin may also have immunorestorative effect on elderly humans
manifesting reduced T cell-dependent immune functions according to a
recent preliminary report showing that the number of T cells of old
individuals can be increased by exposing their white blood cells to
thymosin in vitro (71). However, before assessing the effect of thymosin on elderly individuals, it would seem prudent to carry out
animal studies; i.e., assess the effects of repeated injection into
aging short-lived and long-lived mice on their normal immune functions, disease patterns and life spans.

The use of free radical inhibitors stems from the hypothesis that
aging is caused by somatic mutation (72), and, consequently, excess
formation of free radicals should enhance aging, and the use of
inhibitors delay aging (73). It was further reasoned that since the
immune system plays a major role in aging (12), these agents should
enhance immune functions of aging individuals. This notion was
tested by Harman et al. (74) who incorporated these chemical agents
into the diet of aging mice. Their preliminary results indicate that
vitamin E and other free radical inhibitors can enhance the antibody

response of adult and middle-aged (88 weeks) mice. These studies are
being extended to assess the effectiveness of these agents on immune
functions, disease pattern and life span of older mice. In a related
study, Bliznakov (75) found that coenzyme Q_{10}, a nonspecific stimu-
lant of mitochondrial electron transport, can enhance the level of
antibody response of 2-year-old mice to that approaching adult mice.
Both of these studies will require further investigation to identify
the target cell(s) and the mechanism of action of these agents.

Braun et al. (76) were the first to demonstrate that double-
stranded polynucleotides (e.g., polyadenlic-polyuridylic acid complexes) can restore the T cell-dependent antibody response of middle
aged long-lived mice to that of young adult mice. Han and Johnson
(77) not only confirmed this observation, but proceeded to demonstrate that the supernatant of cultures of thymocytes treated with
double-stranded polynucleotides is equally effective as a immunorestorative agent. This suggests that the double-stranded polynucleotide restores immunologic vigor to aging mice by acting on T cells.
Further studies are required to determine its mechanism of action on
T cells and other immune cells, on both disease pattern and life
span. One insight into a possible mechanism of action at the membrane level comes from an observation by Schmidt and Douglas (78),
who found that double- and triple-stranded, but not single-stranded,
polynucleotides increase the IgG binding activity of human monocytes
in vitro. This would indicate that multi-stranded polynucleotides
stimulate either by unmasking or by stimulating more synthesis of
surface IgG binding receptors.

About a decade ago, when we became interested in intervention, we
decided on the restorative method. We felt that a successful immunorestorative method would lend itself more effectively to the study of
both cellular and molecular mechanisms responsible for the decline in
normal immunologic activities with age. In our initial effort,
immunorestoration of old mice was attempted by replacing their immune
cells with those from syngeneic young mice (65). This was done by
injecting spleen cells from young donors which had been previously
immunized with Salmonella typhimurium vaccine into old mice that had
received no prior treatment. Following this procedure, the old mice
were able to resist lethal doses of virulent Salmonella typhimurium
for an extended period of time. We then found that the combined
treatment of old mice with 400 R of X-rays to destroy most of their
radiosensitive immune cells, followed by injection of bone marrow
cells and implantation of thymic tissues from young syngeneic donors
can elevate the T cell dependent antibody response and T cell proliferative activity of the old mice to levels approaching those of young
adult mice for an extended period (64). These results suggest that a
cell replacement method could be used as a probe to identify the
cell(s) responsible for the decline in immunologic vigor with age.
However, its effectiveness as a molecular probe appears to be limited.

We therefore decided to focus our effort on chemically defined agents that are effective at the cellular level. We chose 2-mercaptoethanol (2-ME) because sulfhydryl compounds have been employed effectively in enhancing various nonimmunologic and immunologic cel lular activities in vitro (79-85), and because 2-ME is a simple 2-carbon compound effective at very low concentrations. We found that the reduced in vitro T cell-dependent antibody forming activities of spleen cells from four out of four genetically-defined old long-lived mice strains can be restored to levels approaching those of young adult mice by exposing the cells to 2-ME at very low concentration (4 μg/ml) (86-88). We demonstrated that the enhancing effect of 2-ME on old spleen cells is greater than that on young spleen cells, as judged by 2 different criteria. That is, the effect of 2-ME on old spleen cells was an order of magnitude greater than that on young spleen cells, in terms of its magnitude of enhancement of the antibody forming capacity of an optimum number of spleen cells, (i.e., 500 versus 30% enhancement). In terms of its ability to transform antigen-stimulated, nonantibody-responding cultures containing limiting numbers of spleen cells into antibody-responding cultures, the effect of 2-ME on old spleen cells was 6.5 times greater than that on young spleen cells.

We demonstrated that 2-ME is an effective immunorestorative agent in intact old mice by restoring the T cell-dependent antibody responding capacity of long-lived old mice to the level of young mice with appropriate doses (87-89). These results suggest that 2-ME and related chemicals may have practical applications.

The mode of action of 2-ME is not known. This is not surprising in view of the multitude of possible biochemical effects sulfhydryl compounds can have on cell structure and functions, ranging from SH/SS exchange reactions at the membrane level to the antioxidant and metal chelating effects (79,80,84). Moreover, various types of immunologic processes have been shown to benefit from the presence of 2-ME, including antibody response (81), mitogentic response of T and B cells to plant lectins (80,82,90), B cell colony formation (91), mixed lymphocyte reaction (83,92) and cytolytic killer T cell formation (93,94).

All three major cell types have been implicated as the target of 2-ME (80-83,90-95), as well as serum factor(s) in the tissue culture medium (90,95). Finally, it should be emphasized that in previous immunoenhancing studies of 2-ME, the source of immune cells has been limited to young adult donors whose magnitude of response in the presence of 2-ME, as demonstrated here, is not enhanced by more than two-fold (100%). Logistically, this could make it difficult to resolve the molecular mechanism of the enhancing action of 2-ME. The use of immune cells of old donors is therefore of obvious advantage, for, at a concentration as low as 4 μg/ml, 2-ME can enhance the primary antibody response of old spleen cells by as much as 11-fold

(1100%) (86-88). For these reasons, we are using 2-ME as a molecular
probe to study the nature and mechanism of age-associated decline in
normal immunologic activities.

CONCLUSION

The field of immunogerontology is still in its scientific
infancy, but the immune system has already shown tremendous promise
both as an experimental model for cellular and molecular aging and as
a clinical model for diseases of the elderly.

What emerges from studies on the etiology of immunologic aging is
that as individuals become old they lose their immunologic vigor
primarily as a result of changes affecting the normal differentiation
pathway of T cells. Consequently, aging individuals become susceptible to attack by microbial and other naturally occurring intrinsic
and extrinsic agents (e.g., mutated cancer cells) that are routinely
destroyed by T cells in healthy adults.

Six model intervention approaches have been used in attempts to
prevent immunologic aging and to restore normal immunologic vigor.
These studies are preliminary, but overall, the findings are most
encouraging. Of the six approaches, genetic manipulation and
chemical therapy appear to be most promising to use as probes in
understanding the biochemical nature and mechanism(s) of the immune
decline. The genetic approach should enable us to determine which
gene(s) is primarily responsible for the decline in normal immune
functions with age and the diseases associated with it. The chemical approach should enable us to determine the cell type(s) that is
most severely affected functionally as well as the nature of associated changes at the subcellular level. However, dietary manipulation
and chemical therapy appear to be the most promising in controlling
immunologic aging, in terms of practical application. Cell grafting
also appears to be promising. Perhaps the most effective approach in
controlling immunologic aging is a combination of dietary manipulation, chemical therapy and cell grafting.

We still do not know what triggers the loss of immunologic vigor
as individuals age. We may know in the near future, however, judging
by the recent advances in areas such as genetic and chemical manipu-
lations of immune functions. While the former approach is not appropriate in humans, no doubt clinical applications will arise from a
better understanding of the specific genetic determinants of immunologic aging and its many consequences. The latter approach not only
offers an understanding of age-related changes in cellular and subcellular function, but direct clinical applications as well. As we
are now in the process of unravelling these puzzles, it is not
unreasonable to predict that either retardation of immune decline or
restoration of immune vigor in humans will be clinically feasible in
the not too distant future.

REFERENCES

1. I. R. Mackay, Ageing and immunological function in man,
    Gerontologia 18:285 (1972).
2. H. Baer and R. T. owser, Antibody production and development
    of contact skin sensitivity in guinea pigs of various ages,
    Science 140:1211 (1963).
3. G. E. Bilder, Studies on immune competence in the rat: Changes
    with age, sex, and strain, J. Gerontol. 30:641 (1975).
4. B. N. Jaroslow, K. M. Suhrbier, and T. E. Fritz, Decline and
    restoration of antibody forming capacity in aging beagle
    dogs, J. Immunol. 112:1467 (1974).
5. T. Makinodan, and W. J. Peterson, Relative antibody-forming
    capacity of spleen cells as a function of age, Proc. Nat.
    Acad. Sci. U.S. 48:234 (1962).
6. M. Mathies, L. Lipps, G. S. Smith, and R. L. Walford, Age
    related decline in response to phytohemagglutinin and
    pokeweed mitogen by spleen cells from hamster and a long-
    lived mouse strain, J. Gerontol. 28:425 (1973).
7. T. A. Nomaguchi, Y. Okuma-Sakurai, I. and Kimura, Changes in
    immunological potential between juvenile and presenile
    rabbits, Mech. Ageing Dev. 5:409 (1976).
8. H. H. Fudenberg, R. A. Good, H. C. Goodman, W. Hitzig, H. G.
    Kunkel, I. M. Roitt, F. S. Rosen, D. S. Rowe, M.
    Seligmann, and J. R. Soothill, Primary immunodeficiencies,
    Bull. WHO 45:125 (1975).
9. I. Penn, and T. E. Starzl, Malignant tumors arising de novo in
    immunosuppressed organ transplant recipients,
    Transplantation 14:407 (1972).
10. M. M. B. Kay, and T. Makinodan, Immunobiology of aging:
    Evaluation of current status, Clin. Immunol. Immunopathol.
    6:394 (1976).
11. "Tolerance, Autoimmunity and Aging," M. M. Seigel, and R. A.
    Good, eds., Charles C. Thomas, Springfield, Ill. (1972).
12. R. L. Walford, The immunologic theory of aging, current
    status. Fed. Proc. 33:2020 (1974).
13. "Immunology and Aging," T. Makinodan, and E. J. Yunis, eds.,
    Plenum Medical Book Company, New York (1977).
14. D. Segre, and M. Segre, Age-related changes in B and T lympho-
    cytes and decline of humoral immune responsiveness in aged
    mice, Mech. Ageing Dev. 6:115-129 (1977).
15. G. B. Price, and T. Makinodan, Immunologic deficiencies in
    senescence. II. Characterization of extrinsic
    deficiencies. J. Immunol. 108:413 (1972).
16. B. Rivnay, A. Globerson, and M. Shinitzky, Viscosity of
    lymphocyte plasma membrane in aging mice and its possible
    relation to serum cholesterol, Mech. Ageing Dev. 10:71
    (1979).

17. F. J. Bach, M. Dardenne, and J. C. Solomon, Studies on thymus products. IV. Absence of serum thymic activity in adult NZB and (NZB x NZW)F1 mice, Clin. Exp. Immunol. 14:247 (1973).

18. G. E. Bilder, and W. D. Denckla, Restoration of ability to reject xenografts and clear carbon after hypophysectomy of adult rats, Mech. Ageing Dev. 6:153 (1977).

19. L. Hayflick, and P. S. Moorhead, The serial cultivation of human diploid cell strains, Exp. Cell Res. 25:585 (1961).

20. P. C. Brennan, and B. N. Jaroslow, Age-associated decline in theta antigen on spleen thymus-derived lymphocytes of B6CF$_1$ mice, Cell. Immunol. 15:51 (1975).

21. P. A. Jacobs, and W. M. Court Brown, Distribution of human chromosome counts in relation to age, Nature 191:1178 (1961).

22. A. M. Preumont, P. Van Gansen, and J. Brachet, Cytochemical study of human lymphocytes stimulated by PHA in function of donor age, Mech. Ageing Dev. 7:25 (1978).

23. Y. H. Oh, and R. A. Conrad, Effect of aging on acetate incorporation in nuclei of lymphocytes stimulated with phytohemagglutinin. Life Sciences 11:677 (1972).

24. M. G. Chen, Impaired Elkind recovery in hematopoeitic colony-forming cells of aged mice. Proc. Soc. Exp. Biol. Med. 145:1181 (1974)

25. D. J. Scribner, H. L. Weiner, and J. W. Moorhead, Anti-immuno-globulin stimulation of murine lymphocytes. V. Age-related decline in Fc receptor-mediated immunoregulation. J. Immunol. 121:377 (1978).

26. C. F. Tam, and R. L. Walford, Cyclic nucleotide levels in resting and mitogen-stimulated spleen cell suspensions from young and old mice, Mech. Ageing Dev. 7:309 (1978).

27. G. B. Price, and T. Makinodan, Immunologic deficiencies in senescence. I. Characterization of intrinsic deficiencies. J. Immunol. 108:403 (1972).

28. R. E. Callard, and A. Basten, Immune function in aged mice. IV. Loss of T cell and B cell function in thymus-dependent antibody response, Eur. J. Immunol. 8:552 (1978).

29. T. Makinodan, J. W. Albright, P. I. Good, C. P. Peter, and M. L. Heidrick, Reduced humoral immune activity in long-lived old mice: An approach to elucidating its mechanisms, Immunology 31:903 (1976).

30. D. Segre, and M. Segre, Humoral immunity in aged mice. II. Increased suppressor T cell activity in immunologically deficient old mice, J. Immunol. 116:735 (1976).

31. N. L. Gerber, J. A. Hardin, T. M. Chused, and A. D. Steinberg, Loss with age in NZB/W mice of thymic suppressor cells in the graft-versus-host reaction, J. Immunol. 113:1618 (1974).

32. H. M. Hallgren, and E. J. Yunis, Suppressor lymphocytes in young and aged humans, J. Immunol. 118:2004 (1977).

33. S. Gupta, and R. A. Good, Subpopulations of human T lympho-
    cytes. X. Alterations in T, B, third population cells, and
    T cells with receptors for immunoglobulin M(tγ) or G(Tμ) in
    aging humans, J. Immunol. 122:1214 (1979).

34. R. L. Krogsrud, and E. H. Perkins, Age-related changes in T
    cell function, J. Immunol. 118:1607 (1977).

35. G. Doria, G. D'Agostaro, and A. Poretti, Age-dependent
    variation of antibody avidity, Immunology 38:601 (1978).

36. R. K. Liu, and R. L. Walford, Mid-life temperature-transfer
    effects on life span of annual fish, J. Gerontol. 30:129
    (1975).

37. J. Furth, Prolongation of life with prevention of leukemia by
    thymectomy in mice, J. Gerontol. 1:46 (1946).

38. J. W. Albright, T. Makinodan, and J. W. Deitchman, Presence of
    life-shortening factors in spleens of aged mice of long life
    span and extension of life expectancy by splenectomy, Exp.
    Gerontol. 4:267 (1969).

39. F. Chino, T. Makinodan, W. E. Lever, and W. J. Peterson, The
    immune systems of mice reared in clean and in dirty
    conventional laboratory farms. I. Life expectancy and
    pathology of mice with long life spans, J. Gerontol. 26:497
    (1971).

40. R. L. Walford, The immunologic theory of aging, current status,
    Fed. Proc. 33:2020 (1974).

41. "Immunogenetics and Immunodeficiency," B. Benacerraf, ed.,
    University Park Press, Baltimore (1975).

42. G. S. Smith, and R. L. Walford, Influence of the main histo-
    compatibility complex on aging in mice, Nature 270:727
    (1977).

43. P. J. Meredith, and R. L. Walford, Effect of age on response to
    T and B cell mitogens in mice congenic at the H-2 locus,
    Immunogenetics 5:109 (1978).

44. G. Fernandes, R. A. Good, and E. J. Yunis, Attempts to correct
    age-related immunodeficiency and autoimmunity by cellular
    and dietary manipulation in inbred mice, in:"Immunology and
    Aging," T. Makinodan and E. J. Yunis, eds., Plenum Medical
    Book Company, New York (1977).

45. L. J. Greenberg, and E. J. Yunis, Histocompatibility determi-
    nants, immune responsiveness and aging in mice, Fed. Proc.
    37:1258 (1978).

46. C. M. McCay, M. F. Crowell, and L. A. Maynard, The effect of
    retarded growth upon the length of life span and upon the
    ultimate body size, J. Nutrition 10:63 (1935).

47. M. H. Ross, Aging, nutrition, and hepatic enzyme activity
    patterns in the rat, J. Nutrition Suppl 1, part 2, 97:565
    (1969).

48. M. H. Ross, and G. Bras, Lasting influence of early caloric
    restriction on prevalence of neoplasia in the rat, J. Nat.
    Cancer Inst. 47:1095 (1971).

49. R. L. Walford, R. K. Liu, M. Mathies, M. Gerbase-DeLima, and
    G. S. Smith, Response to sheep red blood cells and to
    mitogenic agents, Mech. Ageing Dev. 2:447 (1974).

50. G. Fernandes, E. J. Yunis, D. G. Jose, R. A. and Good, Dietary
    influence on antinuclear antibodies and cell-mediated
    immunity in NZB mice, Int. Arch. Allergy Appl. Immunol.
    44:770 (1973).

51. B. Fernandes, E. J. Yunis, J. Smith, and R. A. Good, Dietary
    influence on breeding behavior, hemolytic anemia, and
    longevity in NZB mice, Proc. Soc. Exp. Biol. Med. 139:1189
    (1972).

52. G. Fernandes, E. J. Yunis, and R. A. Good, Influence of diet on
    survival of mice, Proc. Nat. Acad. Sci. USA 73:1279 (1976).

53. W. D. Denckla, Role of pituitary and thyroid glands in the
    decline of minimal O_2 consumption with age, J. Clin. Invest.
    53:572 (1974).

54. N. Fabris, W. Pierpaoli, and E. Sorkin, Lymphocytes, hormones
    and aging, Nature 240:557 (1972).

55. P. O. Teague, and G. J. Friou, Antinuclear antibodies in mice.
    II. Transformation with spleen cells, inhibition or
    prevention with thymus or spleen cells, Immunology 17:665
    (1969).

56. E. J. Yunis, and L. J. Greenberg, Immunopathology of aging,
    Fed. Proc. 33:2017 (1974).

57. S. Kysela, and A. D. Steinberg, Increased survival of NZB/W
    mice given multiple syngeneic young thymus grafts, Clin.
    Immunol. Immunopath. 2:133 (1973).

58. E. J. Yunis, G. Fernandes, and O. Stutman, Susceptibility to
    involution of the thymus-dependent lymphoid system and
    autoimmunity, Am. J. Clin. Path. 56:280 (1971).

59. J. F. Albright, and T. Makinodan, Growth and senescence of
    antibody-forming cells, J. Cell Comp. Physiol. 67(Suppl. 1):
    185 (1966).

60. D. Metcalf, R. Moulds, and B. Pike, Influence of the spleen and
    thymus on immune responses in aging mice, Clin. Exp.
    Immunol. 2:109 (1966).

61. T. Makinodan, and W. H. Adler, The effects of aging on the
    differentiation and proliferation potentials of cells of the
    immune system, Fed. Proc. 34:153 (1975).

62. J. W. Albright, and T. Makinodan, Decline in the growth
    potential of spleen-colonizing bone marrow stem cells of
    long lived aging mice, J. Exp. Med. 144:1204 (1976).

63. K. Hirokawa, and T. Makinodan, Thymic involution: Effect on T
    cell differentiation, J. Immunol. 114:1659 (1975).

64. K. Hirokawa, J. W. Albright, and T. Makinodan, Restoration of
    impaired immune functions in aging animals. I. Effect of
    syngeneic thymus and bone marrow cells, Clin. Immunol.
    Immunopathol. 5:371-376 (1976).

65. E. H. Perkins, T. Makinodan, and C. Seibert, Model approach to immunological rejuvenation of the aged, Infect. Immunity 6:518 (1972).

66. D. Friedman, V. Keiser, and A. Globerson, Reactivation of immunocompetence in spleen cells of aged mice, Nature 251:545 (1974).

67. M.-A. Bach, Lymphocyte-mediated cytotoxicity: Effects of ageing, adult thymectomy and thymic factor, J. Immunol. 119:641 (1977).

68. M. E. Weksler, J. B. Innes, and G. Goldstein, G. Immunological studies of aging. IV. The contribution of thymic involution to the immune deficiencies of aging mice and reversal with thymopoietin, J. Exp. Med. 148:996 (1978).

69. D. Martinez, A. K. Field, H. Schwam, A. A. Tytell, and M. R. Hilleman, Failure of thymopoietin, ubiquitin and synthetic serum thymic factor to restore immunocompetence in T cell deficient mice, Proc. Soc. Exp. Biol. Med. 159:195 (1978).

70. A. L. Goldstein, G. B. Thurman, T. L. Low, G. E. Trivers, and J. L. Rossie, Thymosin: The endocrine thymus and its role in the aging process, in:"Physiology and Cell Biology of Aging," A. Cherkin, C. E. Finch, N. Kharasch, T. Makinodan, F. L. Scott, and B. L. Strehler, eds., Raven Press, New York (1979).

71. J. Rovensky, A. L. Goldstein, P. J. L. Holt, J. Pwkarek, and T. Mistina, Obnova funkcie T lymfocytor tymosinom u klinicky zdravych asob vyssieho veku, Cas. Lek. Ces. 116:1063 (1977).

72. B. Strehler, "Time, Cells and Aging," Academic Press, New York (1977).

73. D. Harman, Prolongation of life: Role of free radical reactions in aging, J. Am. Geriatrics Soc. 17:721 (1969).

74. D. Harman, M. L. Heidrick, and D. E. Eddy, Free radical theory of aging: Effect of free-radical-reaction inhibitors on the immune response, J. Am. Geriatrics Soc. 25:400 (1977).

75. E. G. Bliznakov, Immunological senescence in mice and its reversal by coenzyme Q_{10}, Mech. Ageing Dev. 7:189 (1978).

76. W. Braun, Y. Yajima, and M. Ishizuka, Synthetic polynucleotides as restorers of normal antibody formation capacities in aged mice, J. Reticuloendothel. Soc. 7:418 (1970).

77. I. H. Han, and A. G. Johnson, Regulation of the immune system by synthetic polynucleotides. VII. Amplification of the immune response in young and aged mice, J. Immunol. 117:423 (1976).

78. M. E. Schmidt, and S. D. Douglas, Effects of synthetic single and multistranded polynucleotides on human monocyte IgG receptor activity in vitro, Proc. Soc. Exp. Biol. Med. 151:376 (1979).

79. W. Braun, W. M. Lichtenstein, and C. Parker, eds., "Cyclic AMP, Cell Growth and the Immune Response," Springer-Verlag, New York (1974).

80. J. D. Broome, and M. W. Jeng, Promotion of replication in lymphoid cells by specific thiols and disulfides in vitro, J. Exp. Med. 138:574 (1973).

81. C. Chen, and J. G. Hirsch, The effects of mercaptoethanol and of peritoneal macrophages on the antibody forming capacity of nonadherent mouse spleen cells in vitro, J. Exp. Med. 136:604 (1972).

82   M. W. Fanger, D. A. Hart, J. V. Wells, and A. Nisonoff, Enhancement by reducing agents of the transformation of human and rabbit peripheral lymphocytes, J. Immunol. 105:1043 (1970).

83. E. Heber-Katz, and R. E. Click, Immune responses in vitro. V. Role of mercaptoethanol in the mixed-leukocyte reaction, Cell. Immunol. 5:410 (1972).

84. N. Johnson, R. Jessup, and P. W. Ramwell, The significance of protein disulfide and sulphonyl groups in prostaglandin action, Prostaglandins 5:125 (1974).

85. W. Lands, R. Lee, and W. Smith, Factors regulating the biosynthesis of various prostaglandins, Ann. N.Y. Acad. Sci. 180:107 (1971).

86. T. Makinodan, J. W. Deitchman, G. H. Stoltzner, M. M. Kay, and K. Hirokawa, Restoration of the declining normal immune functions of aging mice, Proc. 10th Internat. Cong. Gerontol. 2:23 (1975).

87. T. Makinodan, Control of immunologic abnormalities associated with aging, Mech. Ageing Dev. 9:7 (1979).

88. T. Makinodan, and J. F. Albright, Restoration of impaired immune functions in aging animals. II. Effect of mercaptoethanol in enhancing the reduced primary antibody responsiveness in vitro, Mech. Ageing Dev. 10:325 (1979).

89. T. Makinodan, and J. F. Albright, Restoration of impaired immune functions in aging animals. III. Effect of mercaptoethanol in enhancing the reduced primary antibody responsiveness in vivo, Mech. Ageing Dev., in press.

90. M. G. Goodman, and W. O. Weigle, Nonspecific activation of murine lymphocytes. I. Proliferation and polyclonal activation induced by 2-mercaptoethanol and a-thioglycerol, J. Exp. Med. 145:473 (1977).

91. D. Metcalf, Role of mercaptoethanol and endotoxin in stimulation of B lymphocyte colony formation in vitro, J. Immunol. 116:635 (1976).

92   M. J. Bevan, R. Epstein, and M. Cohn, The effect of 2-mercapto-ethanol on murine mixed lymphocyte cultures, J. Exp. Med. 139:1025 (1974).

93. H. D. Engers, H. R. MacDonald, J. C. Cerottini, and K. T. Brunner, Effect of delayed addition of 2-mercaptoethanol on the generation of mouse cytotoxic T-lymphocytes in mixed leukocyte cultures, Eur. J. Immunol. 5:223 (1975).

94. T. Igarashi, M. Okada, T. Kishimoto, and Y. Yamamura, In vitro
     induction of polyclonal killer T cells with 2-mercapto-
     ethanol and the essential role of macrophages in this
     process, J. Immunol. 118:1697 (1977).
95. H. G. Opitz, U. Opitz, H. Lemke, H. D. Flad, G. Hewlett, and
     H. D. Schlumberger, Humoral primary immune response in vitro
     in a homologous mouse system: Replacement of fetal calf
     serum by a 2-mercaptoethanol or macrophage-activated
     fraction of mouse serum, J. Immunol. 119:2089 (1977).

NEUROENDOCRINE FUNCTION AND AGING

Arthur V. Everitt

Department of Physiology
University of Sydney
Sydney, Australia

The life program from conception through growth, development, physiological aging, and the onset of terminal diseases leading to death is determined by both genetic and environmental factors. The course of aging and duration of life are affected by environmental factors such as temperature (1), food supply (2), and stress (3). These factors affect body functions by mediations of the neuroendocrine and autonomic nervous systems. For example, a rat or mouse living in a cold environment secretes more thyroxine (4) and catecholamines (5), which increase heat production and enable the animal to survive under these conditions (6). Survival in a hostile or rapidly changing environment is dependent upon adequate functioning of both the autonomic nervous and endocrine systems. The secretions of these two systems, neurotransmitters and hormones, regulate the vast majority of physiological activities throughout the body. Obviously, a deficiency of a specific neurotransmitter or hormone will have far-reaching effects on body function. This forms the basis of the neuroendocrine regulatory failure hypothesis of aging.

THE NEUROENDOCRINE REGULATORY FAILURE HYPOTHESIS

This hypothesis states that peripheral aging phenomena are due to failure of neuroendocrine regulatory mechanisms. There is little doubt that impairments occur in old age in many functions. For example, the ability to maintain constant body temperature is greatly reduced in old age, both in man and in laboratory animals. When young adult mice (aged 10 months) are kept in a cool room at $9\text{-}10^{\circ}C$, body temperature decreased slightly (about $1^{\circ}C$) over a 3 hour period; whereas, in old mice (30 months) body temperature falls markedly (about $8^{\circ}C$) (7). The cause of this impairment of temperature regulation in old mice may be due to single or multiple defects in the thermoregulatory system. Impairments may develop in the temperature receptors (in skin, abdomen, spinal cord, or brain), the afferent nerves which relay information from the receptors to the hypothalamus, the thermoregulatory centers in the hypothalamus, the efferent autonomic nerves, and the neuroendocrine system which transmit instructions from the hypothalamus to the effector organs that control heat production (the liver and muscles) and the organs that control heat loss from the skin. At present, it is not possible to estimate the contribution of these different nervous and endocrine components to the age decrement in thermoregulation.

In a similar manner, age decrements are found in most endocrine functions in old age, and there is an increasing volume of evidence suggesting that central regulatory deficiencies in the rat contribute to the peripheral aging in the ovary (8,9,10), the testis (11), and the adrenal cortex (12). Aging of the regulatory mechanisms has been studied most extensively in relation to the aging ovary.

AGING OF THE HYPOTHALAMIC-PITUITARY-OVARIAN AXIS

This is a very complex system with environmental inputs, hypothalamic surge and tonic centers, hypothalamic release and release inhibitory factors, pituitary gonadotropic hormones (FSH and LH) and prolactin, and the negative and positive feedback of both ovarian hormones (estrogen and progesterone) producing 4 or 5 day cycle of changes in the ovary and accessory reproductive organs.

With increasing age (starting at 10 months) estrous cycle irregularities appear, the cycles cease, pseudopregnancies (estrus every 12-14 days) develop, permanent estrus (anovulatory state) occurs, and then, finally, anestrus, which indicates cessation of ovarian function (8,10).

ROLE OF THE HYPOTHALAMUS

Most evidence indicates that, in the rat, the primary age lesion is in the hypothalamus. The elegant transplant study of Peng and Huang (13) clearly showed that in old non-cycling rats, neither the pituitary nor the ovaries are responsible for the loss of cycles. They found that a young rat with old ovaries and an old pituitary is able to cycle normally. The site of the primary age defect is probably the preoptic area of the hypothalamus, which is the surge or cyclic area controlling the large preovulatory rise in luteinizing hormone (LH) secretion. This is supported by the work of Clemens and Bennett (9), who found that lesions in the preoptic area of young rats reproduced the pseudopregnancy state seen in old rats. These

workers were able to restore normal estrous cycles in these lesioned
rats by injecting lergotrile mesylate, which is a dopamine agonist.
It is also possible to achieve partial restoration of estrous cycles
in old rats by electric stimulation of the preoptic area (14) or by
injections of epinephrine, L-dopa, or iproniazide (15). Both L-dopa
and iproniazide increase catecholamine levels in the brain (16).
These pharmacological studies implicate catecholamines in the
age-related loss of estrous cycles, as suggested by other workers
(17,18). In the basal medial hypothalamus of the old rat, there is a
fall in the content of dopamine and norepinephrine, and the
metabolism of these catecholamines is depressed, while the metabolism
of serotonin is increased (17). These authors suggest that these
changes in biogenic amine metabolism may in part account for the
age-related increase in serum prolactin (secretion stimulated by
serotonin) and decrease in serum LH and FSH (most data indicate that
NE stimulates LH secretion).

The responsiveness of the hypothalamus to the negative feedback
of ovarian steroid hormones is also impaired in old age. Dilman (19)
has presented evidence suggesting that elevation of the hypothalamic
threshold to feedback control is a signficant factor in aging. In
the rat, an age-related elevation of the hypothalamic threshold to
negative feedback has been demonstrated for corticosteroids (12) and
gonadal steroids (20). The hypothalamus becomes less responsive to
changes in ovarian hormones with increasing age. For example, a
deficiency of ovarian hormones created by ovariectomy produces a much
smaller rise in plasma LH in old rats than in young (21).

These studies generally emphasize the importance of the hypothalamus rather than the pituitary as the primary determinant of
ovarian aging.

ROLE OF THE PITUITARY

Age changes in pituitary gonadotropic function may also contribute to the loss of estrous cycles. Pituitary responsiveness to LRH
(luteinizing hormone releasing hormone) is reduced in old female
rats, as shown by a smaller increase in serum LH in aged rats
compared with young animals (22). This means that for the same
amount of LRH secreted by the hypothalamus, less pituitary LH is
secreted. Hence, there is less likelihood of the LH surge being
large enough to initiate ovulation in the aged rat. LH is the
pituitary hormone most concerned with cyclic behavior in the ovary.
Of course, it can be argued that the loss of pituitary responsiveness
to LRH is secondary to age changes in the hypothalamus.

There have been relatively few long-term studies which attempt to
manipulate the course of ovarian aging. At least three different
studies suggest that pituitary gonadotropins regulate the rate of
ovarian aging.

Hemiovariectomy in the young rat produces a compensatory increase in both FSH and LH secretion, which stimulates the remaining ovary to enlarge (23). In the mouse the reproductive performance is halved; the total number of offspring is halved; and the duration of reproduction is halved (24). That is, the life span of the ovary is halved. In women, there is also evidence that after hemiovariectomy the remaining ovary becomes exhausted before the normal age of menopause (25). In the hemiovariectomized rat, the duration of breeding is normal (26), but the onset of senile deviations of the estrous cycle occurs prematurely (27). It is tempting to suggest that the high secretion of gonadotropins is responsible for aging of the remaining ovary.

Complete removal of gonadotropins by hypophysectomy in CBA mice is found to retard the age-related loss of oocytes from the ovary (28), but does not abolish the loss. Although such animals are sterile due to lack of pituitary gonadotropins, ovaries from old hypophysectomized mice well beyond the normal age of reproduction are quite fertile when transplanted into young ovariectomized mice. Thus, a lack of pituitary hormones has delayed the onset of sterility.

Caloric restriction acts in a similar manner to hypophysectomy because it reduces the plasma levels of pituitary gonadotropins (29). Starvation reduces hypothalamic LRH stimulation of the pituitary and so decreases LH secretion (30). The reproductive life of the underfed female rat is prolonged. Berg (31) obtained litters from 16 out of 24 food-restricted rats aged 730 to 790 days, an age when fully-fed rats are sterile.

THE PITUITARY HYPOTHESIS

According to this hypothesis, pituitary hormones accelerate aging processes and lead to an early onset of age-related pathology (32). This hypothesis is supported by the observation that hypophysectomy in the rat retards the rate of aging in tail tendon collagen, kidney, heart muscle, aorta, skeletal muscle, bone, and ovary (32,33).

The effects of hypophysectomy on aging are profound when operations are performed on young rats at age 70 days. Tail tendon collagen in a senescent 1000-day-old (33 months) hypophysectomized rat has the physical properties (breaking time in 7M urea) of a 500-day middle-aged control rat. Similarly, the kidney of the 1000-day-old hypophysectomized rat corresponds to that of a 200-day young adult control, in terms of the excretion of protein in urine. There are no histological signs of renal disease in old hypophysectomized rats. The wall thickness of the thoracic aorta of the 1000-day-old hypophysectomized rat is similar to that of a 100-day young adult control. The 1000-day-old senescent hypophysectomized rat is able to walk normally, whereas 70% of controls of that age have hind leg paralysis causing them to drag their hind legs; and in the remainder,

walking is impaired. The incidence of tumors at autopsy in old
hypophysectomized rats (800-1300 days) averages 5%, whereas in age-
matched controls it is 64%. The tissues of the old hypophysectomized
rat are almost free of obvious pathological changes, such as renal
and cardiac hypertrophy, tumors, and hind leg paralysis. This
suggests that hypophysectomy has delayed the immunologic decline,
usually seen in old age, which is associated with the emergence of
disease (34).

These studies clearly show that hypophysectomy in the rat at an
early age (70 days) produces a general slowing of aging phenomena in
many tissues. The effects of hypophysectomy performed in middle age
(at 400 days) are not quite so dramatic, but still lead to significant retardation of both collagen and renal aging. This study indicates that pituitary hormones are accelerating aging phenomena at all
ages, and not merely turning on an aging program in early life.

One serious problem with hypophysectomy studies is that food
intake is markedly reduced. The anti-aging effects could be due to
either the loss of pituitary hormones or to the lowered food intake.
Food restriction is known to prolong life (35), to delay the onset of
the diseases of old age (36,37), and to retard the aging of collagen
fibers in tail tendon (38,39). Since the anti-aging effects of
hypophysectomy and food restriction are almost identical, a common
mechanism is suggested. The only real difference is in life
duration. The untreated hypophysectomized rat has a significantly
reduced life duration (40,41). However, hypophysectomized rats
receiving corticosteroid replacement (1 mg cortisone acetate per week
subcutaneously) have mean life duration equal to that of food-
restricted rats eating the same amount of food. Their life duration
is significantly greater than that of controls consuming almost three
times the quantity of food. These obvservations have been confirmed
by Denckla (personal communication), who found 20/95 survival at 34
months (1000 days) in hypophysectomized rats receiving cortisone
succinate, desoxycorticosterone acetate and thyroxine in their
drinking water, compared with only 2/125 for controls.

These studies indicate that there are several pituitary factors
concerned in aging phenomena: 1) factors which prolong life (such as
ACTH and TSH, which respectively stimulate corticosteroid and
thyroxine secretion) probably acting by an immunological mechanism,
and 2) factors which increase aging (such as excessive secretion of
TSH, ACTH, and growth hormone), probably acting by some metabolic
mechanism such as crosslinking. Since the secretion of these
hormones is controlled principally by hypothalamic centers, it is
tempting to postulate that the hypothalamus is the ultimate regulator
of these aging phenomena and the duration of life. A number of
workers have discussed the possibility that the aging program is
timed or regulated by a clock or center in the hypothalamus. For
example, Denckla (42) has proposed that the life span is regulated by

a biological clock which acts on endocrine glands to produce failure
of the immune and circulatory systems.

THE HYPOTHALAMIC CLOCK HYPOTHESIS

This hypothesis states that there is a clock or center in the
hypothalamus which regulates the rate of peripheral aging by
mediation of the nervous and endocrine systems (32,43,44). The
proposed center would be analogous to the thermoregulatory, feeding,
satiety, thirst, sleep, and vasomotor centers in the hypothalamus,
which specifically regulate temperature, feeding, etc. It is largely
because of the multiplicity of functions performed by the
hypothalamus that this organ has been proposed as a central regulator
of aging (32). Possibly even more important is its unique
anatomophysiological position, which enables the hypothalamus to
mediate many of the effects of environmental factors, and so adjust
the rate of aging according to the demands of the environment.

Biological clocks have been postulated to regulate endocrine
cyclic phenomena, such as the circadian rhythm of ACTH and
corticosteroid secretion, where the highest plasma level occurs just
before waking, and decreases throughout the day to the lowest level
when going to bed late at night (45). The suprachiasmatic nucleus in
the anterior hypothalamus has been implicated in the diurnal rhythm
of corticosteroid secretion (45,46). This nucleus appears to be
implicated in many biological rhythms, such as periodicity in
locomotor behavior, periodicity of feeding and drinking activity,
periodicity of body temperature, and estrous cycle periodicity.
Since the suprachiasmic nucleus area appears to control a great
number of biological cycles, perhaps it also controls life's major
cycle--that from birth to death. This is probably unlikely, because
the role of this area is apparently to initiate the cycle. The clock
or regulator which we are searching for is that which controls the
duration of the cycle. The duration of most biological cycles is
relatively resistant to change by altering environmental conditions.
This is certainly not true of the life cycle when one considers the
enormous effect of temperature on life duration in poikilothermic
animals like Drosophila (47) and the large increases possible in rat
life duration by manipulating the diet (48). Again, in the case of
the estrous cycle, exposure to continuous light (49) leads to failure
of ovulation and the development of the constant estrous pattern as
seen in old age. Furthermore, rats exposed to low temperatures
(2°C) have longer estrous cycles due to increased duration of
estrus or proestrus (50). These experiments show how the environment
can influence an intrinsic biological process. In a clock or biological rhythm mechanism, there are three components: 1) a receptor
to detect light, heat, etc.; 2) a clock to measure time and integrate
the information received; 3) an effector system to modify body
functions. In the hypothalamic-pituitary thyroid axis, Ooka-Souda et
al. (51) have shown how light deprivation from birth delays the

maturation of the pituitary-thyroid axis. Ooka-Souda (personal communication) has also shown that when the day length is reduced to 18 hours, the pituitary-thyroid axis develops more rapidly, the rats grow faster and have shorter estrous cycles. Is the whole program of aging accelerated?

It is clear that environmental factors can modify the rate of development and aging. Quite a number of these factors appear to be acting by mediation of the hypothalamus. It is tempting to suggest that the state of the environment is detected by the appropriate receptors, which delay this information to an aging center or clock, most probably located in the hypothalamus. After integration of all information received, the clock adjusts the level of body functions and the rate of aging by altering the quantities of hormones and neurotransmitters delivered to the tissues concerned. The rate of aging in a given tissue is presumed to be regulated by the hormones and neurotransmitters stimulating or depressing that tissue.

ACKNOWLEDGEMENTS

I am especially grateful to Mr. Frank Jones, who performed most of the hypophysectomies, and to Roussel Pharmaceuticals, Sydney, who generously supplied the cortisone acetate used in these studies. The hypophysectomy studies reported here were supported, in part, by grants from the Consolidated Medical Research Fund of the University of Sydney and the University Research Grant.

REFERENCES

1. R. K. Liu and R. L. Walford, The effect of lowered body temperature on life span and immune and non-immune processes, Gerontologia 18:363 (1972).
2. C. H. Barrows and L. M. Roeder, Nutrition, in:"Handbook of the Biology of Aging," C. E. Finch and L. Hayflick, eds., Van Nostrand Reinhold, New York (1977).
3. H. Selye and B. Tuchweber, Stress in relation to aging and disease, in:"Hypothalamus, Pituitary and Aging," A. V. Everitt and J. A. Burgess, eds., Charles C. Thomas, Springfield, Illinois (1976).
4. H. D. Johnson, H. H. Kibler, and H. Silsby, The influence of ambient temperature of 9°C and 28°C on thyroid function of rats during growth and aging, Gerontologia 9:18 (1964).
5. J. Ledvic, Catecholamine production and release in exposure and acclimation to cold, Acta Physiol. Scand. 53(Suppl. 183):1 (1961).
6. T. R. Bauman and C. W. Turner, The effect of varying temperatures on thyroid activity and the survival of rats exposed to cold and treated with L-thyroxine or corticosterone, J. Endocrinol. 37:355 (1967).

7. C. E. Finch, J. R. Foster, and A. E. Mirsky, Ageing and the regulation of cell activities during exposure to cold, J. Gen. Physiol. 54:690 (1969).

8. P. Aschheim, Resultats fournis par la greffe heterochrone des ovaires dans l'etude de la regulation hypothalamo-hypophyso-ovarienne de la ratte senile, Geontologia 10:65 (1964/5).

9. J. A. Clemens and D. R. Bennett, Do aging changes in the preoptic area contribute to loss of cyclic endocrine function? J. Gerontol. 32:19 (1977).

10. H. H. Huang and J. Meites, Reproductive capacity of aging female rats, Neuroendocrinology 17:289 (1975).

11. C. D. Riegle, J. Meites, A. Miller, and S. M. Wood, Effect of aging on hypothalamic LH-releasing and prolactin inhibiting activities and pituitary responsiveness to LHRH in the male laboratory rat, J. Gerontol. 32:19 (1977).

12. C. D. Riegle, Chronic stress effects on adrenocortical responsiveness in young and aged rats, Neuroendocrinology 11:1 (1973).

13. M. T. Peng and H. H. Huang, Aging of hypothalamic pituitary-ovarian function in the rat, Fert. Ster. 23:535 (1972).

14. J. A. Clemens, Y. Amenomorri, T. Jenkins, and J. Meites, Effects of hypothalamic stimulation, hormones, and drugs on ovarian function in old female rats, Proc. Soc. Exp. Biol. Med. 132:561 (1969).

15. S. Quadri, G. Kledzik, and J. Meites, Reinitiation of estrous cycles in old constant estrous rats by central acting drugs, Neuroendocrinology 11:248 (1973).

16. J. H. Dowson and I. Laszlo, Quantitative histochemical studies of formaldehyde-induced parenchymal fluorescence following L-DOPA administration, J. Neurochem. 18:2501 (1971).

17. J. W. Simpkins, G. P. Mueller, H. H. Huang, and J. Meites, Evidence for depressed catecholamine and enhanced serotonin metabolism in aging rats: Possible relation to gonadotropin secretion, Endocrinology 100:1672 (1977).

18. C. E. Finch, Monamine metabolism in the aging male mouse, in: "Development and Aging in the Nervous System," M. Rockstein and M. L. Sussman, eds., Academic Press, New York (1973).

19. V. M. Dilman, Age-associated elevation of hypothalamic threshold to feedback control and its role in development, ageing and disease, Lancet 1:1211 (1971).

20. C. J. Shaar, J. S. Enker, G. D. Riegle, and J. Meites, Effects of castration and gonadal steroids on serum LH and prolactin in old and young rats, J. Endocrinol. 66:45 (1975).

21. R. G. Gosden and L. Bancroft, Pituitary function in reproductively senescent female rats, Exp. Gerontol. 11:157 (1976).

22. B. E. Watkins, J. Meites, and C. D. Riegle, Age related changes in pituitary responsiveness to LHRH in the female rat, Endocrinology 97:543 (1975).

23. B. E. Howland and C. Preiss, Effects of aging on basal levels of
    serum gonadotropins, ovarian compensatory hypertrophy and
    hypersecretion of gonadotropins after ovariectomy in female
    rats, Fert. Ster. 26:271 (1975).

24. E. C. Jones and P. L. Krohn, The effect of unilateral
    ovariectomy on the reproductive lifespan of mice, J.
    Endocrinol. 20:129 (1960).

25. M. Magendie, I. Bernard, M. Kolenc, and Partimbene, Le
    comportment hormonal de l'ovaire restant! C.R. Soc. Franc.
    Gynec. 23:201 (1953).

26. C. E. Adams, Ageing and reproduction in the female mammal with
    particular reference to the rabbit, J. Reprod. Fert., Suppl.
    12:1 (1970).

27. P. Aschheim, Aging in the hypothalamic-hypophyseal ovarian axis
    in the rat, in:"Hypothalamus, Pituitary and Aging," A. V.
    Everitt and J. A. Burgess, eds., Charles C. Thomas,
    Springfield, Illinois (1976).

28. E. C. Jones and P. L. Krohn, The effect of hypophysectomy on the
    number of oocytes in the adult albino rat, J. Endocrinol. 21,
    497 (1961).

29. B. E. Howland, Effect of restricted feed intake on LH levels in
    female rats, J. Anim. Sci. 34:445 (1972).

30. G. A. Campbell, M. Kurcz, S. Marshall, and J. Meites, Effects of
    starvation in rats on serum levels of FSH, LH, thyrotropin,
    growth hormone and prolactin; response to LH-releasing
    hormone and thyrotropin releasing hormone, Endocrinology
    100:580 (1977).

31. B. N. Berg, Nutrition and longevity in the rat. I. Food intake
    in relation to size, health and longevity, J. Nutrition
    71:242 (1960).

32. A. V. Everitt, The hypothalamic-pituitary control of aging and
    age-related pathology, Expl. Gerontol. 8:265 (1973).

33. A. V. Everitt, Hypophysectomy and aging in the rat, in:
    "Hypothalamus, Pituitary and Aging," A. V. Everitt and J. A.
    Burgess, eds., Charles C. Thomas, Springfield, Illinois
    (1976).

34. T. Makinodan, Immunity and aging, in:"Handbook of the Biology of
    Aging," C. E. Finch and L. Hayflick, eds., Van Nostrand
    Reinhold Co., New York (1977).

35. C. M. McCay, M. F. Crowell, and L. A. Maynard, The effect of
    retarded growth upon the length of life span and upon the
    ultimate body size, J. Nutrition 10:63 (1935).

36. J. A. Saxon, Jr., Nutrition and growth and their influence on
    longevity in rats, Biological Symposia 11:177 (1945).

37. B. N. Berg and H. S. Sims, Nutrition, onset of disease and
    longevity in the rat, Can. Med. Assoc. J. 93:911 (1965).

38. M. Chvapil and Z. Hruza, The influence of aging and
    undernutrition on chemical contractility and relaxation of
    collagen fibres in rats, Gerontologia 3:241 (1959).

39. A. V. Everitt, Food intake, growth and the ageing of collagen in
     rat tail tendon, Gerontologia 17:98 (1971).
40. F. Verzar and H. Spichtin, The role of the pituitary in the
     aging of collagen, Gerontologia 12:48 (1966).
41. A. V. Everitt and L. M. Cavanagh, The ageing process in the
     hypophysectomized rat, Gerontologia 11:198 (1965).
42. W. D. Denckla, A time to die, Life Sciences 16:31 (1975).
43. M. Hasan, P. Glees, and E. El-Ghazzawi, Age-associated changes
     in the hypothalamus of the guinea pig: Effect of
     dimethylaminoethyl p-chlorophenoxyacetate. An electron
     microscopic and histochemical study, Exp. Gerontol. 9:153
     (1974).
44. T. Samorajski, Central neurotransmitter substances and aging: A
     review, J. Amer. Geriatrics Soc. 25:337 (1977).
45. D. T. Krieger, Factors influencing the circadian periodicity of
     ACTH and corticosteroids, Medi. Clin. North Am. 62:251 (1978).
46. M. A. Slusher, Effects of chronic hypothalamic lesions on
     diurnal and stress corticosteroid levels, Amer. J. Physiol.
     206:1161 (1964).
47. J. V. Burcombe and M. J. Hollingsworth, The relationship between
     environmental temperature and longevity in Drosophilia,
     Gerontologia 16:172 (1970).
48. M. H. Ross, Length of life and caloric intake, Amer. J. Clin.
     Nutr. 25:834 (1972).
49. I. E. Lawton and N. B. Schwartz, Pituitary-ovarian function in
     rats exposed to constant light: A chronological study,
     Endocrinology 81:497 (1967).
50. M. E. Denison and M. X. Zarrow, Changes in the estrous cycle of
     rat during prolonged exposure to cold, Proc. Soc. Exp. Biol.
     Med. 89:632 (1955).
51. S. Ooka-Souda, D. J. Draves, and P. S. Timiras, Developmental
     patterns of plasma TSH, T_4 and T_3 in rats deprived of
     light from birth, Mech. Ageing Dev. 6:287 (1977).

EFFECT OF ADULT THYMECTOMY ON IMMUNE POTENTIALS, ENDOCRINE ORGANS AND TUMOR INCIDENCE IN LONG-LIVED MICE

Katsuiku Hirokawa and Yoshio Hayashi

Department of Pathology
Medical Research Institute
Tokyo Medical and Dental University
Yushima, Bunkyo-ku, Tokyo-113
Japan

INTRODUCTION

The thymus is known to be a central lymphoid tissue playing an important role in the ontogenic development of the immune system. Neonatal thymectomy causes severe immunodeficiency in mice, which usually die from wasting disease in the conventional environment (1). In contrast, thymectomy performed at the adult state results in no immediate effect on the immune potentials of the mice (2). However, since the thymic functions to promote T cell-differentiation are known to be maintained in the thymus of mice of any age, although these functions decline progressively with age (3), it would be expected that removal of the adult thymus would result in a delayed impairment of T cell-dependent immune potentials (4,5). The T cell-dependent component of the immune system is also said to play an important role in immune surveillance (6). If so, the incidence of naturally occurring tumors would increase in adult thymectomized mice. Moreover, growth and involution of the thymus is said to be closely interrelated with normal function of the other endocrine organs (7). If so, adult thymectomy would also influence the function of the other endocrine organs.

METHODS

To test these questions, B6C3F$_1$ female mice were thymectomized at 6 weeks of age and then studied at 6, 12, and 24 months of age. Non-thymectomized B6CF$_1$ female mice were used as controls. Immunological assessment of the spleens of both groups was performed as described previously (3), and the organs were examined pathohistologically.

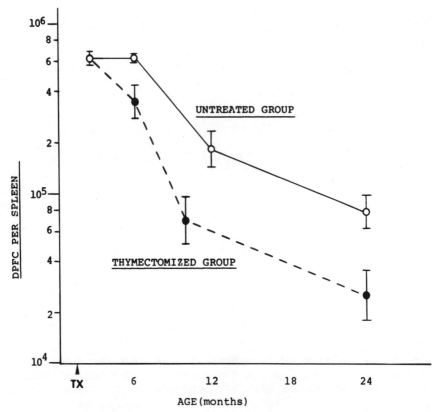

Fig. 1.   Anti-SRBC antibody response measured by number of direct
          plaque forming cells (DPFC) per spleen in untreated control
          (open circles and solid lines) and thymectomized group
          (solid circles and broken lines). DPFC was assessed 5 days
          after i.p. injection of 3×10^8 SRBC. Each point,
          average of 3 to 6 samples. Vertical bars, one standard
          error of the mean. TX, thymectomy, performed at 6 weeks of
          age.

RESULTS AND DISCUSSION

Antibody response to sheep red blood cells (SRBC)

     The level of anti-SRBC antibody response in untreated group
declined gradually after 6 months of age, reaching the level of about
10% of the peak response at 24 months of age, as shown in Figure 1.
In the thymectomized group, a significantly accelerated decline of
this response was observed, showing 10% of the peak response at 12
months of age and 4% level at 24 months of age.

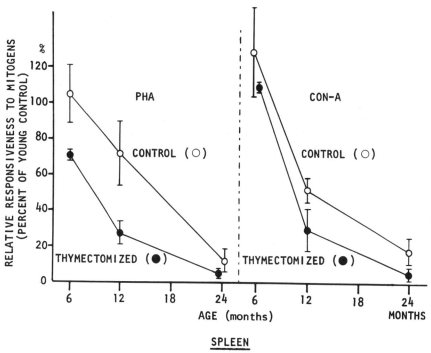

SPLEEN

Fig. 2.   Responsiveness of spleen cells to phytohemagglutinin (PHA)
           and concanavalin A (Con A), expressed by percent of the
           responsiveness of 3-month-old young control. Spleen
           cells, 5 x 10⁵, in 0.2 ml of RPMI 1640 were cultured
           with 1.0 μg of either PHA or Con A in a microplate, pulsed
           66 hr later with 0.25 μCi of ³H-thymidine (sp. act. 8
           Ci/mM) for 6 hr and processed. The responsiveness was
           expressed by cpm/culture. Open circles, untreated
           age-matched control. Solid circles, thymectomized group.
           Vertical bars, one standard error of the mean.
           TX, thymectomy performed at 6 weeks of age.

Mitogenic responsiveness of the spleen cells

Responsiveness of spleen cells to phytohemagglutinin (PHA) also
progressively declined with age in controls (Fig. 2). An accelerated
decline of this responsiveness in the thymectomized group was thought
to be observed at 6 and 12 months of age, but the difference became
marginal at 24 months of age. Responsiveness of the spleen cells to
concananvalin A (Con A) also showed a similar pattern of age-associated decline, as observed in PHA-responsiveness in both treated and
non-treated animals, but the acceleration of the declining responsiveness to Con A in the thymectomized group was not apparent until
12 and 24 months of age. These results suggest that PHA- and Con A-

Table I. Effect of Adult Thymectomy on the Incidence of
          Spontaneously Occurring Tumors in B6C3F$_1$ (♀)

Age.	6m	12m	24m
Control	0/3	0/6	2/7
Thymecto-mized at 6 wks old	0/3	1/6	4/6

responsive T cells in the spleen do not belong to the same subpopu-
lation of T cells. The data in Figures 1 and 2 indicate that the
thymus is necessary throughout the course of the life for continuous
recruitment of T cells, although the T cell-inducing capacity
progressively declines with age (3).

Incidence of spontaneously occurring tumors

   In BC3F$_1$ mice, reticulum cell sarcoma (Dunn's A type) occurs in
50% of mice at 30 months of age (8). In the thymectomized group of
B5C3F$_1$ mice, which are genetically almost identical to BC3F$_1$ mice, an
increased incidence of reticulum cell sarcoma was observed as early
as 12 months of age (1/6). This incidence further increased to 4/6
at 24 months of age. This incidence is significantly higher than
that of the control group, which is 2/7 at 24 months of age (Table
I). These results appeared to be compatible with the concept that
the thymus-dependent component of the immune system does indeed
perform the task of immune surveillance (6).

Weight of endocrine organs

   The weight of adrenal and pituitary glands in the thymectomized
group appeared to be less than that of the same endocrine organs in
the age-matched control (Fig. 3). A significant difference was
observed in the weight of the adrenal glands at 6 and 24 months of
age. This difference might be ascribed to higher susceptibility of
the thymectomized group to infection and tumor as compared with the
control. However, at 6 months of age, both thymectomized and control
mice were revealed to be healthy by pathological examination. Therefore, presence of the weight difference suggested that function of
the adrenal and pituitiary glands is closely interrelated with the
normal function of the thymus.

SUMMARY

   The data presented here indicate that the thymus plays an
important role not only in the early ontogenic development of the
immune system, but also in the maintenance of the immune potentials

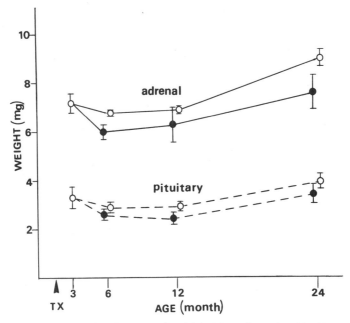

Fig. 3. Net weight of adrenal (solid lines) and pituitary glands
        (broken lines) in untreated, age-matched control (open
        circles) and thymectomized group (solid circles). TX,
        thymectomy, performed at 6 weeks of age. Vertical bars, one
        standard error of the mean.

throughout the course of life. Moreover, thymic function is closely
interrelated with functions of the other endocrine organs.

REFERENCES

1. J. F. A. P. Miller, Lancet ii:748 (1961).
2. J. F. A. P. Miller and D. Osoba, Physiol. Rev. 47:437 (1967).
3. K. Hirokawa and T. Makinodan, J. Immunol. 114:1659 (1975).
4. D. Metcalf, Nature 208:1336 (1965).
5   L. C. Robson and M. R. Schwarz, Transplantation 11:465 (1971).
6. M. Burnet, "Immunological Surveillance," Pergamon Press, Oxford
        (1970).
7. N. Fabris, W. Pierpaoli, and E. Sorkin, Nature 240:557 (1972).
8. F. Chino, T. Makinodan, W. E. Lever, and W. J. Peterson, J.
        Gerontol. 26:497 (1971).

ENVIRONMENT AND AGING: AN APPROACH TO THE ANALYSIS OF AGING MECHANISMS USING POIKILOTHERMIC VERTEBRATES

Nobuo Egami

Zoological Institute, Faculty of Science
University of Tokyo
Hongo, Tokyo 113, Japan

INTRODUCTION

Epidemiological data and various circumstantial evidence suggest that the rate of aging in humans is influenced by many environmental conditions, such as nutrition, climate, or more complicated factors, including social conditions. Research designed to analyze the relationship between each environmental factor and the aging of organisms has been carried out using laboratory animals, particularly mice and rats. However, it is difficult to draw either specific or general conclusions regarding these relationships, since, in mammals, homeostatic mechanisms are well developed, and cells within the individuals are not always directly exposed to environmental conditions. One possible approach toward solving this problem would be to reevaluate the use of simple animal models, together with that of using cultured cells of animals and poikilothermic vertebrates. These animals reflect environmental conditions more directly than mammals do (Fig. 1). Data or comments on environmental effects, such as temperature, nutrition, photoperiod, radiation and chemical trace elements on the life span of small laboratory fish will be presented.

TEMPERATURE

It is difficult to analyze the effect of temperature on the life span of mammals directly, since body temperature is regulated by complicated mechanisms. However, animal longevity at various temperatures has been examined, and many zoologists have recorded long life spans in hibernators. In the case of poikilothermic animals, the situation is simpler. The life span of fish is, in general, longer at low temperatures, within a limited range. Under natural conditions, some fish species which live in cooler

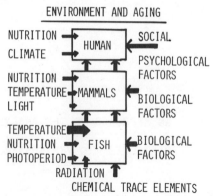

Fig. 1.   Diagram showing relationsip between environment and aging
           in different classes of animals.

environments live longer than other members of the same species
living in warmer localities. In 1970, Liu and Walford (1) used
several species of Cynolebias as model animals in the laboratory.
They concluded that the longer survival at low temperatures is due to
a decrease in the rate of aging, since the slope of the survivorship
curve at low temperatures decreased at about the same ratio as the
increase in the mean survival time. Further studies using this model
were performed by them in 1972, from an immunological perspective (2).

The small teleost fish Oryzias latipes, native to Japan, is a
temperature-tolerant species. The fish is known to live in hot
springs at 40°C, but the same species can survive under ice at
1°C. We have previously reported that if the fish are irradiated
with 8 kR of X-rays, the proliferation of cells in the intestine is
completely inhibited. Following this, the cell population of the
intestinal epithelium decreases day by day, since the intestinal
epithelium is a typical cell renewal system, and the life span of the
epithelial cells is limited. Finally, so-called "intestinal death
induced by radiation" occurred (3,4). The rate of development of
this syndrome is temperature-dependent because the cell cycle time
and life span of the cells are determined by the water temperature
(Fig. 2). In other words, the survival time after irradiation with 8
kR is clearly dependent upon the water temperature (Fig. 3). We
believe from autoradiographic examination that dependency of survival
time of fish on the temperature is a reflection of the temperature
dependency of the rate of the aging process in the differentiated
intestinal epithelial cells.

Moreover, during the period between 1970 and 1974, I observed
that the life span of non-irradiated fish is longer if the fish are
kept in cool thermal surroundings in summer, and shorter if the fish
are heated in winter (5) (Fig. 4). Furthermore, it was demonstrated

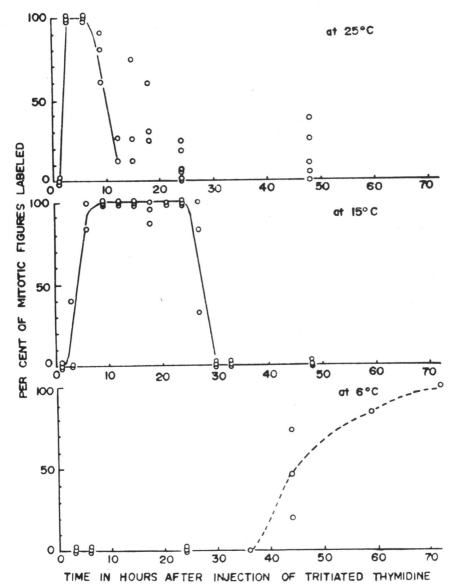

Fig. 2.   Percent of labeled mitotic figures of intestinal
           epithelial cells of goldfish kept at different
           temperatures (Hyodo-Taguchi).

in these fish that a delay in the development and promotion of
hepatic tumor nodules contributed to some extent to longevity at low
temperature (Fig. 5) (6,7,8).

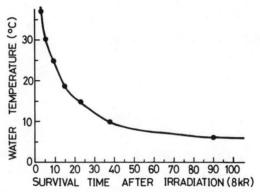

Fig. 3.   Effects of temperature on rate of development of acute
radiation injury in Oryzias latipes.

The behavior at different temperatures of cultured fish cells in
vitro has also been studied by Shima, Etoh, Mano and Mitani. Details
will be reported by Shima in his paper. These experimental results
indicate that more can be learned from the use of fish and cultured
fish cells to analyze the effects of temperature on the aging process
of cells and organisms.

QUALITY AND QUANTITY OF FOOD

Comfort reported in 1963 that the restriction of food prolonged
the life span of the female guppy (9). Similar experiments were
repeated by him using fish of various ages, and the relationship
between the growth rate and aging was discussed. Our experience
using Oryzias latipes has been similar; however, no quantitative
results have yet been obtained. The growth rate of fish is easy to
control by controlling the food conditions, and fish can survive even
if the growth rate is markedly modified. Therefore, the control of

TEMPERATURE	MEAN SURVIVAL TIME AFTER IRRADIATION	
	0 R	1000 R
NATURAL TEMPERATURE	725	320
10°C OR LESS	1042	431
20°C OR MORE	430	102

Fig. 4.   Temperature effects on mortality of irradiated fish and
non-irradiated fish.

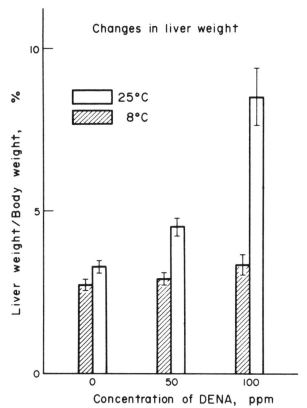

Fig. 5.   The ratios of liver weight to body weight in DENA-treated
          fish kept at different temperatures. The weight indicates
          the development of the tumor.

longevity in fish is more easily accomplished than that of mammals.
Recent developments in fish cultivation, particularly in Japan, have
stimulated the scientific study of the nutrient value of feed. Many
reports on the effects of the quantity and quality of food on growth,
maturation, and the induction of various fish diseases, including
tumors, have been published. Moreover, further fundamental studies
of fish nutrition will be necessary before its relationship to the
aging process of fish can be completely understood.

PHOTOPERIODICITY

     If animals are exposed to short or long photoperiods over a
considerable period, what happens to their aging rate? In an attempt
to answer this question, Noumura and his co-workers are keeping mice
exposed to artificial illumination for 20-, 24-, or 30-hour days. A
similar type of experiment has been tried by our group with normal,

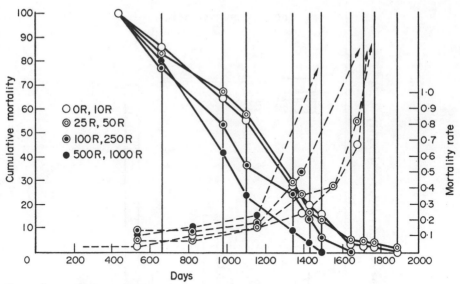

Fig. 6.   Mortality rate and cumulative mortality of fish exposed to
X-rays during embryonic stage.

blind, and pinealectomized fish. It was found, in the preliminary
experiment, that a small number of blind fish survived longer than
intact fish. In some fish, it is known that the pineal body
functions as a photoreceptor. Using Oryzias latipes, Urasaki
demonstrated in 1976 that photoperiods influence the pineal by way of
the eyes (10). Positive effects of the photoperiods on the behavior
and on the maturation of intact, but not pinealectomized, fish were

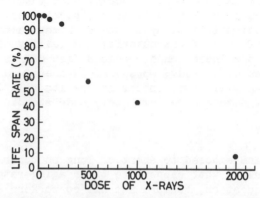

Fig. 7.   Effect of X-irradiation of embryos on life span in Oryzias
latipes.

Table 1. Important Histological Characteristics in Senile Fish

---

(1) Degenerative changes (cerebrum)

(2) Decrease in cell number (liver, kidney)

(3) Enlargement of cells (liver, kidney)

(4) Increase of conective tissue (testis)

(5) Deposition of lipofuscin (cerebrum)

(6) Degeneration of the thymus

---

recognized by a series of Urasaki's papers. The results on the
effects of aging rate, however, are not yet conclusive.

RADIATION

The life-span-shortening effect of ionizing radiation has been
well demonstrated in fish as well as in mammals (11). However, it is
not yet certain that radiation does accelerate the non-specific aging
process; nor that a low dose, or a low dose rate, of radiation exerts
hormetic effects.

I have examined the effects of X- and γ-rays on the life span in
Oryzias latipes, after establishing the life span table. Our results
were reported at the symposium of the XIth International Congress of
Gerontology. The conclusion we reached was that dose-dependent
life-shortening effects of X-rays were demonstrated if these X-rays
were given at high dose rates (11,12) (Figs. 6,7). However, under
low-dose-rate conditions (less than 20 R/day), no significant effects
on longevity were demonstrated.

Our histological studies of senile fish revealed various
characteristics peculiar to them (Table 1). Most age-specific
histo-cytologic changes in the liver, the spleen, the brain, and the
testis occurred in irradiated fish. However, in some organs, the
senile changes were not always felt to be stimulated by radiation
(13). In addition, an examination of the effects of radiation on
tumorigenesis is now in progress. Generally speaking, the nature of
the radiation effects on fish is the same as that on mammals, so fish
can be used as model animals (Table 2).

The data of the fish experiments show that radiation has clear
life-shortening effects, but further quantitative study is necessary
before we can conclude that radiation stimulates the non-specific
aging processes.

Table 2. Summary of the Radiation Effects on Life Span in
Oryzias latipes

---

(1) Life span shortening effects of radiation was
clearly demonstrated at high dose-rate.

(2) At 320-35 R/day, accumulated dose for 50%
mortality was 10-17 KR.

(3) At lower dose-rate, no clear effects were observed.

(4) Histological observation did not always demonstrate
"radiation accelerates all non-specific aging
processes".

MUTAGENIC, CARCINOGENIC, AND OTHER TRACE SUBSTANCES

The so-called "somatic mutation theory" as a mechanism for the
aging process seems one of the most attractive. Therefore, the
effects on tumorigenesis, mutagenesis, and lethality of compounds
that specifically bind to DNA and interfere with DNA metabolism, such
as actinomicin D, ethidium bromide, 5-bromodeoxyuridine (BUdR), and
some alkylating agents and nitrosamine compounds, caffeine and
urethane were examined in our laboratory. In addition, the effects
of trace elements and trace metals, particularly $HgCl_2$ and CH_3HgCl in
water, on mortality and mutagenicity were examined in our laboratory
using Oryzias latipes by Sakaizumi. The effects of these substances
were compared to those of ionizing radiation.

Some effects were measured by examining the chromosome aberration
and DNA content distribution of cultured fish cells (Shima). We
tried to demonstrate change in the template-primer activities of
nuclear DNA to various types of DNA-polymerase by autoradiography,
with sections of ethanol-fixed fish tissue treated with some drugs by
a method similar to that reported by Price, Modak, and Makinodan
(14). However, at the present time, no clear age-related changes
have been demonstrated (15).

At any rate, aquatic organisms are very suitable for ascertaining
the effects of Na and K, and their ion balance, (Ca, Mg, Zn, Fe, and
some trace metals like Pb, Cd, and Hg) and of water-soluble mutagenic

and carcinogenic substances on histological characteristics which are generally felt to indicate tumor formation and aging.

DISCUSSION

In order to properly study environmental effects on organisms, the organisms should be genetically homogeneous. Recently, at least eight pure inbred strains of Oryzias have been established by Hyodo-Taguchi. In addition, the very strange Amazon molly and Japanese silver tuna fish, which show gynogenetic reproduction, have been found, and genetically pure populations have been obtained. These fish have also been used as a model system of aging study by Setlow and our groups (16). Furthermore, the cultivaton in a germ-free environment of some fish has been successfully accomplished. Thus, the use of pathogen-free fish for gerontological research is also possible.

In order to obtain fundamental knowledge of the mechanism of the aging process in animals, comparative studies of the effects of environmental factors on aging process in different animals and their cells are essential. For instance, if the basic causes of biologial aging were related to somatic mutation, including chromosome aberration, or accumulation of errors in genetic information in the critical cells, ionizing radiation and some radiomimetic substances might accelerate the rate of aging process in all animals, even at cellular levels. If mesenchymal tissue changes were key causes of animal aging, the effects of temperature and of drugs interfering with collagen might be great on the aging rate in all animals in tissue, organ, or organism levels.

If the pineal body or homeostatic regulatory systems, such as hypothalamus, were the time keeper or biological clock of aging process in higher organisms, environmental factors which affect such systems, including photoperiod or administration of some exogenous hormonic substances, might change the rate of aging process only in vertebrate animals, and at whole animal levels. These effects might appear more markedly in higher species, in accord with the evolutionary development of the regulatory system. If more complicated factors, like psychological or social conditions play a more important role in human aging process, the effects might appear only in the more advanced societies.

I would like to re-emphasize the significance of using various animals, including poikilothermic species in which homeostatic mechanism is simple, and environmental factors act more directly, as a way to approach this complicated problem. In conclusion, I will add that in order to analyze environmental effects on aging, the reevaluation of interrelationship among aging phenomena occurring in different animal species is also important, as well as that in different levels of organization (Fig. 8).

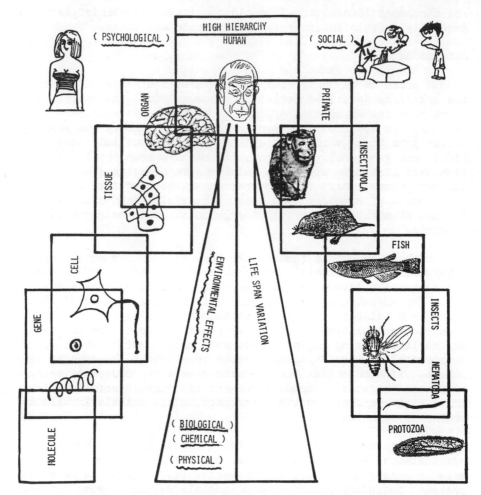

Fig. 8. Diagram showing approaches to analyze environmental effects
on aging by reevaluation of interrelationships among aging
phenomena occurring in different animal species and in
different levels of organization.

REFERENCES

1. R. K. Liu and R. L. Walford, Observations on the life spans of
    several species of annual fishes and of the world's smallest
    fishes, Exp. Gerontol. 5:241 (1970).
2. R. K. Liu and R. L. Walford, The effect of lowered body
    temperature on life span and immune and non-immune processes,
    Gerontologia 18:363 (1972).

3. Y. Hyodo, Effect of X-irradiation on the intestinal epithelium
   of the goldfish Carassius auratus II. Influence of
   temperature on the development of histological changes in
   the intestine, Rad. Res. 24:133 (1965).
4. Y. Hyodo-Taguchi and N. Egami, Development of intestinal
   radiation injury and recovery at different temperatures in
   fish, in:"Comparative Cellular and Species
   Radiosensitivity," T. Suguhara and Y. P. Bond, eds.,
   Igakushoin, Tokyo (1969).
5. N. Egami, Long-term observations of mortality of irradiated fish
   at different temperatures, Rad. Res. 59:132 (1974).
6. Y. Kyono and N. Egami, The effect of temperature during the
   diethylnitrosamine treatment on liver tumorigenesis in the
   fish, Oryzias latipes, Eur. J. Cancer 13:1191 (1977).
7. Y. Kyono, Temperature effects during and after the
   diethylnitrosamine treatment on liver tumorigenesis in the
   fish, Oryzias latipes, Eur. J. Cancer, 14:1089 (1978).
8. Y. Kyono, A. Shima, and N. Egami, Changes in the labeling index
   and DNA content of liver cells during liver tumorigenesis in
   the fish, Oryzias latipes, J. Natl. Cancer Inst., 63:71
   (1979).
9. A. Comfort, Effect of delayed and resumed growth on the
   longevity of a fish (Lebistes reticulatus, Peters) in
   captivity, Gerontolgia 8:150 (1963).
10. H. Urasaki, The role of pineal and eyes in the photoperiodic
    effects on the gonad of the Medaka, Oryzias latipes,
    Chronobiologica 3:228 (1976).
11. N. Egami, Radiation effects on life span of the fish, Oryzias
    latipes, in:"Proc. XI Int. Congress Gerontology," 314 (1978).
12. N. Egami and H. Etoh, Effect of X-irradiation during embryonic
    stage on life span in the fish, Oryzias latipes, Expt.
    Gerontol. 8:219 (1973).
13. N. Egami, M. M. H. Ghoneum, A. Kikuta, and K. Ijiri, Effects of
    radiation on life span and lymphoid tissues in the fish,
    Oryzias latipes, in:"Abst. 2nd Radiation Biology Center Int.
    Symp.," 20.
14. G. B. Price, S. P. Modak, and T. Makinodan, Age-associated
    changes in the DNA of mouse tissue, Science 171:917 (1971).
15. M. Matsui, A. Shima, and N. Egami, Autoradiographic detection of
    the template-primer activities of DNA by exogenous DNA
    polymerase in fixed mouse tissues, J. Fac. Sci., Univ.
    Tokyo, IV, 13:399 (1976).
16. A. D. Woodhead, Ageing changes in the liver of two Poeciliid
    fishes, the guppy, Poecilia (Lebistes) reticulata and the
    Amazon molly, P. formosa, Expt. Gerontol. 13:37 (1978).

CENTRAL VS. PERIPHERAL AGING[*]

Richard G. Cutler

Gerontology Research Center
National Institute on Aging
National Institutes of Health
Baltimore City Hospitals
Baltimore, Maryland 21224

INTRODUCTION

The slow but progressive deterioration of man's health, followed by an increased onset frequency of diseases, results mostly from a complex spectrum of time-dependent changes collectively called aging (1). There is agreement that substantial prolongation of useful and enjoyable life span would require a _uniform_ decrease in the rate of expression of most of these aging processes (2,3). However, there is much disagreement on the probability and advisability of slowing down man's aging rate, a process often considered to be incredibly complex (4,5).

At the present time, we know little about the biological nature of aging or about the genetic and biochemical complexity of processes which may be governing the aging rate. However, the hypothesis that specific processes may exist that govern the aging rate is fairly new and may, as we shall see later, be less complex than the aging process _per se_ (5). In this regard, it must be determined whether the aging rate of man is controlled by a special set of genes. If so, we must also determine the number and informational complexity of these genes, and that of possible regulatory genes (6,7,8,9). Consideration of the evolutionary processes that gave rise to all living forms of life, and eventually to the unusually long period of longevity that man enjoys today (3,6,9,10), is likely to yield useful

---

[*]A similar lecture has also been presented for publication in "Biology of Aging," C. Borek and D. W. King, eds., Stratton Intercontinental Medical Book Corp., New York.

information toward this objective. Moreover, this endeavor requires
a study of biology at its most general and fundamental level. The
author believes that a clear understanding of all living processes,
past and present, is not likely to be obtained without also an
understanding of the basic nature of aging processes and how these
processes are controlled (3,9). This paper presents highlights of
such an evolutionary study of human longevity--and as part of this
study, central vs. peripheral factors in aging are evaluated.

MAMMALIAN SPECIES HAVE DIFFERENT INNATE AGING RATES

There is little doubt that different mammalian species have substantial differences in their innate aging rates, even species that
are genetically closely related. The major evidence supporting this
concept is the different maximum life span potentials (MLP) found for
different species. MLP is the life span of the last surviving member
of a given population. Under conditions where the species' natural
hazards have been largely removed and reasonable medical and sanitary
conditions are observed (such as in modern zoos), this value
approaches the innate biological ability of a species to survive.
Obviously, the larger the initial young population observed, the more
accurate the value obtained. For a number of primates and other animals, a reasonable MLP is known now that is probably no more than 20%
underestimated (11,12,13). More importantly, from a comparative
viewpoint, the different MLP's are probably even more accurate proportionally.

In Table 1, estimates of MLP's are given for some primate species. Man lives about 14 times longer than the shortest-lived of the
primate species, the Phillipine tree shrew. Man appears to be the
longest-lived of all living mammalian species, and probably of all
mammalian species that ever lived.

Differences in ability to survive, or MLP, do not necessarily
imply corresponding differences in aging rate. However, when rate of
decline of physiological function is compared to MLP, an excellent
correlation is observed. These studies have mainly been confined to
mice, rats, guinea pigs, dogs, Rhesus monkeys, chimpanzees, and man
(3,6,11). For example, the rate of loss of immune function in man
and mouse is inversely proportional to MLP. This is also true for
physical vigor, resistance to disease, and the rate of decline in
mental function. Thus, MLP appears to be related to the innate ability of the animal to maintain its general mental and physical
health. The different MLP's and the excellent correlation found with
the rate of decline of common physiologic functions, mental abilities, and in the susceptibility to common diseases, strongly support
the thesis that different aging rates exist which reflect a constitutive biological characteristic of an animal. It is emphasized,
however, that very few comparative physiological and pathological
studies have been carried out for the purpose of relating MLP, aging

Table 1.   Maximum Life Span Potentials for Some Primates

Homo sapiens	man	113
Pan troglogytes	chimpanzee	55
Cebus capucinus	capucin	40
Galago senegalensis	galago	25
Saimiri sciureus	squirrel monkey	21
Tarsius syrichta	tarsier	12
Perodicticus potto	potto	12
Urogale everetti	Phillipine tree shrew	8

Taken from (11). MLP is in years.

rate, and onset frequency of disease, or the qualitative differences
in these processes that may exist in different mammalian species.
Clearly, much more comparative information is required.

WHY ANIMALS HAVE DIFFERENT MLP'S

If different mammalian species do have different innate capacities to maintain their physiology and mental health for a given
period of time, then an evolutionary reason for it is likely to
exist. An understanding of why animals have different MLP's would
help clarify the concept of different aging rates and how these rates
evolved mechanistically.

One possibility is that some type of biological limitation
exists, unique to each species, preventing further increase in MLP
regardless of how advantageous it might be to have a longer life
span. Another possibility is that each species maintains its health
for a characteristically optimum period of time because further
increase would have no significant evolutionary selective advantage.
This latter possibility appears at present to have more support. For
example, mammalian species are essentially identical in their
biological makeup, which is probably why mammals age qualitatively in
a similar manner. It seems reasonable that similar metabolic and
general physiological processes would give rise to similar aging
processes. Also, an excellent correlation appears to exist between
the intensity of a species' environmental hazards and its MLP--the
life span observed when most of these environmental hazards are

Table 2.   Correlation Between Mortality Rate in the Wild
           and Maximum Life Span Potential for Some Birds

Common name	Average annual adult mortality (fraction that is killed)	Maximum life span potential (yrs)
Blue tit	0.72	9
European robin	0.62	12
Lapwing	0.34	16
Common swift	0.18	21
Sooty shearwater	0.07	27
Herring gull	0.04	36
Royal albatross	0.03	45

Taken from (9).

removed.   Typical data showing this correlation are shown in Table 2
for some birds and in Table 3 for some rodents.   However, more data
is needed to establish this correlation as a general phenomenon.   If
true, it could be hypothesized that animals in the wild seldom
undergo significant senescence in their natural environment as a
result of the balance of nature.   Most animals would be killed by
their natural predators or by accident before their performance is
seriously reduced by their innate aging processes.   Thus, there would
be no evolutionary selective advantage for a mouse to be able to
maintain optimum physical and mental health for 10 years if, on the
average, 95% of the population could not survive beyond one year.
Only animals at the top of the food chain, such as the elephant and
man, appear to undergo senescence in the wild.

Not too many years ago, man's average life span (not MLP) was
much shorter, and the problem of senescence was minor compared to
other causes of death.   In Table 4, the average life span of man is
seen to be about 30 to 40 years under conditions of natural
environmental hazards.   Only after the age of 30 or 40 years did
man's mental and physical health begin to show significant decline.

Table 3. Mortality Rate of Some Rodent Species in their
          Natural Ecological Environment

Species	Average mortality rate	Maximum life span potential	Maximum calorie consumption (MCC) (Kilocalories/g/MLP
Peromyscus manicu-latus (deer mouse)	63-94% in 1 yr (rarely live over 2 yrs)	3040 days	703
Peromyscus leucopus (white-footed mouse)	rarely live over 2-3 yrs	3300 days	672
Mus musculus (field mouse)	99% in 1 yr (rarely live over 1 yr)	1200 days	250
Tamias striatus	50% in 1.5 yrs	12 yrs	561

Taken from (9).

The good correlation found between mortality rate and MLP indicates that MLP evolved to the point where it was no longer advantageous. The almost total absence of senescence in the population of
wild animals in their natural environment is also consistent with the
idea that sensescence has no evolutionary advantage, and is postponed
to an age that insures its non-occurrence.

Would MLP always increase if the environmental hazards permitted
it? Clearly, there are advantages to limited life span, such as
enhancing turnover in the population, thus increasing the rate of
evolutionary selective processes. However, for mammlian species, it
appears that natural turnover rate in the population has been sufficient. The need to evolve a genetic program to terminate it is
bypassed.

A great number of variables are involved in determining the
resultant evironmental hazards of a species. One important parameter
is the ability of the organism to learn from its environment in order
to better adapt, protect, and feed itself. A rough correlation
appears to exist between the amount of learned vs. instinctive behavior a given species demonstrates and its innate MLP (10,11,14).
Apparently, longer lived mammalian species have been able to lower
their environmental hazards by taking advantage of their ability to
learn and reason. This implies, of course, that longer lived species
in general have superior intelligence capabilities, which also
appears to be true (11,14). Longer life spans could provide more
time for an individual to achieve a certain degree of mental

Table 4.   Average Mortality Rate of Present-Day Man in His
           Past and Present Environment

Time period	Average chrono- age at 50% survival (yrs)	Maximum life span potential (yrs)
Würm (about 70,000-30,000 yrs ago)	29.4	69-77
Upper Paleolithic (about 30,000-12,000 yrs ago)	32.4	95
Mesolithic (about 12,000-10,000 yrs ago)	31.5	95
Neolithic Anatolian (about 10,000-8000 yrs ago)	38.2	95
Classic Greece (1100 B.C.-1 A.D.)	35	95
Classic Rome (753 B.C.-476 A.D.)	32	95
England (1276 A.D.)	48	95
England (1376-1400)	38	95
United States (1900-1902)	61.5	95
United States (1950)	70.0	95
United States (1970)	72.5	95

Taken from (9).

development and knowledge, and to pass this on to the young. Thus, a
slower aging rate would be essential to take advantage of a superior
cognitive ability. In this manner, the great differences in MLP and
mental capacities that exist among the mammalian species can be
explained by the conventional chance and necessity mechanisms of evolution. In this case, adaptive and learned behavior with increased
MLP marks the evolutionary success of the mammalian species, and in
particular for the primates.

THE BIOLOGICAL BASIS OF THE DIFFERENT MLP'S OF MAMMALIAN SPECIES

As was previously mentioned, differences in MLP do not seem to
involve fundamental qualititative differences in biological makeup.
Nevertheless, species that are remarkably similar at the biological

level age at significantly different rates. The chimpanzee, having
an MLP one-half that of man, appears to age twice as fast in all
biological aspects, in spite of remarkable similarities to man at the
biological level. The whole gamut of aging processes, such as
changes in hearing, taste, smell, heart and kidney capacities, function of the immune system, mental function, as well as the onset
frequency of age-dependent diseases, including cancer, would be
expected to uniformly run at twice the rate in the chimpanzee as in
man. It this proves true, then how is man able to maintain his
mental and physical health so much longer? Further, can we enhance
man's health for an even longer period of time by using means similar
to those that have evolved in the past? This question represents a
completely new approach in biomedical science: to discover the basis
of general health maintenance and the origin of age-related
dysfunctions of man.

Of course, some genetic differences must exist between species
having different MLP's; but how much difference is there, and can we
estimate an upper limit to the genetic complexity governing the aging
rate of man? Two approaches have been used to make this estimate.
The first was a biological comparison of the nucleic acids and proteins known in genetically closely related species having substantial
differences in MLP. A study of about 50 major proteins of man and
chimpanzee indicates that 99% of the amino acid sequences were identical, and many of the differences found were trivial in terms of
biological function (15,16,17). Also, the nucleic acid sequence differences were found to be only about 1% between man and chimpanzee.
In fact, man and chimpanzee are so similar at the genetic level that
they are classified as sibling species (species that are remarkably
similar in appearance) (15). Yet, man and chimpanzee are placed in
different families on the basis of their obvious morphological and
behavioral differences.

The second approach was to determine how quickly longevity can
change, and to compare this value with how rapidly useful genetic
alterations are known to occur. Two different methods were used to
estimate this value (5,11). The first method compares the MLP
between living species with the time when they had a common ancestor. For example, man and chimpanzee, with MLP's of about 100 and 50
years, respectively, had a common ancestor 15 x 10^6 years ago, the
time the evolutionary lines of man and chimpanzee diverged. Thus, a
minimum change of 50 years of MLP occurred with a time period of 15 x
10^6 years, or a change of 1.6 years MLP per 10^6 years of evolution.
Tables 5, 6, and 7 show how this method was used to estimate the
direction and speed MLP changed during the evolution of the primate
species. The results show that MLP tended to always increase; the
rate of increase of MLP increased as the higher-order primate species
emerged; and the maximum rate of increase occurred during the emergence of the Hominidae-Pongidae families.

Table 5. Estimates of the Evolutionary Rate of Increase in Maximum Life Span Potential within the Superfamilies of the Primates

Order	Suborder	Superfamily	Mean MLP within a superfamily	MLP differences within a superfamily	Common divergence time ($\times\ 10^{-6}$ yrs) (Fossil dates)	Change in MLP per 10^6 yrs (Fossil)
Primates	Prosimii	TUPAIOIDEA	6	1.5	65	0.02
		LORIDOIDEA	14	18	30	0.6
		LEMUROIDEA	19	24	30	0.8
		CEBOIDEA	22	25	30	0.83
		CERCOPITHECOIDEA	30	27	25	1.1
	Anthropoidea	HOMINOIDEA	52	63	30	2.1

Taken from (11). MLP is in years.

Table 6. Estimates of the Evolutionary Rate of Increase in Maximum
Life Span Potentials Between Closely Related Superfamilies
of the Primates

Superfamily	Mean MLP of the two superfamilies	Difference in mean MLP between superfamilies	Common divergence time $(x\ 10^{-6}$ yrs) (Fossil dates)	Increase in MLP (yrs) per 10^6 yrs (Fossil)
LORISOIDEA-TUPAIOIDEA	10.3	8	65	0.12
LEMUROIDEA-LORISOIDEA	16.8	5	40	0.13
CERCOPITHECOIDEA-CEBOIDEA	25.6	8	55	0.15
HOMINOIDEA-CERCOPITHECOIDEA	40.8	22	40	0.55

Taken from (11). MLP is in years.

Table 7. Estimates of the Evolutionary Rate of Increase in Maximum
Life Span Potential between the Closely Related Families
of Hominoidea

Family	Largest difference in MLP between families	Common Divergence time $(x\ 10^{-6}$ yrs) (Fossil dates)	Increase in MLP (yrs) per 10^6 yrs (Fossil)
PONGIDAE-HYLOBATIDAE	18	30	0.6
HOMINIDAE-PONGIDAE	55	15	4.0

Taken from (11). MLP is in years.

The second method estimates the MLP of extinct fossil species
using the empirical correlation found between MLP and brain and body
weights for living species. This method was used by Cutler (5,11)
and Sacher (13). The equation used is taken from Sacher's work in
this area (18) and is:

$$MLP = (10.839)\ (\text{brain wt., g})^{0.636}(\text{body wt., g})^{-0.225}$$

The stongest rationale for using this equation to predict MLP for
extinct species is that the prediction works equally well for living
fossil species and for progressive species (11). Sacher did not
support his findings using this rationale (13). Estimates of MLP
using the brain and body weights for living fossils are shown in
Table 8, and agree with known MLP's. The equation is also shown to
predict MLP for mammals in general and primates, shown in Tables 9
and 10, respectively.

MLP was predicted for 59 ungulates, 32 carnivores, 24 primates,
and 156 Hominidae fossil species. Knowing when the fossil species
existed, a phylogenetic tree for the evolution of MLP was construc-
ted. The results found were similar to that using the first method.
Table 11 summarizes the ungulate and carnivore data, and Figure 1
illustrates that, although MLP generally increased, an increase in
dispersion of MLP also occurred, reaching a maximum for present
living species.

Table 8.   Estimation of Maximum Life Span Potential for Living Fossil
           and Recent Mammals Living in a Mesozoic Niche

Common name	Cranial capacity (cm^3)	Body Wt (g)	MLP Pred.	MLP Obs.	Time of appearance (x 10^{-6} yrs)
Short tailed shrew	0.347	17.4	2.9	3.3	14-0
Pygmy shrew	0.11	5.3	1.8	1.5	14-0
European shrew	0.2	10.3	2.3	1.5	14-0
long tailed shrew	0.12	5.7	1.9	1.5	14-0
tenrec	2.75	832	4.5	2	10-0
Madagascar hedgehog	1.51	248	4.1	3	10-0
streaked tenrec	0.83	110	3.3	3	5.5-0
Norwegian rat (wild)	1.59	200	4.4	3.4	5.5-0
field mouse	0.45	22.6	3.2	3.5	5.5-0
vole	0.66	23.7	4.1	2-3	3-0
vole	0.74	27.9	4.2	2-3	3-0

Taken from (12). MLP is in years.

Table 9. Prediction of Maximum Life Span Potential on the Basis of
Body and Brain Weight for Some Mammalian Species

Common name	Cranial capacity (cm^3)	Body wt (g)	Maximum life span potential (MLP)	
			Observed	Predicted
Pigmy shrew	0.11	5.3	1.5	1.8
Field mouse	0.45	22.6	3.5	3.2
Opossum	7.65	5000	7.0	5.8
Mongolian horse	587	260,000	46	38
Camel	570	450,000	30	33
Cow	423	465,000	30	27
Giraffe	680	529,000	34	35
Elephant (India)	5045	2,347,000	70	89
Mountain lion	154	54,000	19	23
Domestic dog	79	13,400	20	21

Taken from (9,12). MLP is in years.

The phylogenetic tree of MLP for the primate species is shown in
Figure 2. The general increase in MLP is clearly evident, indicating
maximum rate of increase along the ancestral-descendant-sequence
leading to modern man. This latter observation is illustrated in
Figure 3, showing the entire hominid ancestral-descendant-sequence
lineage over the 60×10^6 years of primate evolution. More detailed
data was obtained from the analysis of the 156 hominid species, and
is shown in Figure 4, indicating an exponential rise of increased MLP
and the sudden stop in the increase of MLP about 100,000 years ago.
The rate of change in MLP over the past 2 million years is shown in
Figure 5 for both MLP and the number of neurons for the hominid
species. Richard Leakey's recent findings of a Homo habilis species
existing 2×10^6 years ago are compatible with these conclusions (19).

The main conclusions of these studies are that: (1) increased
longevity and not increased senescence evolved during the evolutionary history of mammals, and (2) the maximum rate of increased MLP for
the primate species, which is about 14 years of MLP per 100,000
years, occurred along the hominid ancestral-descendant-sequence about
100,000 years ago.

Table 10.   Prediction of Maximum Life Span Potential on the Basis of
Body and Brain Weight for Some Primates

Common name	Cranial capacity (cm^3)	Body wt (g)	Maximum life span potential (MLP)	
			Observed	Predicted
Tree shrew	4.3	275	7	7.7
Marmoset	9.8	413	15	12
Squirrel monkey	24.8	630	21	20
Rhesus monkey	106	8719	29	27
Baboon	179	16,000	36	33
Gibbon	104	5500	32	30
Orangutan	420	69,000	50	41
Gorilla	550	140,000	40	42
Chimpanzee	410	49,000	45	43
Man	1446	65,000	95	92

Taken from (11). MLP is in years.

The increase in MLP is predicted to be the result of a uniform
decrease in the aging rate of the entire spectrum of aging processes
as we observe the spectrum of aging processes to exist in primate
species living today. The basis of this argument is that, although
different primates living today have different MLP's, they
nevertheless appear to have qualitatively similar biological makeup,
aging processes, and age-dependent diseases.

The next question is how fast adaptive point mutations can occur
over a 100,000 year period. Three different methods were used to
make this estimate (5,10,13). The first is based on Haldane's
approximation that the maximum genomic load of harmful recessive
mutations that can exist in germ cells limits the mutation rate that
can occur to one substitution per genome per 300 generations. Using
this, the mutation rate is calculated to be 44 adaptive amino acid
substitutions per 40,000 genes per 100,000 years (where 40,000 genes
are taken to be the average number of functional genes in a typical
primate cell). Sacher arrived at a similar conclusion using
Haldane's approximation, but made no calculations (13).

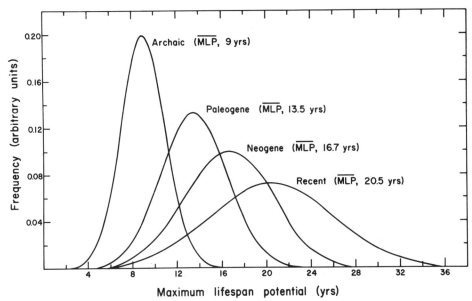

Fig. 1. Increase in mean MLP and dispersion of MLP in the archaic
and progressive ungulates. Archaic species became extinct
but progressive ones did not. Data represents analysis of
about 10 species at each time era. Similar results were
found for the carnivores. Taken from (12).

The second method is based on the DNA and protein sequence
differences measured between the different primate species. These
data are used to calculate the average change in nucleotide sequence
of the DNA that actually did occur throughout the evolutionary
history of the primates. From this data, an adaptive mutation rate
is calculated at about 250 amino acid substitutions per 40,000 genes
per 100,000 years for the hominid species 100,000 years ago.

The last method is based on a theoretical calculation to predict
how rapidly adaptive mutations can occur. Using a spontaneous
mutation rate of 10^{-9} per cell and a selective value parameter of
10^{-2}, the adaptive mutation rate calculated is 160 amino acid substitutions per 40,000 genes per 100,000 years.

Thus, all three methods used to estimate the number of adaptive
mutations occurring during hominid evolution 100,000 years ago
indicate that about 40 to 250 adaptive amino acid substitutions per
genome occurred over a period of 100,000 years. This change has to
account not only for the 14 years of uniform increase in the general
maintenance of physical and mental health (a slowing down of aging
rate by about 20%), but also for the morphological and cognitive
changes that occurred during the recent evolution of man. Could this

Table 11. Average Values of Maximum Life Span Potential Along the
Evolutionary Ancestral-Descendent Sequence of the
Ungulates and Carnivores and Their Corresponding
Archaic Species

Order	Average time of presence (x 10^6 yrs) and epoch		Average MLP
CONDYLARTHRA (archaic)	52	Paleogene	12
PERISSODACTYLA	44	Paleogene	16
	5	Neogene	29
	-	Recent	34
AMBLYPODA (archaic)	55	Paleogene	7
ARTIODACTYLA	34	Paleogene	13
	14	Neogene	18
	-	Recent	26
CREODONTA (archaic)	41	Paleogene	11
CARNIVORA	26	Paleogene	13
	17	Neogene	17
	-	Recent	20

Taken from (12). MLP is in years.

be true, or did some genetic parameter other than point mutation
underlie this change? One important assumption made in these calculations is that the total number of functional genes is only 40,000
out of a potential maximum number of about 3.5 x 10^6, if all the
genome is utilized. If more genetic information is utilized (over
40,000), then the possible number of adaptive mutations would
increase proportionally.

Similar calculations and results to those described here have
been made by other investigators (15,16,17,20,21,22,23,24). The
general conclusion has been that it is difficult to account for the
evolutionary changes that have occurred in mammals as being a result
of point mutations in structural genes. Instead, the major genetic
changes that best account for mammalian evolution are at the

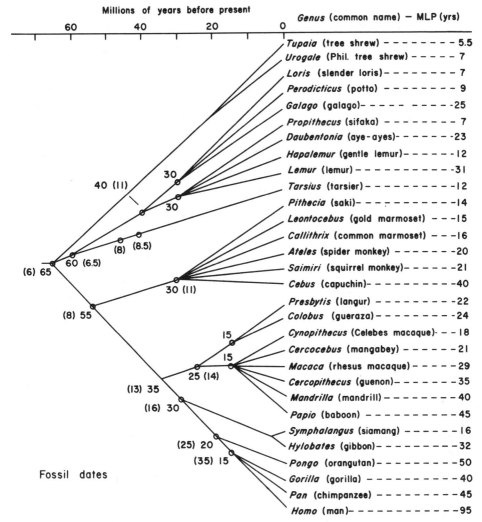

Fig. 2. Maximum life span potential phylogenetic tree for the
        primate species. Numbers in parenthesis are estimates of
        MLP of the species existing at that time. Neighboring
        numbers are millions of years according to geological
        dating. Taken from (11).

regulatory gene level (14,15,16). That is to say, mammalian evolution occurred as a result of changes in the expression of regulatory
genes governing the same set of structural genes, either by a few
point mutations or by chromosomal rearrangements.

There is major support for this new concept. It underlies the
finding of little correlation between the rate of change in amino

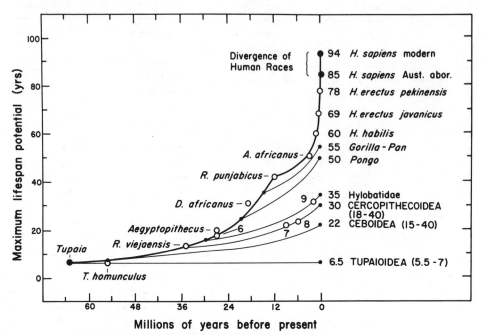

Fig. 3. Evolution of maximum life span potential along the ances-
       tral-descendent-sequence leading to modern man. (O) MLP
       calculated from fossil estimates of brain capacity and body
       weight; (●) MLP of living species. Taken from (11).

acid sequences of proteins or nucleotide sequences of DNA and the
rate of change occurring in morphology or the appearance of new
species. This is illustrated in some of the data shown in Table 12,
where the change in nucleotide pairs (NTP's) per increase in MLP is
not a constant. Indeed, the former appears to decrease as MLP
increases. In addition, a good correlation has been found between
morphological change and the change in chromosomal morphology, which
indicates that perhaps chromosomal rearrangement played an important
role in governing timing and levels of gene expression during the
differentiation and development of the organism. Also, adaptive
studies with microorganisms and recently with Drosophila demonstrate
that the type of genetic change involved, when the organism adapts to
a new food source or to environmental condition, is almost always a
regulatory change in existing genes, and not the appearance of new
gene products. Finally, morphological differences occurring during
the evolution of man and other primates have an underlying similarity.

Many of the changes in the morphology of primates with increasing
MLP can be explained by a general retardation of development, a
process called neoteny. Man is more fetal and child-like at all

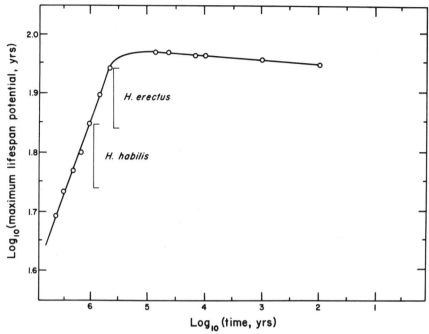

Fig. 4. Evolution of maximum life span potential for the hominid
       species calculated from a regressive analysis of 156
       independent estimates of brain capacity and body weight.
       Open circles represent typical data indicating spread of
       data. Taken from (11).

stages of development than is the chimpanzee. Thus, different rates
of development are also likely to be governed by regulatory genes and
not by different types of structural genes (9,17,25,26).

     To summarize, there is now substantial evidence indicating a
surprisingly high rate of increase of MLP during the evolutionary
appearance of man. Few point mutational changes occur during this
period. Moreover, morphological changes cannot be accounted for
easily by the accumulation of point mutational changes in structural
genes. This concept is supported by the conservation of molecular
and cellular biology, physiology and morphology among different
species. The differences that are found can be explained as a result
of timing and degree of expression of a common set of genes. The
author has therefore suggested that the genetic differences between
man and other primates that account for their innately different
aging rates and mental capacities are not different types of structural genes but rather a common set of genes being expressed at different times and to different degrees (3,5,9,11). This common set of
genes governing aging rate is postulated to be internally governed by

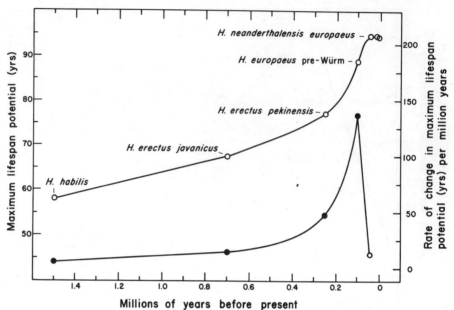

Fig. 5(a).   Evolution of maximum life span potential and number of
              extra cortical neurons (encephalization quotient)
              during the recent emergence of the hominid species.
              (0) MLP; (●) rate of change of MLP.   Taken from (11).

a common set of regulatory genes. These regulatory genes have under-
gone a few simple genetic modifications which have resulted in
changes in the timing and level of expression of the genes they control and that determine the aging rate.

How many regulatory genes are involved in controlling aging rate,
and to what extent and speed were these genes altered to give rise to
man's rapid increase in MLP? If point mutational changes were the
major source of change, and there is a random distribution of regulatory genes along the genome, then the estimate remains at about 40 to
250 amino acid substitutions per 14 years of increased MLP per
100,000 years. On the other hand, if chromosomal rearrangements are
involved, we have no way at present to estimate how rapidly these
changes can occur. Comparative analysis is now being undertaken at
the chromosomal level between man and the chimpanzee, and the differences do not appear to be outstanding at this time (22). Nevertheless, we have to consider that, although the likelihood of changes at
the point mutation level affecting the aging rate appear to be low,
chromosomal rearrangement superimposed on these changes could sub-
stantially increase the complexity of the regulatory processes
governing the aging rate of man.

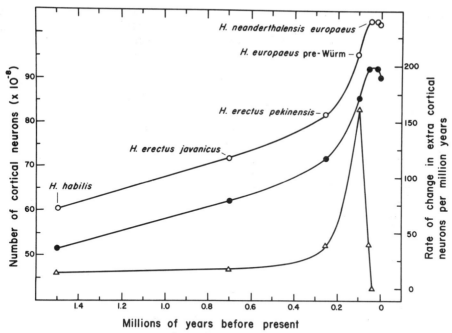

Fig. 5(b).   Evolution of maximum life span potential and number of
              extra cortical neurons (encephalization quotient)
              during the recent emergence of the hominid species.
              (O) MLP; (●) number of cortical neurons; (Δ) rate of
              change of cortical neurons. Taken from (11).

GENERAL AND SPECIAL HYPOTHESES OF AGING AND LIFE MAINTENANCE

The data and ideas presented above can be summarized most clearly
in a general hypothesis for all forms of life and a special
hypothesis for the mammalian species (3,6,9). Both hypotheses are
based on the notion that two opposing processes, aging and life
maintenance, played major roles in the origin and evolution of all
living systems.

Life maintenance processes are broadly defined as any characteristics or properties of a living system that act to increase the
probability of its survival. Two major types of life maintenance
processes exist. The first is related to the maintenance of the
organism relative to external environment hazards. This includes
morphological and the common house-keeping functions, plus special
biological functions unique to a species. The second type of life
maintenance process relates to internal environmental hazards, or to
the intrinsic aging processes. This includes the finite functional
life span of biological constituents making up the organism and the
side-effects of metabolic reactions evolved to provide the life

Table 12. Estimates of the Evolutionary Rate of Increase in Maximum
Life Span Potential per Percent Change in Unique DNA
Sequences Between Closely Related Primate Genuses

Genus	Percent change in nucleotide pairs	Increase in MLP	Increase in MLP per percent change in nucleotide pairs
Galago ↓ Cebus	54	26	0.5
Cercopithecus ↓ Pan	11	10	0.9
Hylobates ↓ Pan	6.5	13	2.0
Pan ↓ Homo	2.5	50	20.0

Taken from (11). MLP is in years.

maintenance properties of the constituents. The side-effects of
metabolic reactions, the harmful pleiotropic nature of metabolism and
development, are considered by many to be the major aging processes.
Special life-maintenance processes are postulated to exist solely to
reduce these long-term detrimental effects.

The general hypothesis postulates that much of the morphology and
biochemistry of cells and organisms today reflects the co-evolution-
ary history of these aging and life maintenance processes. Most of
these two opposing processes emerged during the 3 to 4 billion year
period leading to the evolution of the free-living eukaryotic cell.
Some additional aging and life maintenance processes were added
during the remaining evolutionary history of multicellular organisms,
and were associated with their differentiation and developmental
characteristics. From the appearance of mammalian species about 150
million years ago to the emergence of primate species 60 million
years ago, few different aging and life maintenance processes evolved. Even fewer have evolved during the 15 to 4 million year period
of hominid evolution. For these reasons, in addition to the remarkable biochemical similarities between the primate species, the recent
increase in MLP is postulated not on the appearance of new structural

genes or radically new biochemical pathways, but rather on a difference in the timing and degree of expression of a common set of life
maintanance genes found in all primate species.

These conclusions, expressed in a general hypothesis for all life
forms on the origin and evolution of aging and life maintenance
processes, lead to a special unified hypothesis for the evolution of
mammals, and in particular for the evolution of the primates. This
special hypothesis unifies the aging and life maintenance processes
of the mammalian species in seven major postulates, which are as
follows:

1. All mammalian species express the same qualitative specturm of
aging processes at the genotypic and phenotypic levels.

2. All mammalian species' aging processes are of a pleiotropic
nature and are of two major types: (a) Continuously-Acting Aging
Processes and (b) Developmentally-Linked Aging Processes.

3. All mammalian species express the same qualitative and
time-dependent patterns of general physiological decline in
function and increased sensitivity to disease as the result of
these two common pleiotropic-acting aging processes.

4. All mammalian species express the same set of life maintenance
processes or genes acting to control the rate of expression of
the Continuously-Acting and Developmentally-Linked Aging
Processes.

5. Differences in the time period in which each mammalian species
is intrisically capable of maintaining its optimal physical and
mental health (MLP) are a result of the timing and degree of
expression of the common set of life maintenance processes.

6. The timing and degree of expression of this common set of life
maintenance processes is controlled by a common set of regulatory
genes that may constitute a small fraction of the functional
genetic material of the cell.

7. Evolution of increased MLP was the result of changes, either
by rearrangement within the genome and/or by point mutations of a
common set of regulatory genes. These mechanisms are considered
to be of a nature similar to those involved in the recent
evolution of different morphological, developmental, and
behavioral features of the primate species.

The ideas presented here as general and special hypotheses were
first published in general form in 1972 (6) and later expanded
(3,9). The hypotheses are unique so far as this author can determine, and should not be confused with the related and interesting

Table 13.

Accumulation of Damage or Dysfunctions that are or may be a
Function of MLP

1. Chromosomal aberration frequency
2. Age pigments
3. Physiological functions
4. Mental or cognitive functions
5. Resistance to pathogenic diseases
6. Onset frequency of degenerative diseases
7. Physico-chemical alteration of chromatin (protein and DNA)*
8. Alteration of enzyme induction kinetics*
9. Ability of cells to maintain a given state of differentiation*
10. Accumulation of methionine sulfoxide residues in protein*

Repair or Protective Processes that are or may be a Function of MLP

1. DNA repair (UV, depurination, DNA-protein adducts)
2. Selective protein degradation*
3. Superoxide dismutase level*
4. Glutathionine peroxidase*
5. Catalase*
6. Vitamin E*
7. Vitamin C*
8. Activation of precarcinogen agents
9. Ratio of B/A lactate dehydrogenase
10. Metabolic rate
11. Encephalization index
12. Reduction of developmental rate
13. Neoteny
14. Free radical scavanger and antioxidant levels*
15. Rate of general nucleic acid and protein synthesis and
    degradation*
16. Fidelity of DNA and protein synthesis*
17. Interferon levels*
18. Methionine sulfoxide reductase*

----

*Under investigation in our laboratory
Taken from (3,6,8,9).

work of Sacher (13,18,27).

The most important role of the special hypothesis is to suggest
meaningful experiments that might elucidate the biological nature of
human aging and the processes determining the period during which
optimum physical and mental health is maintained. A new experimental
approach is suggested that would search for the "natural" differences
governing aging rate by using a comparative analysis of species
closely related genetically but having significant differences in
their innate aging rate. A comparision of age-dependent changes, as
well as other innate characteristics of the organism, as a function

of MLP would give important insights as to which are important aging
and life maintenance processes. Table 13 summarizes some data that
is already known and areas where experiments are planned that relate
to MLP.

DEDIFFERENTIATION AS THE PRIMARY SENESCENT PROCESS

A common idea in gerontology is that organismal aging is related
to the time-dependent accumulation of some type of damage, be it cellular or extracellular (8,28,29). This damage is usually predicted
to interfere with the proper function of the cell or lead to cell
death. According to this idea, time-dependent accumulation of damage
would be expected where the rate of accumulation is proportional to
the characteristic aging rate of the species (8,30).

However, a completely different and more recent idea is that
aging is primarily a result, not of accumulation of damage, at least
primarily (31), but instead is the result of an inherent instability
of organs or cells in terms of their ability to maintain their properly differentiated state, or the ability of the organism to maintain
proper homeostatic processes. For example, the advent of sexual
maturity brings a new set of hormones which could affect the long-
term functional stability of many different cells, and not merely the
immediate changes in the target tissues. This developmentally-linked
type of aging process is of an epigenetic nature.

It is not necessary to observe any time-dependent accumulation of
damage as the result of the Continuously-Acting or Developmentally-
Linked Action Processes. Although it is possible that some type of
accumulation of damage occurs, the author suggests a new concept in
which a constant time-independent pool of defective or damaged cellular constituents exists within the cell or organism. A simple model
follows, illustrating this idea, and is coupled with the hypothesis
that the key primary aging process results from a slow
dedifferentiation of cells.

Continuously-Acting and Developmentally-Linked Aging Processes
are suggested to act by slowly destabilizing and altering the proper,
differentiated states of cells following sexual maturation. Every
type of differentiated cell is postulated to have a characteristic
level, or pool, of agents that cause damage. This, in turn, produces
a characteristic level (pool) of damaged cellular constituents. However, counteracting processes exist that reduce the level of these
damaging agents and remove or repair the damaged cellular components. Thus, an equilibrium is maintained. The net rate of turnover,
and the resultant "pool of damage," is determined by the cells' characteristic rates of input and removal of damage.

It is proposed that the degree and rate of turnover of this complex spectrum of damage within the cell determine the time-dependent

probabilty that dedifferentiation or epigenetic-like cell alterations will occur.

Thus, cells from an organism which has a long MLP would be expected to have a higher differentiated stability state as the result of a lower constitutive pool of damage. This lower pool of damage would be the result of higher levels of protective and repair processes, as well as initially lower levels of production of damaging agents.

Aging is produced by Developmentally-Linked Aging Processes by a similar mechanism. It is proportional to the length of time cells are exposed to the developmentally-related harmful agents, as well as to the amounts of these substances to which cells are exposed. The agents would not result in an accumulation of damage, but would simply increase the time-dependent probability that a dedifferentiation-like cellular alteration would occur.

Aging would not necessarily be a result of a time-dependent loss of repair or protective processes. Each cell would have an innate and characteristic probability of dedifferentiating on the basis of its constitutive levels of damage. Different cell types within an organism would be expected to have different probabilities of dedifferentiation. Of course, the original state of dedifferentiation would direct the probability of what types of dedifferentiation events would most likely occur.

The idea of a correlation existing between MLP and the constitutive level of damage within a cell leads to the question of how this level is controlled. A feedback relationship probably exists between the levels of damage within a cell and the level of repair and protective processes that are expressed. Thus, the sensitivity of such a feedback loop may determine the species' innate levels of Continuously-Acting Anti-Aging Processes and would therefore be a key regulatory process governing aging rate.

What evidence supports the innate loss of ability of cells to maintain their proper post-maturational state of differentiation as a primary aging process? There is at present very little positive data (33), and perhaps the most convincing aspect of the dedifferentiation hypothesis is that it can satisfactorily explain, as a causative process, many of the different physiological problems and diseases associated with aging. For example, the slow loss of a particular physiological function could be the result of a higher fraction of the cells in a tissue not producing the optimum spectrum of enzyme levels, hormone receptors, structural proteins, hormones, and so forth. A detailed search for something radically wrong with the cells making up the tissue, such as an accumulation of defective proteins, reduced protein synthesis capacity, or defective structures in the genetic apparatus of the cell, would be fruitless. Yet, significant loss of proper function is evident.

More damaging to the organism could be the synthesis of a protein with high biological activity from a certain cell type that should not normally be synthesizing that protein. For example, suppose a liver cell began to synthesize small amounts of a hormone that inhibited proper homeostatic regulation of thyroid or immune function.

Strong evidence for such dedifferentiation processes occurring more frequently as a function of increased physiological age is found on analysis of the proteins present in many types of tumors (34-37). A common finding is a complex appearance of gene derepression, where often a tumor of an adult synthesizes proteins normally found in fetal development, such as alpha-fetal protein, or when non-endocrine cancerous tissue synthesizes hormones. In this sense, the age-dependent increase in at least some types of cancers may represent a special case of the general much broader age-dependent dedifferentiation process apparently occurring in all cells with time (38). A slight change in a cell's differentiated state would not be noticed, particularly in post-mitotic tissue. However, if the change in differentiation represents a reverse back to a dividing state, then the process of simple uncontrolled growth would amplify this type of dedifferentiation until it is readily detected and results in the early death of the organism.

Any protein synthesized by a cell that was not present when general immunocompetence occurred in early life could be antigenic. Thus, dedifferentiation could be the basis for many of the autoimmune diseases associated with increased age (39,40). Furthermore, the well known age-dependent changes in hair growth, density and appearance of wild coarse hair, blemishes such as age-spots and moles in skin, the decrease of response time of cells to hormones or other types of stimuli, the loss of hormone receptor sites and the appearance of abnormal protein in the brain (41,42), all can be accounted for by a slight alteration in the cells' differentiated state, and without proposing that the cell operates improperly because of a high accumulation of some type of damage or basic impairment to cell life-maintenance functions.

It is also known that viruses and/or virus-related genetic material is endogenous in the normal genome of cells by a vertical transfer mechanism (through germ cells) (43,44). The role of such viral-related genetic information is not known—but it may be related to cancer and slow-type virus diseases (45,46). The age-dependent loss of a cell's ability to maintain repression of these genes by random dedifferentiation events could also be an important component of the aging process (47,48).

We have recently investigated the dedifferentiation aging model in our laboratory by searching for the age-dependent expression of genes in cells where these genes are not expected to be expressed (38). Specifically, the possible expression of α and β globin genes and the endogenous mouse leukemia virus genes (MuLV) as a function of increased age in liver and brain of mouse was investigated. The assay system utilized a highly radioactive synthesized probe called complementary DNA (cDNA), produced by a purified preparation of globin mRNA or MuLV RNA and reverse transcriptase enzyme. The cDNA probe was mixed with RNA preparations obtained from liver and brain at different ages and examined for the presence of cDNA-RNA hybrid complexes. The presence of a cDNA-RNA hybrid would show that RNA complementary to that specific cDNA probe was present in the RNA preparation. The results, shown in Table 14, reveal an age-dependent two-fold increase in the levels of α and β globin in liver and brain. Results shown in Table 15 for the MuLV show a two-fold increase in the amount of MuLV-related RNA, which is related to an increased fraction of RNA complementary to the entire virus genome found present. More experimentation along these lines should be undertaken to evaluate the role dedifferentiation might play in aging.

EXTENSION OF HUMAN MENTAL AND PHYSICAL HEALTH--POSSIBILITY AND ADVISABILITY

Most persons prefer good health, with mental health as the most prized possession (49). But would people prefer a short healthy life span or a long healthy one? Recent surveys on this question clearly indicate that, although many social, economical and theological problems would surface upon any substantial extension of human mental and physical health, most of the people of the United States at least favor the opportunity of having a choice (50-54).

The most serious difficulty in discussing this subject is that of evaluating whether a significant extension of human health is a real possibility in the near future (55-57). The subject is brought up here because the unified hypothesis of aging and life maintenance processes as presented in this chapter suggests that, although a reasonable understanding of the vast complexity of the biological nature of the aging process may lie in the distant future, some significant control of the aging rate may be possible in the near future. For example, processes which govern aging rate are likely to be far less difficult to investigate than aging processes. If the unified hypothesis presented here proves correct, then we should be prepared for a substantial increase in our knowledge in the near future about these specific life maintanance processes and how their effectiveness to slow aging may be enhanced. Progress in this area would almost be impossible to stop, for it could come not only from laboratories primarily interested in the biological nature of aging, but also from cancer and environmental toxicology groups.

One interesting idea that may result in our first significant reduction of innate aging rate is based on the notion that levels of repair and protective processes are governed by a cell's characteristic level, or pool, of damaged cellular constituents. It may prove

Table 14. Amount of Globin Sequences in Brain and Liver as a Function of Age[a]

	6-month old animal		20-month old animal		27-month old animal	
	Nucleus	Cytoplasm	Nucleus	Cytoplasm	Nucleus	Cytoplasm
Brain						
$\dfrac{\text{globin RNA (g)}}{\text{total RNA (g)}} \times 10^6$	5.3	11.3	11.2	14.4	12.0	20.6
$\dfrac{\text{globin RNA}}{\text{cell}}$	15	282	32	360	34	515
Liver						
$\dfrac{\text{globin RNA (g)}}{\text{total RNA (g)}} \times 10^6$	3.8	1.9	7.5	4.7	9.5	8.6
$\dfrac{\text{globin RNA}}{\text{cell}}$	12	111	23	274	30	502

[a]Taken from Ono and Cutler (38).

Table 15. Amount of Murine Leukemia Virus-Related RNA in Brain and
          Liver Nuclei as a Function of Age[a]

	6 month animal	27 month animal
Brain		
$\dfrac{\text{virus RNA}}{\text{total RNA}}$ X 10^5	5	9
percent genome transcribed	42	70
Liver		
$\dfrac{\text{virus RNA}}{\text{total RNA}}$ X 10^5	9	16
percent genome transcribed	50	74

[a]Taken from Ono and Cutler (38).

possible to induce higher levels of a complex spectrum of repair and
protective processes within a cell, without knowing what they are or
the details of how they are controlled, by simply compelling a cell
to incorporate a complex spectrum of damaged cellular components (9).

In terms of Developmentally-Linked Aging Processes, means to
induce a slower rate of development, or to selectively remove or
inhibit hormone secretions after their useful period is over, may
also prove practicable in the near future.

Thus, I believe the possibility of developing life-extension
technology, such that the aging rate is slowed down by a factor of
two or so, should be taken seriously. Consequently, consideration as
to whether life-extension would be advisable should begin now
(56,57). Too frequently in the past, such possibilities were thought
unrealistic and were readily discarded (53). Hence, life span extension has not been sufficiently considered either in terms of its
possible benefits or problems. Resolute decisions in this area are
essential for proper distribution of funds supporting research that
is more oriented toward the development of life-extension technology.

If significant life extension is a real possibility in the near
future, say over the next 50 years, what about advisability? People
seem more capable of picking out the problems rather than the benefits. Some obvious problem areas are (1) population growth control,

(2) economic institutions, such as the Social Security System, which now depends on existing MLP, (3) the fair distribution of life extension technology to the poor and rich, and (4) the conflict extended life span might cause for different ethnic and religious groups.

And what about the benefits? At the individual level, a longer period of good physical and mental health is usually associated with a correspondingly greater enjoyment of life, but this, of course, could be highly debated. However, one could have less fear that many of the enjoyments of life would pass him by simply because there was not enough time. Moreover, a postponement of death and the suffering that frequently accompanies it would be welcome.

Less obvious are social and economic benefits for the entire human race. If we reflect on why increased longevity of man evolved in the first place and how this played a key role in his evolutionary success, I believe the benefits for man will become more obvious. It is disappointing to find even in recent and popular publications on the evolutionary history of man a complete lack of coverage on the role longevity may play in the evolutionary success of man. We learn of the importance of bipedalism, of the importance of the thumb and fingers, of the ability to talk, of the spoken and written language and, of course, of man's other remarkable mental abilities. But could man have possibly survived without a corresponding extension of his years of good physical and mental health? I doubt it very much.

Further extension of life span may produce more of the same type of benefits that occurred in the past. If so, there would be more time for learning, resulting perhaps in a higher qualitative increase in our knowledge, not only about the universe, but also of ourselves. With more time to explore and discover, with greater understanding of life and the control over it, would not this lead to a better world? In terms of economics, would not increased productivity, as well as creativity, offset an increase in the length of time an individual might spend in the senescent period of life?

This last question bears importantly on just how life extension might be achieved. If life is extended in a way similar to how it evolved in the past, then an increased period of health would bring a proportional increase in the period of senescence. Would this be acceptable?

It is unrealistic to believe that some type of treatment may be developed to maintain health up to, say, 100 years, and then for the organism suddenly to grow older overnight and die, thus eliminating the senescent phase of life. Such an idea is frequently stated as an interpretation of a further squaring of the percent survival curve (53,58). But, as noted before, this idea simply conveys the incorrect concept that the declining slope of the survival curve is related to the rate of aging.

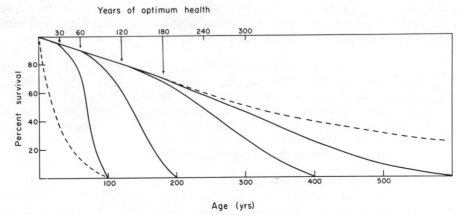

Fig. 6. Percent survival curves for man in the past, present and
        possible future. Dotted lines represent the two exponential
        decline curves where smallest fraction of senescent individ-
        uals occurs, first curve with MLP of about 100 years about
        10,000 years ago and second curve, with infinite MLP. For
        the various curves shown, number of years of optimum health
        is taken to be when the curve breaks for the theoretical
        maximum level of percent survival where aging rate of zero
        or MLP is infinite.

   What happens instead as the curve becomes squared is that the
percent of senescent individuals increases. For example, let us go
back several thousand years, where man, as a Homo sapien with a MLP
of 100, had an average life span (50% mean) of 30 years. This is
shown in Figure 6 for percent survival and Figure 7 for the corresponding rate of mortality curve. The exponential decline in percent
survival, or a constant rate of death with time, determined how long
man lived under the natural environmental hazards that led to his
evolution. An increased probability of death with time, where death
becomes more related to senescence, was an exception.

   As man becomes able to diminish his environmental hazards, but
unable to reduce his innate aging rate correspondingly, the 50% mean
survival increased, as well as did the percent senescent individuals
in the population (see Figs. 6,7). This trend continued to what we
have today, where average life span has reached about 75 years in the
developed nations, and MLP has remained constant. Further significant squaring of the curve in the future is unlikely. Even if it
does occur, it would only further increase the high level (about 50%)
of people over 35 years of age that we now have in the population.

   However, one result not frequently considered is that, given the
present intensity of environmental hazards and medical care, a

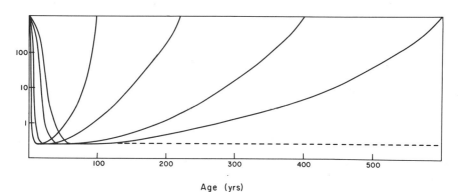

Age (yrs)

Fig. 7. Rate of mortality for man in the past, present and possible
       future. Curves correlate to the present survival curves in
       Fig. 6, including the dotted lines where probability of
       death is independent of physiological age.

reduction in aging rate or an increase in MLP would reduce, not
increase, the percent of senescent individuals in the population.
Examples of how an increase in MLP would affect future percent
survival curves are shown in Figures 6 and 7 for 200, 400, 600 and
infinite MLP's. In effect, increasing MLP would bring the cycle back
to normal, to a balance between probability of death and innate
capacity to maintain health--the way it originally was several
thousand years ago. Thus, if MLP begins to increase again, an
individual would have more of a chance of being killed before he
reached a given level of senescence. For example, if the aging
process can be stopped so that the probability of death does not
exceed that for a 30-year-old man today in the U.S., then MLP would
be about 1246 years and 50% mean survival would be 374 years. Of
course, if environmental hazards began to reduce in proportion to
increased MLP, then the percent of senescent individuals in the
population would remain constant.

    The population problem may also not become as serious as is
frequently believed. Increased MLP does not imply a correspondingly
increased reproduction rate. Couples today could have up to 20
children, but instead they usually have 2 or 3. Even further birth
control measures are being undertaken in some nations today. As long
as the rate of birth is balanced by the rate of death, any population
would be stable, regardless of the longevity of its members. A more
immediate problem is the initial size to which the population would
increase before such an equilibrium came into play. Estimates of
this equilibrium value, if MLP were doubled today and maintained for
100 years, appear to be small compared to the normal population
growth that is expected under no change in MLP.

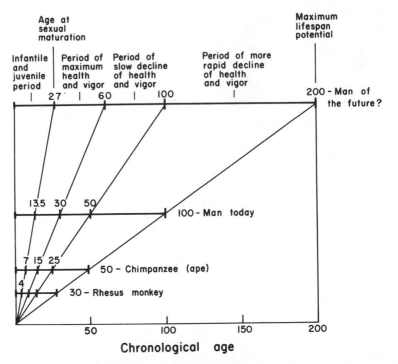

Fig. 8.   Stages of development of the primate species relative to
one another and the projection of these stages to man with
a maximum life span potential of 200 years. Taken from (9).

Life extension up to a MLP of 200 or more years, if achieved by
similar processes as those that have recently evolved, would likely
require a uniform prolongation of the stages of development. Figure
8 shows the different developmental periods of life span in Rhesus,
chimpanzee, and man; and from these values an extrapolation is made
as to what the extended time-period of these various phases of life
span would be for man with a MLP of 200 years. In the example, the
period of maximum health and vigor increases from 16.5 years to 33
years, and the period of rapid decline in vigor and health increases
from 50 years to 100 years. It appears that more years of senescence
would be gained than years of youth. However, it should be clear
from our previous discussion and Figures 6 and 7 that, in spite of an
increased period of senescence, the percent of the population in such
a phase of life would decrease.

Another remarkable change occurring during the recent evolutionary history of man is his increase in brain size with the accompany-
ing increase in mental ability (59,60). Figure 9 illustrates the
correlation of brain weight to MLP during recent hominid evolution.
If such a trend continued, a brain size increase from about 1450 g to
5000 g would evolve for a corresponding increase of MLP from 100 to

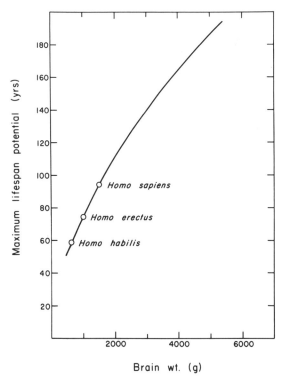

Braln wt. (g)

Fig. 9. Evolutionary trend of increased brain size in relation to
         increase in MLP for man in his recent evolutionary past and
         a projection for the future. Equation for this projection
         is:

$$\text{MLP (yrs)} = 1.607 \, (\text{Brain wt., g})^{.5579}$$

200 years. Whether such an increase also would result in higher
mental functions, remains to be determined (61,62), but recent
comparative studies on neuron networks between man and chimpanzee
show few qualitative differences. It may very well be that higher
brain functions, as evident in man, result from a relatively small
amount of genetic information, where there is much redundancy in its
design. This would be consistent with such a high evolutionary rate
of development of the brain, along with an increased MLP.

    An interesting hypothesis on the mechanism of how the morphologi-
cal functions of man evolved, known as neoteny, is that certain
stages of early development were retarded, as compared to similar
stages of development in the apes (63-66). In this sense, adult man
has many fetal characteristics that are found only in the infant
developmental stages of man's hominid ancestors, as well as some of
the living ape species (67,68). This idea suggests that the general

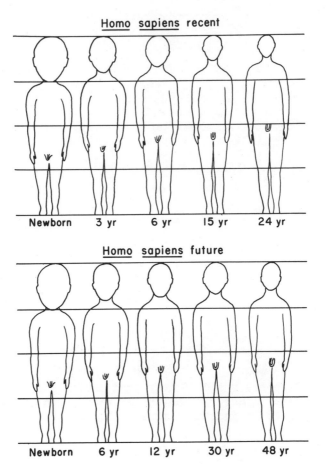

Homo sapiens recent

Newborn   3 yr   6 yr   I5 yr   24 yr

Homo sapiens future

Newborn   6 yr   12 yr   30 yr   48 yr

FURTHER RETARDATION OF DEVELOPMENT AND FETALIZATION
OF CHARACTERISTICS AS A MODEL FOR THE FUTURE
EVOLUTION OF MAN

Fig. 10.   The proportional changes in body and brain sizes during
postnatal developmental stages of man and how these stages
might appear in a man whose MLP has evolved to a level of
200 years. Taken from (9).

morphology of man, such as large brain size and his unusually slow
pattern of development, evolved as a result of small alterations in
the regulatory processes governing developmental rate (69).

The general morphological appearance of postnatal developmental
stages of man today, and what it may be in the future if continued
along similar lines, is shown in Figure 10. Table 16 summarizes some
of the major developmental and physical characteristics of man with a

Table 16.   Model of Continued Evolution of Human Longevity[a]

MLP, yrs	92	150	200
Brain capacity, cm^3	1446	3396	5688
EQ	7.5	15.2	22.6
N_c X 10^{-8}	91	168	240
Body wt, g	65	81	97
SMR, c/g/d	23	21.8	20.8
MCC, Kc/g	780	1198	1523
ASM, yr	14-17	22-27	30-37
% Br wt/Body wt, g/g	2.2	4.2	5.8

[a]The assumption is made that these parameters continued to evolve along the same equation as they have during the past 2.5 million years of hominid evolution.

MLP of 100 and 200 years.

Just as man thought his earth to be the center of the universe, so he has also thought his body to be nearly perfect and improvement to be impossible. We are now closer to challenging this idea directly by inquiring about what biological processes determine the innate duration of health, how these processes might be improved, and what might be the consequences if significant life extension occurs. If the potential benefits of extended physical and mental health are realized, man may be nearing a quantum jump in his evolution--a self-evolutionary process that is perhaps as natural as his evolutionary past, and as inescapable.

REFERENCES

1. C. E. Finch and L. Hayflick, eds., "Handook of the Biology of Aging," Van Nostrand Reinhold, New York (1977).
2. P. S. Timiras, ed., "Developmental Physiology and Aging," Macmillan Co., New York (1972).
3. R. G. Cutler, in:"Interdisciplinary Topics in Gerontology," Vol. 9, R. G. Cutler, ed., Karger, Basel (1976).
4. P. Weiss, in:"Perspectives in Experimental Gerontology," Charles C. Thomas, Springfield, Illinois (1966).
5. R. G. Cutler, Proc. Natl. Acad. Sci. USA 72:4664 (1975).
6. R. G. Cutler, in:"Advances in Gerontological Research, Vol. 4," B. L. Strehler, ed., Academic Press, New York (1972).
7. R. G. Cutler, Mech. Ageing Dev. 2:381 (1974).

8. R. G. Cutler, in:"Genetic Effects on Aging," D. Bergsma, D. E. Harrison, and N. W. Paul, eds., Alan R. Liss, New York (1978).
9. R. G. Cutler, in:"The Biology of Aging," J. A. Behnke, C. E. Finch, and G. B. Moment, eds., Plenum Press, New York (1978).
10. K. M. Weiss, J. Human Evol. (in press).
11. R. G. Cutler, J. Human Evol. 5:169 (1976).
12. R. G. Cutler, Gerontology 25:69 (1979).
13. G. A. Sacher, in:"Primate Functional Morphology and Evolution," R. Tuttle, ed., Mouton, The Hague (1975).
14. H. J. Jerison, "Evolution of the Brain and Intelligence," Academic Press, New York (1973).
15. M. C. King and A. C. Wison, Science 188:107 (1975).
16. F. J. Ayala, "Molecular Evolution," Sinauer Pub., Sunderland, Mass. (1976).
17. G. B. Kolata, Science 189:446 (1975).
18. G. A. Sacher, in:"Ciba Foundation Colloquium on Aging," Vol. 5 (1959).
19. R. E. Leakey and R. Lewin, "Origins," E. P. Dutton (1977).
20. A. C. Wilson, L. R. Maxson, and V. M. Sarich, Proc. Natl. Acad. Sci. USA 71:2843 (1974).
21. A. C. Wilson, V. M. Sarich, and L. R. Maxson, Proc. Natl. Acad. Sci. USA 71:3028 (1974).
22. A. C. Wilson, S. S. Carlson, and T. J. White, Ann. Rev. Biochem. 46:573 (1977).
23. G. L. Bush, S. M. Case, A. C. Wilson, and J. L. Patton, Proc. Natl. Acad. Sci. USA 74:3942 (1977).
24. J. F. MacDonald, G. K. Chambers, J. David, and F. J. Ayala, Proc. Natl. Acad. Sci. USA 74:4562 (1977).
25. D. Pilbeam and S. J. Gould, Science 186:892 (1974).
26. S. J. Gould, "Ontogeny and Phylogeny," Belknap Press of Harvard University Press, Cambridge, Mass. (1977).
27. G. A. Sacher, Exp. Geront. 3:265 (1968).
28. R. G. Cutler, in:"Aging, Carcinogenesis and Radiation Biology," K. C. Smith, ed., Plenum Press, New York (1976).
29. J. P. Ogrodnik, J. H. Wulf, and R. G. Cutler, Exp. Geront. 10:119 (1975).
30. R. G. Cutler, Exp. Geront. 10:37 (1975).
31. C. E. Finch, Quart. Rev. Biol. 51:49 (1976).
32. U. Reiss and D. Gershon, Eur. J. Biochem. 63:617 (1976).
33. H. Ursprung, "The Stability of the Differentiated State," Springer-Verlag, New York (1968).
34. C. L. Markert, Cancer Res. 28:1908 (1968).
35. A. D. Braun, "The Biology of Cancer," Addison-Wesley, Reading, Mass. (1974).
36. J. H. Goggin and N. G. Anderson, Adv. Cancer Res. 19:105 (1974).
37. J. Uriel, in:"Cancer, A Comprehensive Treatise," F. Becke, ed., Plenum Press, New York (1975).
38. T. Ono and R. G. Cutler, Proc. Natl. Acad. Sci. USA 75:4431 (1978).
39. R. L. Walford, Gerontologia 21:184 (1975).

40. R. L. Walford, "The Immunologic Theory of Aging," Williams and Wilkins, Baltimore (1969).
41. K. Nandy, in:"The Aging Brain," K. Nandy and I. Sherwin, eds., Plenum Press, New York (1976).
42. R. D. Terry, in:"A New Look at Biological Aging," J. A. Behnke, C. E. Finch, and G. B. Moment, eds., Plenum Press, New York (1978).
43. R. J. Huebner and G. J. Todaro, Proc. Natl. Acad. Sci. USA 64:1087 (1969).
44. H. M. Temin, Science 192:1075 (1976).
45. J. Uriel, Cancer Res. 36:4269 (1976).
46. M. R. Ahuja and R. Anders, in:"Recent Advances in Cancer: Cell Biology, Molecular Biology, and Tumor Virology, Vol. 1," R. C. Galli, ed. (1977).
47. E. J. Field and A. Peat, Gerontologia 17:129 (1971).
48. E. J. Field and B. K. Shelton, Gerontologia 19:211 (1973).
49. G. J. Gruman, Trans. Amer. Phil. Soc. New Series, Part 9:56 (1966).
50. B. L. Strehler, Fed. Proc. 34:5 (1975).
51. P. G. Goldschmidt and I. H. Jillson, "A Comprehensive Study of the Ethical, Legal, and Social Implications of Advances in Biomedical and Behavioral Research and Technology," Policy Research Inc., Baltimore, Md.
52. B. L. Neugarten and R. J. Havighurst, "Extending the Human Life Span: Social Policy and Social Ethics," Committee on Human Development, University of Chicago, Chicago (1977).
53. B. L. Neugarten and R. J. Havighurst, "Social Policy, Social Ethics and the Aging Society," Committee on Human Development, University of Chicago, Chicago (1977).
54. H. Gerjuoy, in:"Frontiers in Aging: Life Extension," F. M. Lassman, ed., International J. Aging and Human Development, in press.
55. Life-Span Conference: The Center for the Study of Democratic Institutions/The Fund for the Republic, Inc., Santa Barbara, CA (1970).
56. R. G. Cutler and R. A. Kalish, Gerontologist 17:141 (1977).
57. R. G. Cutler, in:"Frontiers in Aging: Life Extension," R. M. Lassman, ed., International J. Aging and Human Development, in press.
58. L. Hayflick, Nat. Hist. 86:22 (1977).
59. P. V. Tobias, "The Brain in Hominid Evolution," Columbia University Press, New York (1971).
60. R. E. Leakey and R. Lewin, "Origins," E. P. Dutton, New York (1977).
61. B. Rensch, Amer. Naturalist XC:81 (1956).
62. L. Van Halen, Amer. J. Phys. Anthrop. 40:417 (1974).
63. A. H. Schulz, Proc. Amer. Phil Soc. 94:428 (1950).
64. S. J. Gould, Nat. Hist. 85:22 (1976).
65. S. J. Gould, Nat. Hist. 85:18 (1976).

66. S. J. Gould, "Ontongeny and Phylogeny," Harvard University
    Press, Cambridge, Mass. (1977).
67. A. H. Schultz, Quart. Rev. Biol. 1:465 (1926).
68. G. F. R. S. DeBeer, "Embryos and Ancestors," Oxford University
    Press, London (1971).
69. S. J. Gould, "Ever Since Darwin," W. W. Norton & Co., New York
    (1977).

LONGEVITY POTENTIAL, PHYLOGENETIC

AND ECOLOGICAL CONSTRAINTS IN MAMMALS

François Bourliére

INSERM Gerontology Research Unit
Paris, France

The dependence of mammalian life span on some constitutional variables, adult body weight, brain body weight, specific metabolic rate and deep body temperature, has been repeatedly discussed by Sacher (1,2). Furthermore, having found, in his 1976 paper, a relationship between the rate of entropy production and the duration of life when body weight is constant, Sacher goes so far as to conclude that "everything we know about the neurological concomitants of mammalian longevity--sensory, intellectual, and motor--supports the intuition that the length of life of a species is closely related to its intelligence and, indeed, that longevity is a major teleonomic purpose and manifestation of animal intelligence."

Such a view is hard to substantiate when one considers the numerous data on mammalian longevity recently made available in the literature (3,4,5,6,7). The maximum recorded life span of a number of small animals is given in Table 1, together with the adult body weight, and the capability of the species to undergo hibernation (H) or periods of daily torpor (T).

The extreme longevity potential of bats (Chiroptera) stands out at once, despite the fact that the behavioral performances of this mammalian order are not particularly sophisticated, and in spite of a brain/body weight ratio not very different from that of the short-lived and non-heterothermic small rodents. It is also to be noted that within a given taxonomic category--whether it be Marsupialia, Insectivora, Chiroptera, Primates, or Rodentia--all the species sharing a similar body weight which are also able to lower their body temperature when environmental conditions become unfavorable, are at the same time those which enjoy the greater longevity potential. This is quite obvious when one compares murids and heteromyids among the Rodentia.

Table 1. Adult Body Weight (g), Maximum Recorded Life Span
          (years), Ability to Hibernate or Estivate (H) and to
          Enter Daily Torpor (T), Among Small Mammals

	Adult body weight	Maximum longevity	Hibernation or Torpor
Marsupialia			
Planigale sp.	5	1	
Sminthopsis crassicaudata	10-15	3	T
Acrobates pygmaeus	12-14	4	T
Cercartetus caudatus	15-25	>5.5	T
Antechinus stuartii	24-49	>3	T
Petaurus norfolcensis	90-130	12	
Dasycercus cristicaudata	120-170	>5	T
Caluromys derbianus	190-220	>5	
Caluromysiops irrupta	ca 200	>7.5	
Dasyuorides byrnei	ca 200	>5	
Macrotis lagotis	300-1600	>7	T ?
Dasyurus viverrinus	680-1130	7	
Potorous tridactylus	1360-1810	>9.5	
Insectivora			
Suncus etruscus	1.25-2.3	>2	
Sorex araneus	6-10	1.5	
Crocidura russula	6-10	4	
Neomys fodieus	10-22	1.5	
Blarina brevicauda	14-22	2.5	
Chiroptera			
Pipistrellus pipistrellus	3.8-6.5	11	H.T
Myotis mystacinus	4-8	18	H.T
Rhinolophus hipposideros	4-9	>18	H.T
Myotis daubentoni	6-12	18	H.T
Plecotus auritus	6-12	13	H.T
Barbastella barbastellus	6-13	18	H.T
Myotis nattereri	7-12	17	H.T
Plecotus austriacus	7-14	12	H.T
Rhinolophus ferrum-equinum	13-34	>22	H.T

Another constitutional variable that must be taken into consideration is the reproductive potential of species. Those with a high
reproductive rate (large litter-size and several litters per year),
like rodents of the microtine or murine type, have a low longevity
potential. In contrast to these "r-strategists," the "K-strate-
gists," such as bats and primates with a low reproductive potential,
have a much longer life span (8,9).

"Intelligence" as such has, therefore, quite probably very little
to do with the longevity potential of mammals. Those species which

Table 1. (Continuation). Adult Body Weight (g), Maximum Recorded
         Life Span (years), Ability to Hibernate or Estivate (H)
         and to Enter Daily Torpor (T), Among Small Mammals

	Adult body weight	Maximum longevity	Hibernation or Torpor
Chiroptera (continued)			
Myotis myotis	20-45	18	H.T
Desmodus rotundus	33-47	12.5	
Eidolon helvum	250-310	21.5	
Primates			
Microcebus murinus	45-170	>11	H.T
Galago demidovii	50-90	10	H.T
Cebuella pygmaea	110-160	10	
Galago senegalensis	150-300	>10	
Callithrix jacchus	260-320	12.5	T
Microcebus coquereli	300-400	15.5	H.T
Cheirogaleus major	340-600	11	H.T
Saguinus fuscicollis	370-436	> 7	T ?
Leontopithecus rosalia	430-654	10	
Perodictitus potto	600-1600	11	
Calimico goeldi	645-680	10	
Miopithecus talapoin	800-900	28	
Galago crassicaudatus	1000-1800	14	
Rodentia			
Micromys minutus	7-10	4	
Perognathus longimembris	7-19	>8	T
Perognathus fallax	14-17	>8	T
Mus musculus	14-25	3.5	
Peromyscus leucopus	14-30	>8	T
Microtus arvalis	16-51	>1.5	
Apodemus sylvaticus	16-30	>4	
Peromyscus maniculatus	17-35	8	T
Apodemus flavicollis	18-40	5	
Microtus agrestis	20-47	>1.5	
Muscardinus avellanarius	23-43	6	H
Rattus rattus	150-250	4.5	
Rattus norvegicus	240-360	3	

are endowed with the longest life span appear to be basically those
most capable of efficiently adapting to environmental changes, both
at the individual and at the population levels. Such a high degree
of adaptability can actually be achieved in two different (and not
forcibly exclusive) ways, through adaptive behaviors (i.e., "intelligence," according to Sacher) as well as through physiological mechanisms like heterothermy which enable an organism to temporarily
withstand adverse environmental conditions.

A relationship between an extended longevity potential and a high degree of physiological and/or behavioral adaptability to changing environmental conditions might also help to explain why, in a toxonomic category like bats, long-lived species are more frequently ecountered in temperate than in tropical areas. The more adaptable, thus, the potentially more longevous species would in our view have a better chance to be selected by the extreme seasonality or the impredictability of climatic conditions in northern latitudes.

REFERENCES

1. G. A. Sacher, Relations of lifespan to brain weight and body weight in mammals, in:"The Lifespan of Animals," G. E. W. Wolstenholme and M. O'Connor, eds., Churchill, London (1959).
2. G. A. Sacher, Evaluation of the entropy and information terms governing mammalian longevity, Interdis. Top. Gerontol. Basel 9:69 (1976).
3. L. R. Collins, "Monotremes and Marsupials. A Reference for Zoological Institutions," Smithsonian Institution, Washington (1973).
4. G. B. Corbet and H. N. Southern, eds., "The Handbook of British Mammals, Second Edition," Blackwell, Oxford (1977).
5. Th. Haltenorth and H. Diller, "Bestimmungsbuch. Saugetiere Afrikas und Madagascars," BLV Verlagsgesellschaft, Munchen (1977).
6. P. Hershkovitz, "Living New World Monkeys (Platyrrhini). Volume I," University of Chicago Press, Chicago (1977).
7. J. Niethammer and F. Krapp, "Handbuch der Saugetiere Europas, Band I," Akademische Verlagsgesellschaft, Wiesbaden (1978).
8. F. Bouliere, Lifespans of mammalian and bird populations in nature, in:"The Lifespan of Animals," G. E. W. Wolstenholme and M. O'Connor, eds., Churchill, London (1959).
9. F. B. Golley, K. Petruscewicz, and L. Ryszkokwski, "Small Mammals: Their Productivity and Population Dynamics," Cambridge University Press, Cambridge (1975).

POPULATION DOUBLING NUMBERS IN CELLS

WITH GENETIC DISORDERS

Osamu Nikaido, Sadayuki Ban[*] and Tsutomu Sugahara

Radiation Biology Center and Department of Experimental
Radiology, Faculty of Medicine[*], Kyoto University
Kyoto 606, Japan

INTRODUCTION

The limited life spans of fibroblasts derived from human embryonic lungs were first reported by Hayflick (1). Then, the correlation between doubling potentials of cells and maximal life spans of
donor animals (2) as well as the inverted correlation between doubling potentials of human fibroblasts and ages of donors were established (3). Thus, it has been thought that cells age as donors age,
or cells in vitro at least mimic parts of various processes of in
vivo aging, although the mechanisms of cellular aging are not yet
known.

Comparative evolutionary studies on the relationship between the
extent of unscheduled DNA synthesis (UDS) induced in the cells by
exposure to ultraviolet light (UV), and maximal life spans in various
placental animals from which the cells were derived, offered the
hypothesis that the ability of cells to repair DNA damage induced by
various environmental agents determines the life spans in animals
(4). On the other hand, cells obtained from patients with a genetic
disease, Hutchinson-Gilford progeria, were reported to be defective
in repairing single strand breaks formed in cellular DNA by gamma-
irradiation (5,6) and to have low doubling potentials in culture
(7). A contradictory result was also reported, however, for the same
disease (8). Nevertheless, these results have called the attention
of many investigators to the role of DNA repair in cellular aging.

Ontogenetic analyses are necessary to elucidate the role of a
cell's ability to repair DNA damage in its aging process. Results of
the alterations in this cellular reparability throughout in vitro
life spans, as obtained by many workers, are controversial (9,10,11).

For example, it was recently reported that the extent of UDS in mouse embryonic fibroblasts gradually decreased as in vitro age increased (12). A similar decrease in the extend of UDS as cells proceed through their life spans has never been reported for human cells. This decrease is seen in human cells only at very late passages (13).

By applying the repair hypothesis to in vitro aging, one can suggest that the limited life spans of cultured human cells result from the accumulation of DNA damage introduced by various environmental agents present in culture conditions. At the moment, it is unknown what sorts of and to what extent DNA damage accumulates in cells during their life spans. The biological characterization and identification of these damages is necessary before it will be possible to establish causal relationship between "cellular reparability" and cellular aging.

Cells obtained from patients with recessive genetic diseases, such as xeroderma pigmentosum (XP) and ataxia telangiectasia (AT), are known to be sensitive to UV and X-rays, respectively (14). It is well known that the sensitivity of these cells to various agents is due to their deficient ability to repair specific types of DNA damage (15,16). One might expect early cessation of growth potentials in such repair deficient mutants if the damage accumulated during culture, in ambient conditions, contained at least some damage the cells could not repair. Therefore, evaluation of doubling potentials of cells obtained from patients with XP, AT, and Werner's syndrome (WS), showing "premature" aging, and from healthy donors of various ages, was carried out.

For the assessment of "cellular reparability" to UV-damaged DNA, host-cell reactivation (HCR), using herpes simplex virus irradiated with UV, was applied to various cells as well as to cells at various in vitro ages (17,18). This technique was employed because the UDS induced in cells following treatment with UV, which is usually applied to detect the DNA repair, might not show actual completion of DNA repair. Rather, it might show only insertion of exogenous radioactive bases into the sites of damage. Virus production in host cells, on the other hand, implies complete repair of UV-induced damage in viral DNA.

MATERIALS AND METHODS

Cells, Culture Method and Medium

Fetal lung and heart tissues at five months gestational age were provided by the courtesy of the Human Embryo Center for Teratological Studies, Faculty of Medicine, Kyoto University. Skin biopsies taken from healthy donors of various ages were obtained through Kansai Electric Co. Hospital by courtesy of Dr. Y. Isobe. Skin biopsy

specimens of patients with conditions known to produce defective DNA
repair were provided by the courtesy of Professor Takebe, Radiation
Biology Center, Kyoto University, and those of Werner's syndrome were
offered by Kyoto University Hospital, Chiba University Hospital,
Tenri Hospital, and Obama Municipal Hospital.

Fibroblasts propagated from tissues or biopsy fragments by a
method being published elsewhere (19) were cultured in TD-40 culture
bottle at a concentration of 10^6 cells per 10 ml of Eagle's MEM
medium (Nissui Seiyaku Co , Tokyo) supplemented with 10% calf serum
(Flow Laboratories, Stanmore). The same batches of calf serum were
used throughout this experiment. Three bottles of cells were succes-
sively cultured. Cells were fed every 2 days with fresh medium and
subcultured at the 4th to 7th day, prior to reaching to near confluency. After harvesting the cells with 0.1% trypsin (Difco Laboratories, Detroit) and 0.01% EDTA (Waken Pharmacy Co., Osaka) in phosphate
buffer saline, an aliquot of 10^6 cells was inoculated into a TD-40
culture bottle. The cessation of growth of a cell population was
recognized when lower cell yields than inoculum cell number (10^6
cells) were obtained twice in successive subcultures. The number of
population doublings (PDN) attained by cells was calculated by the
method being published elsewhere (19).

The Virus and its Assay

Herpes simplex virus, type I, a large plaque variant of the +GC
Miyama strain (20), having a titer of 1.7 x 10^7 pfu/ml against
human aminon F1 cell line, was used for all virus experiments. After
diluting viral suspensions with phosphate buffer saline to the appropriate concentration, various doses of UV were given with germicidal
lamps (10 watt x 2, Toshiba GL-10) at a dose rate of 1.7 to 1.8
J/m^2/sec., and monitored at each exposure by Topcon radiometer
(Tokyo Kogaku Co. Ltd., Tokyo). 0.5 ml of UV-irradiated viral suspension was delivered to freshly confluent cells in plastic dishes (6
cm in diameter), which had been previously washed once with phosphate
buffer saline and incubated for 90 min. at 37°C. Virus adsorption
was stopped by adding 4.5 ml of complete medium containing 0.25%
human gammaglobulin (human immunoglobulin, Midorijuji Co., Osaka).
Plaques were scored on the 3rd day of incubation, and survival curves
for successful UV-irradiated herpes simplex virus infection of various cell strains were depicted as the function of UV doses. The survival curves were usually composed of two components (17). D_0 values
were obtained from the first component.

RESULTS

Repair of UV-Damaged Virus DNA by Various Host Cells

When cell progression had reached 20% of usual life spans, various cells were assayed for the UV-survival of herpes simplex

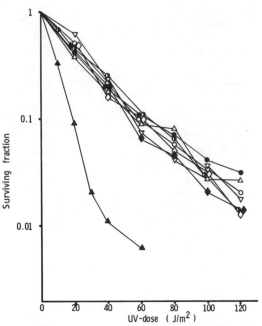

Fig. 1.   Host-cell reactivation of UV-irradiated herpes simplex
          virus in cells derived from healthy donors. △ 1.5-year-old
          female; ▽ 33-year-old female; ◇ 65-year-old female, from
          patient with genetic disorders; ◆ AT1SE, 9-year-old male;
          ▲ XP6NA, 6-year-old female; ● WS10B, 47-year-old male, and
          from fetus; ○ lung; and ◐ heart.

viruses. Cells obtained from healthy donors, patients with ataxia
telangiectasia and those with Werner's syndrome were most efficient
in HCR of UV-irradiated viruses, while cells from xeroderma pigmentosum patients were most reduced in HCR. D_0 values in J/m^2 for the
first component of the survival curves were 25 for normal cells and 8
for XP cells, as shown in Figure 1.

It is noteworthy that the lung and heart fibroblasts obtained
from a single fetus showed the same D_0 values in HCR of UV-irradiated viruses, though they had distinctly different doubling potentials, as shown later. Age-dependent changes of D_0 values were not
observed in three cell strains obtained from healthy donors of various ages.

Relationship Between in Vitro Ages and HCR

Cells cultured for various lengths of time were assayed for HCR
of UV-irradiated herpes simplex viruses. The D_0 values of the

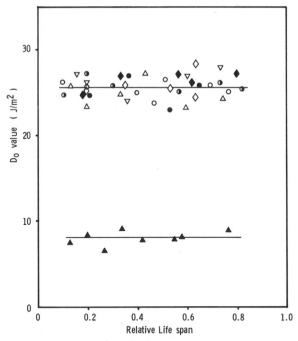

Fig. 2.   Changes of D_0 values of the first component in UV-survival
curves of herpes simplex virus in various cells during
culture. Maximal PDN attained by each cell strain was
assigned a relative life span of 1.0. Various symbols
denote as in legend of Figure 1.

first component in the survival curves plotted against in vitro ages
are shown in Figure 2.

As shown in this figure, no marked changes in D_0 values were
observed in each cell population throughout 80% of its life span,
though low D_0 values were observed in XP cells. It is remarkable
that different D_0 values were not observed among cells derived from
fetal lung and heart having different PDNs, and that WS cells having
lower PDNs as proved in Figure 3 showed the same magnitude of D_0
values as normal cells. This is in agreement with the results
obtained from UDS experiment after UV exposure (21).

Distribution of PDNs in Cells Obtained from Various Donors

Cells derived from donors of various ages and patients with
genetic disorders were assayed in terms of their PDNs. Figure 3
shows the relationship between PDNs in various cells and ages of
donors. Donors with a history of diabetes mellitus and cortisone
medication were carefully excluded from this experiment, with the
exception of those with Werner's syndrome. All patients with

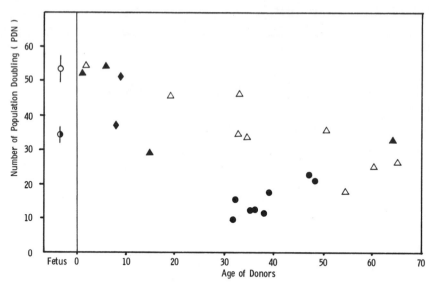

Fig. 3. Distribution of PDNs of cells derived from lung (○) and
         heart (◐) tissues of 6 fetuses, skin of healthy donors (△),
         and of patients with xeroderma pigmentosum (▲), ataxia
         telangiectasia (◆), and Werner's syndrome (●), as a
         function of donors' ages.

Werner's syndrome from which cells were obtained had a history of
diabetes. PDNs of repair-defective cells from patients with XP and
AT, though the latter were few, seemed to distribute normally. It is
not possible to draw a regression line of PDN against donors' ages in
this figure, because not enough cell strains have yet been examined.
However, an apparent tendency in reduction of PDNs as donors' ages
increased may exist among various cells, with the exception of WS
cells. PDNs of WS cells fell well below the range of PDNs for normal
cells.

DISCUSSION

     The aim of the present study was, first, to statistically confirm
the results on the doubling potentials of XP cells previously
reported by Goldstein (22), and then to extend the experiment further
by testing other repair-defective cell strains. Because the number
of population doublings attained by human cells was known to spread
within a wide range (3,23), either repeat cultures of a cell strain
or an increase in the number of cell strains in culture was necessary
to obtain statistically significant results. Our results were in
good agreement with those previously reported (22). XP cells, known
to be defective in the first step of excision repair to UV damage in
DNA (24), showed a low D_0 value in the first component of UV survival

curve of herpes simplex virus. However, their number of population
doublings fell well within the normal range. On the other hand, the
number of population doublings of AT cells, which were defective in
gamma-endonuclease (16), also fell within the range of PDNs attained
by normal cells. These results might suggest that defects in both
UV- and gamma-specific endonucleases in cells do not shorten their
life spans and that the damages accumlated in cellular DNA during
culture does not require both endonucleases for their repair, even if
the accumulation of damage in cellular DNA is a causal event in
cellular aging.

A striking correlation between the extent of UDS in cells derived
from various placental animals, following irradiation with UV as a
model agent, and maximal life spans of donor animals suggested to us
the important role of DNA repair in aging. The present results, however, do not readily establish this correlation in cases of human
cells, because XP cells defective in HCR for UV-irradiated viruses
had age-matched population doubling numbers comparable to those of
normal cells. Furthermore, it is known that cellular sensitivities
to UV do not differ largely among cells derived from various animals
(25), so cells showing low extent of excision repair might have other
compensatory repair mechanisms. Therefore, it is also conceivable
that repair mechanisms other than excision repair play important
roles in cellular aging.

It was recently reported that non-cycling cells in WI-38 cell
population at very late passages had a reduction in the extent of UDS
to UV-induced DNA damages (13). Non-cycling cells, defined as cells
unable to enter the S period for a long time, accumulated in cell
populations with increasing in vitro age (26) and with increasing
donor age (27). The accumulation rates of non-cycling cells per unit
time were higher in both WS and heart cells having low PDNs than in
their counterparts, age-matched normal cells and lung cells, respectively (Nikaido, unpublished). Despite the growing subpopulations of
non-cycling cells, the reparability of whole cell population to
repair UV-damaged DNA, assayed by HCR in the present study, remained
unchanged among the various cell strains, with the exception of XP
cells and cells at various passages up to 80% of their life spans.
One way to explain these results is that non-cycling cells, as well
as cycling cells, are susceptible to virus production. It is also
possible that only the residual cycling cells in a population participate in the production of viruses, which masks the lack of susceptibility of non-cycling cells to viruses. Thus, the increasing
heterogeneity in a cell population as it ages may disturb biological
characteristics such as DNA repair and DNA synthesis in cells. Analyses and purification of subpopulations showing different characteristics in aging cells may increase our knowledge of the mechanisms of
cellular aging. An experiment on this is now in progress.

ACKNOWLEDGEMENTS

The authors wish to express their gratitude to Dr. S. Arase for introducing to us the virus experiment, and to Drs. H. Imura, O. Nagatani, M. Nishikawa, and Y. Tanabe for providing us with specimens obtained from patients with Werner's syndrome. We also wish to acknowledge Professor H. Takebe for his helpful discussions and for providing us with various biopsy specimens. This research was supported in part by a Grant-in-Aid for Cancer Research from the Ministry of Education, Science and Culture, Japan.

REFERENCES

1. L. Hayflick and P. S. Moorhead, The serial cultivation of human diploid cell strains, Exp. Cell Res. 25:585 (1961).
2. L. Hayflick, The longevity of cultured human cells, J. Amer. Geriat. Soc. 22:1 (1974).
3. G. M. Martin, C. A. Sprague, and C. J. Epstein, Replicative life span of cultivated human cells, effect of donor's age, tissue and genotype, Lab. Invest. 23:86 (1970).
4. R. W. Hart and R. B. Setlow, Correlation between deoxyribonucleic acid excision-repair and life span in a number of mammalian species, Proc. Natl. Acad. Sci. USA 71:2169 (1974).
5. J. Epstein, J. R. Williams, and J. B. Little, Deficient DNA repair in human progeroid cells, Proc. Nat. Acad. Sci. USA 70:977 (1973).
6. J. Epstein, J. R. Williams, and J. B. Little, Rate of DNA repair in progeria and normal human fibroblasts, Biochem. Biophys. Res. Comm. 59:850 (1974).
7. S. Goldstein, Lifespan of cultured cells in progeria, Lancet 1:424 (1969).
8. J. D. Regan and R. B. Setlow, DNA repair in human progeroid cells, Biochem. Biophys. Res. Comm. 59:858 (1974).
9. R. B. Painter, J. M. Clarkson, and B. R. Young, Ultraviolet induced repair replication in aging diploid human cells (WI-38), Radiation Res. 56:560 (1973).
10. J. M. Clarkson and R. B. Painter, Repair of X-ray damage in aging WI-38 cells, Mutat. Res. 23:107 (1974).
11. P. D. Bowman, R. L. Meek, and C. W. Daniel, Decreased unscheduled DNA synthesis in nondividing aged WI-38 cells, Mech. Age. Dev. 5:251 (1976).
12. V. Paffenholts, Correlation between DNA repair of embryonic fibroblasts and different life span of 3 inbred mouse strains, Mech. Ageing Dev. 7:131 (1978).
13. R. W. Hart and R. B. Setlow, DNA repair in late passage human cells, Mech. Ageing Dev. 5:67 (1976).
14. J. E. Cleaver, DNA repair and radiation sensitivity in human (xeroderma pigmentosum) cells, Int. J. Radiat. Biol. 18:557 (1970).

15. R. B. Setlow, J. D. Regan, J. German, and W. L. Carrier, Evidence that xeroderma pigmentosum cells do not perform the first step in the repair of ultraviolet damages in their DNA, Proc. Nat. Acad. Sci. 64:1035 (1969).

16. M. C. Paterson, B. P. Smith, P. H. M. Lohman, A. K. Anderson, and L. Fishman, Defective excision repair of X-ray-damaged DNA in human (ataxia telangiectasia) fibroblasts, Nature 260:444 (1976).

17. C. D. Lytle, Host-cell reactivation in mammalian cells. I. Survival of ultraviolet-irradiated herpes simplex virus in different cell lines, Int. J. Radiat. Biol. 19:329 (1971).

18. H. Takebe, S. Nii, M. I. Ishii, and H. Utsumi, Comparative studies of host cell reactivation of Xeroderma pigmentosum, normal human and some other mammalian cells, Mutat. Res. 25:383 (1974).

19. S. Ban, O. Nikaido, and T. Sugahara, Acute and late effects of a single exposure of ionizing radition on cultured human diploid cell populations, Radiat. Res. in press.

20. O. Niwa and S. Nii, Applicability of microbiological technique to selection of HCR- mutants of mammalian cells, Biken J. 15:39 (1972).

21. Y. Fujiwara, T. Higashikawa, and M. Tatsumi, A retarded rate of DNA replication and normal level of DNA repair in Werner's syndrome fibroblasts in culture, J. Cell. Physiol. 92:365 (1977).

22. S. Goldstein, The role of DNA repair in aging of cultured fibroblasts from xeroderma pigmentosum and normals, Proc. Soc. Exp. Biol. Med. 137:730 (1971).

23. R. Holliday, L. I. Huschtscha, G. M. Tarrant, and T. B. L. Kirkwood, Testing the commitment theory of cellular aging, Science 198:366 (1977).

24. K. Tanaka, M. Sekiguchi, and Y. Okada, Restoration of ultraviolet-induced unscheduled DNA synthesis of xeroderma pigmentosum cells by the concomitant treatment with Bacteriophage T4 endonuclease V and HVJ (Sendai virus), Proc. Nat. Acad. Sci. USA 72:4071 (1975).

25. A. M. Rauth, Effects of ultraviolet light on mammalian cells in culture, in:"Current Topics in Radiation Research," Vol. 6, M. Evert and A. Howard, eds., North-Holland, Amsterdam (1970).

26. V. J. Cristofalo and B. B. Sharf, Cellular senescence and DNA synthesis. Thymidine incorporation as a measure of population age in human diploid cells, Exptl. Cell Res. 76:419 (1973).

27. E. Schneider and Y. Mitsui, The relationship between in vitro cellular aging and in vivo human age, Proc. Nat. Acad. Sci. USA 73:3584 (1976).

SUBJECT INDEX

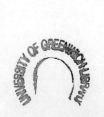